Current Clinical Urology

Eric A. Klein, MD, Series Editor
Professor of Surgery
Cleveland Clinic Lerner College of Medicine Head,
Section of Urologic Oncology
Glickman Urological and Kidney Institute
Cleveland, OH

For further volumes:
http://www.springer.com/series/7635

Gopal H. Badlani
Editor

Minimally Invasive Therapy for Urinary Incontinence and Pelvic Organ Prolapse

Humana Press

Editor
Gopal H. Badlani
Department of Urology
Wake Forest University
Winston-Salem, NC, USA

ISSN 2197-7194 ISSN 2197-7208 (electronic)
ISBN 978-1-4939-0007-7 ISBN 978-1-4939-0008-4 (eBook)
DOI 10.1007/978-1-4939-0008-4
Springer New York Heidelberg Dordrecht London

Library of Congress Control Number: 2014931759

Printed on acid-free paper

Humana Press is a brand of Springer
Springer is part of Springer Science+Business Media (www.springer.com)

Preface

Anything that gives us new knowledge gives us an opportunity to be more rational.

Herbert Simon (1916–2001)

Pelvic floor dysfunction is a major healthcare problem, affecting millions of women throughout the world. Incontinence has a larger economic impact than many chronic conditions and diseases. One in every nine American women will undergo surgery for a pelvic floor disorder in her lifetime, with 30 % of those women requiring additional surgical procedures for recurrence of the same condition. Moreover, it is thought that the demand for surgery for pelvic floor disorders will increase by 45 % in the next 30 years.

Evolving understanding on this subject and technological advancements has led to availability of a number of minimally invasive treatment options. The gap in knowledge base is keeping up with these techniques and their complications. The aim of this book is to provide a detailed insight into "when, why, what and how" of various minimally invasive surgical procedures for surgical management of SUI, OAB and POP. The goal would be to provide detailed diagrammatic/pictorial step-by-step description of the techniques and management of complications related to these procedures. Thus, this book is intended to be an up-to-date, one-stop reference for anything pertaining to MIT of these pelvic disorders.

The book is designed for both urologist and urogynecologist treating patients with urinary disorders and pelvic organ prolapse. The utilisation of kits and devices has expanded; however, the training has lagged behind. There is a relatively large number of urologists and gynaecologists who have not undergone fellowship training, but due to the ease of the kits are entering the field of female urology, male incontinence and prolapse. This book could be a handy guide for them. Improving the quality of life without doing harm should be the goal of every physician or healthcare provider treating women with pelvic floor disorders.

I would like to thank Dr. Mayank Agarwal for helping me put this project together and Dr. David Koslov for putting on the finishing touches. Kathryn Drinkuth, my able administrative assistant, kept me going. Most of all the contributing colleagues have made this a reality and I owe them a debt of gratitude.

Winston-Salem, NC, USA — Gopal H. Badlani

Contents

Contributors

Tamer Aboushwareb, M.D., Ph.D. RSS Urology, Mid Atlantic, Allergan Medical Affairs, Irvine, CA, USA

Oussama El Yazami Adli, M.D. Department of Urology, McGill University, Jewish General Hospital, Montreal, QC, Canada

Mayank Mohan Agarwal, M.S., D.N.B., M.R.C.S.(Ed.), M.Ch. Department of Urology, Postgraduate Institute of Medical Education and Research, Chandigarh, India

Yogesh R. Barapatre, M.S., M.Ch. Department of Urology, Postgraduate Institute of Medical Education and Research, Chandigarh, India

Jerry G. Blaivas, M.D. Department of Urology, Weill Cornell Medical College of Cornell University, New York, NY, USA

Department of Urology, SUNY Downstate College of Medicine, Brooklyn, NY, USA

Institute for Bladder and Prostate Research, New York, NY, USA

Timothy Boone, M.D., Ph.D. Department of Urology, Houston Methodist Hospital, Houston, TX, USA

Jane Cho, M.D. Department of Urology, University of California Irvine, Orange, CA, USA

Denise Chow, M.D. Division of Pelvic Medicine and Reconstructive Surgery, Department of Urology, University of California, Los Angeles, CA, USA

Jacques Corcos, M.D., F.R.C.S.(S). Department of Urology, McGill University, Jewish General Hospital, Montreal, QC, Canada

Anurag K. Das, M.D., F.A.C.S. Department of Urology, Center for Neuro-urology and Continence, Beth Israel Deaconess Medical Center, Boston, MA, USA

Prokar Dasgupta, M.B.B.S., M.Sc. (Urol.), M.D., D.L.S., F.R.C.S. (Urol.), F.E.B.U. Department of Urology, Guy's Hospital, MRC Center for Transplantation, King's College London, King's Health Partners, London, UK

G. Willy Davila, M.D. Department of Gynecology, Cleveland Clinic Florida, Weston, FL, USA

Gamal M. Ghoniem, M.D., F.A.C.S. Department of Urology, University of California Irvine, Orange, CA, USA

Alienor S. Gilchrist, M.D. Department of Urology, Medical University of South Carolina, Charleston, SC, USA

E. Ann Gormley, M.D. Department of Surgery, Dartmouth-Hitchcock Medical Center, Lebanon, NH, USA

Jay Iyer, M.B.B.S., M.D., D.N.B., F.R.C.O.G., F.R.A.N.Z.C.O.G. Division of Urogynecology, Department of Obstetrics and Gynaecology, The Townsville and Mater Hospitals and James Cook University, Townsville, QLD, Australia

Forrest Jellison, M.D. Division of Pelvic Medicine and Reconstructive Surgery, Department of Urology, University of California, Los Angeles, CA, USA

Jaspreet Joneja, M.D. Department of Urology, University of Illinois at Chicago, Chicago, IL, USA

Saad Juma, M.D., F.A.C.S. Incontinence Research Institute, Encinitas, CA, USA

Ravi Kacker, M.D. Division of Urology, Department of Surgery, Beth Israel Deaconess Medical Center, Boston, MA, USA

Michael J. Kennelly, M.D. McKay Department of Urology, Women's Center for Pelvic Health, Charlotte Continence Center, Carolinas Medical Center, Charlotte, NC, USA

Muhammed Shamim Khan, F.R.C.S. (Urol.), F.E.B.U. Department of Urology, Guy's Hospital, MRC Center for Transplantation, King's College London, King's Health Partners, London, UK

Rose Khavari, M.D. Department of Urology, Houston Methodist Hospital, Houston, TX, USA

Kathleen C. Kobashi, M.D. Department of Urology, Virginia Mason Medical Center, Seattle, WA, USA

Ervin Kocjancic, M.D. Department of Urology, Pelvic Health and Reconstructive Urology, College of Medicine, University of Illinois at Chicago, Chicago, IL, USA

Courtney Lee, M.D. Center for Female Urology and Reconstructive Pelvic Surgery, Glickman Urological and Kidney Institute, Cleveland Clinic, Cleveland, OH, USA

Dominic Lee, M.B.B.S. (Hon.), F.R.A.C.S. (Australia) Department of Urology, University of Texas Southwestern Medical Center, Dallas, TX, USA

Karan Motiani, M.D. Department of Surgery, University of Cincinnati, College of Medicine, Cincinnati, OH, USA

Gaspar Msangi, M.D. Department of Urology, Oakland University, William Beaumont School of Medicine, Royal Oak, MI, USA

Bhavin N. Patel, M.D. Department of Urology, Virginia Mason Medical Center, Seattle, WA, USA

Kenneth M. Peters, M.D. Department of Urology, Oakland University, William Beaumont School of Medicine, Royal Oak, MI, USA

Andrew C. Peterson, M.D., F.A.C.S. Division of Urology, Duke University Medical Center, Durham, NC, USA

Leon N. Plowright, M.D. Department of Gynecology, Cleveland Clinic Florida, Weston, FL, USA

Rajveer S. Purohit, M.D., M.P.H. Department of Urology, Weill Cornell Medical College of Cornell University, New York, NY, USA

Ajay Rane, M.B.B.S., M.Sc., M.D., F.R.C.S., F.R.C.O.G., F.R.A.N.Z.C.O.G., C.U., P.H.D., F.I.C.O.G. (Hon.), F.R.C.P.I. (Hon.) Department of Obstetrics and Gynaecology, James Cook University, Townsville, QLD, Australia

Shlomo Raz, M.D. Division of Pelvic Medicine and Reconstructive Surgery, UCLA School of Medicine, Los Angeles, CA, USA

Department of Urology, UCLA School of Medicine, Los Angeles, CA, USA

Eric S. Rovner, M.D. Department of Urology, Medical University of South Carolina, Charleston, SC, USA

Arun Sahai, Ph.D., F.R.C.S. (Urol.) Department of Urology, Guy's Hospital, MRC Center for Transplantation, King's College London, King's Health Partners, London, UK

John P. Selph, M.D. Department of Urology, UNC School of Medicine, Chapel Hill, NC, USA

Jai Seth, B.Sc., M.Sc., M.R.C.S. Department of Uro-Neurology, National Hospital for Neurology and Neurosurgery, London, UK

Martijn A.C. Smits, M.D. Department of Urology, Maastricht University Medical Centre, Maastricht, The Netherlands

Philip E.V. van Kerrebroeck, M.D., Ph.D., M.M.Sc. Department of Urology, Maastricht University Medical Centre, Maastricht, The Netherlands

Sandip Vasavada, M.D. Center for Female Urology and Reconstructive Pelvic Surgery, Glickman Urological and Kidney Institute, Cleveland Clinic, Cleveland, OH, USA

Philippe Zimmern, M.D. Department of Urology, University of Texas Southwestern Medical Center, Dallas, TX, USA

Part I

Introduction/Basics

Basic Urologic History and Questionnaires and the Role of Imaging in Female Pelvic Medicine and Reconstructive Surgery

1

Courtney Lee and Sandip Vasavada

The initial evaluation of a patient with suspect urinary incontinence or pelvic organ prolapse should be quite detailed as there are many aspects to these disorders that tie in to other disease processes throughout the body. A complete and thorough history and physical exam will help the clinician optimize the correct approach to the patient, be it observation or more interventional approaches to management.

Initial assessment of urinary incontinence and pelvic organ prolapse should evaluate a patient's signs and symptoms in order to develop a differential diagnosis, determine need for additional testing, and decide possible treatment options. A thorough history and physical exam is necessary for initial evaluation and subsequent testing should be based on clinical suspicion and treatment goals.

Further tests should be considered if surgical intervention is planned, conservative therapies are not effective, or there is suspicion for pelvic pathology such as stone, cancer, or fistula. In addition, further testing is valuable if there is a prior history of pelvic surgery or radiation, recurrent UTI, neurologic disease, voiding dysfunction, significant prolapse, pain, or hematuria [1].

Important in the assessment of both urinary incontinence and pelvic organ prolapse is an assessment of the impact of the pelvic floor disorder on the patient. Several questionnaires have been developed to assess the severity of the disease, the degree of bother from the disease, and the effect of the disease on quality of life.

History

Urinary symptoms should be evaluated in all patients with urinary incontinence and pelvic organ prolapse. Storage symptoms are symptoms that occur with bladder filling. They include urinary urgency, daytime and nighttime frequency, nocturnal enuresis, and urinary incontinence.

A patient with urinary incontinence should be questioned about the duration of her symptoms and whether the leakage appears to be per urethra or per vagina. The severity of incontinence can be estimated by asking the patient about the frequency of incontinent episodes and pad usage. A micturition diary, which will be described below, is useful to determine the severity of incontinence.

The physician should attempt to determine the precipitating factors of incontinence in order to characterize the incontinence. Stress urinary incontinence (SUI) is an involuntary loss of urine during physical activity; urgency incontinence is leakage of urine associated with urinary urgency; mixed incontinence is a combination of both stress and urgency incontinence. When a patient

C. Lee, M.D. (✉) • S. Vasavada, M.D.
Center for Female Urology and Reconstructive Pelvic Surgery, Glickman Urological and Kidney Institute, Cleveland Clinic, Q-10-1 Urology, 9500 Euclid Avenue, Cleveland, OH 44195, USA
e-mail: Vasavas@ccf.org

G.H. Badlani (ed.), *Minimally Invasive Therapy for Urinary Incontinence and Pelvic Organ Prolapse*, Current Clinical Urology, DOI 10.1007/978-1-4939-0008-4_1,

complains of mixed incontinence, the physician should ask which type of incontinence occurred first and which is more bothersome to the patient.

During questioning regarding urinary incontinence, patients may complain of continuous incontinence or insensate incontinence when the patient is unaware of urinary leakage. Patients may also complain of postural urinary incontinence, which occurs when the patient loses urine when changing positions. The exact mechanism of postural incontinence is unknown and will require further evaluation [2]. Bladder sensation during filling should also be assessed. Bladder sensation can be increased, reduced, or absent.

Both urinary incontinence and pelvic organ prolapse can be associated with urinary obstruction. Therefore, voiding symptoms, such as hesitancy, slow stream, straining to urinate, position-dependent micturition, and inability to pass urine, should be assessed. Patients with prolapse may also complain of a need to reduce the prolapse in order to void.

Other urinary symptoms such as dysuria, gross hematuria, and a history of urinary tract infections are important to ascertain during a history for pelvic floor dysfunction. These symptoms signify a need for additional tests to rule out pelvic pathology.

Defecatory symptoms should be evaluated. A patient should be asked whether vaginal or perineal splinting is required to evacuate her bowels. Constipation is relatively common in the community. A meta-analysis showed the prevalence of chronic idiopathic constipation in North America is about 14 % [3]. It is more common in the elderly and in women and can be exacerbated by anticholinergics used to treat OAB symptoms. A history of fecal incontinence should also be elicited.

Patients with prolapse can present with a variety of symptoms. The most common and specific symptom of prolapse is the sensation or visualization of a vaginal bulge [4–9]. Several studies have shown that visualization or sensation of a vaginal bulge correlates with the degree of pelvic organ prolapse [5–7, 9]. Women with pelvic organ prolapse are more likely to complain of pain and pressure in the lower abdomen, pelvis, and genital region [10]. While low back pain is common in the community, this has been evaluated and thought to not likely be caused by pelvic organ prolapse [11].

Sexual symptoms should be assessed as part of the routing pelvic floor evaluation. Issues including dyspareunia, disorders of vaginal lubrication, and coital incontinence should be further evaluated. As such, coital incontinence can occur during penetration or orgasm yet the pathology of incontinence during sexual activity is likely multifactoral. SUI is common in patients with leakage during penetration and urgency incontinence tends to be more common in patients with incontinence describing leakage during orgasm [12].

One of the most effective adjuncts to the clinical office visit is the use of a fluid or voiding diary. This diary allows the clinician to assess the timing and amount of fluid intake as well as consumption of caffeinated and other bladder stimulant type beverages. Furthermore, the log can be used as an objective measure of a patient's level of frequency and urgency and allows the physician to estimate one's functional capacity. From the voiding diary the physician can calculate daytime and nighttime frequency, number of incontinence episodes, number of urgency episodes, pad usage, total urine volume, maximum voided volume, and nighttime urine volume. It is a good quantitative measure of patients' urinary frequency and incontinence episodes and can be used to track treatment. Perhaps it is most useful for patients who present with nocturnal symptoms as it allows the physician to determine if the patient has nocturnal polyuria—a medical cause of nocturia.

In addition, a good gynecologic history is necessary in pelvic floor disorders and will include obstetric and menstrual history including menopausal status. The medication list should be evaluated for hormone replacements, diuretics, and medications that can affect the urinary tract. Prior medical history should be evaluated for history of trauma, congenital abnormalities, pelvic radiation, neurological diseases, and prior history of treatment for incontinence and pelvic organ prolapse. A history of diabetes mellitus or diabetes insipidus may account for an increase in urine volume leading to urinary incontinence.

Diabetes mellitus may also cause an acontractile bladder and overflow incontinence. Prior surgical history should include prior hysterectomy, pelvic surgery, and past surgical treatment for incontinence or prolapse.

Questionnaires

Diagnostic questionnaires are administered as a tool to determine if a patient has a disease. Furthermore, it can provide a baseline measurement or assessment of symptoms prior to a planned intervention. Currently, two validated questionnaires designed for the diagnosis of OAB are used commonly: the overactive bladder awareness tool (OAB-V8) and the overactive bladder symptom score (OAB-SS). OAB-V8 is an 8-item patient administered questionnaire to identify men and women with bothersome OAB symptoms that may benefit from treatment [13]. This questionnaire is designed ideally for a primary care setting. The OAB-SS is a 7-item patient administered symptom score for men and women [14]. It has 4 items related to urgency and urge incontinence, and two questions related to nighttime and daytime frequency, and one general question regarding "bladder control." The OAB-SS does not address bother or quality of life issues but is designed to grade the severity of urgency using an urgency subscale.

The questionnaire for urinary incontinence diagnosis (QUID) is a 6-item questionnaire to diagnose and differentiate between SUI, UUI, and MUI in women [15]. It has a stress and urge subscale. Patients with a stress subscale greater than or equal to 4 are more likely to have a diagnosis of stress incontinence, and those with an urge subscale greater or equal to 4 are more likely to have a diagnosis of urgency incontinence. Those with both evidence of stress and urge have mixed incontinence.

Urinary incontinence and pelvic organ prolapse do not cause significant morbidity or mortality in a majority of patients suffering from these conditions. The main effect of incontinence and prolapse is on a patient's quality of life. Therefore, it is important to evaluate the effects of UI and pelvic organ prolapse on a patient's quality of life at initial presentation and throughout a patient's treatment course.

Many of quality of life questionnaires have validated short forms with fewer questions to make them easier to use in a clinical setting. The short forms may also be beneficial in a research situation where patients are given numerous questionnaires. While there are a multitude of questionnaires available for use, several more common ones are highlighted below.

The Bristol Female Lower Urinary Tract Symptoms Questionnaire (BFLUTS) measures the severity and bother of urinary incontinence and lower urinary tract symptoms in women [16]. It also evaluates the effects of lower urinary tract symptoms on quality of life. It consists of 33 questions with 4 domains. The domains are incontinence severity, associated lower urinary tract symptoms, quality of life, and sexual function. The BFLUTS-SF is a scored form of the BFLUTS with 19 items and 5 domains. BFLUTS-IS measures urinary incontinence symptoms, BFLUTS-VS measures voiding symptoms, BFLUTS-FS measures urinary storage symptoms, and the BFLUTS-sex and BFLUTS-QoL measure sexual symptoms and quality of life symptoms related to lower urinary tract symptoms [17].

The urinary distress inventory (UDI) and incontinence impact questionnaire (IIQ) are paired measures that evaluate the bother and psychosocial impact of urinary incontinence in women. The UDI evaluates bother from urinary incontinence. It has 19 questions with 3 subscales: irritative symptoms, obstructive/discomfort, and stress symptoms [18–20]. The IIQ measures the psychosocial impact of urinary incontinence. It has 30 items with 4 subscales: physical activity, travel, social relationships, and emotional health [18–20]. The UDI-6 and IIQ-7 are short forms of the UDI and IIQ [21, 22].

The Kings Health questionnaire is a 21-item questionnaire that evaluates the impact of urinary incontinence on a woman's quality of life. It has 8 domains which evaluates perception of severity of incontinence and the effect of urinary incontinence on general health, role, physical interactions, social interactions, personal relationships, emotions, and sleep [23].

The overactive bladder symptoms and health-related quality of life questionnaire (OAB-Q) is an OAB-specific measure that evaluates bother and impact of OAB in men and women [24, 25]. This survey, which is validated for use in continent and incontinent patients, has 33 questions with 2 parts. The first part evaluates symptom bother. The second part has 4 domains that evaluate the impact of OAB in areas of coping, concern, sleep, and social interaction. The OAB-Q SF is a 19 question short form of the OAB-Q with questions related to symptom bother and health-related quality of life [26].

The short form of the International Consultation on Incontinence Modular Questionnaire (ICIQ-SF) is a 4-question measure that evaluates symptom severity and bother from lower urinary tract symptoms in men and women [27]. The York Incontinence Perception Scale (YIPS) is an 8-item questionnaire that evaluates the psychosocial effects of incontinence in women [28].

Single question global measures can be used as a quick tool to evaluate a patient's experience with urinary symptoms. A patient is asked to sum all the effects of a symptom to answer one question. These measures don't allow a physician to determine specifics about a patient's bother or quality of life, but gives a general impression how a symptom affects the patient. The Patient Perception of Bladder Condition (PPBC) is a single-item global index to evaluate the impression of urinary problems in men and women with OAB. It is validated for use in both continent and incontinent patients with OAB [25, 29]. The Patient Global Impression of Severity is a single question global index validated to evaluate the severity of SUI [30].

Two commonly used questionnaires for the evaluation of health-related quality of life in patients with pelvic organ prolapse is the Pelvic Floor Distress Inventory (PFDI) and the Pelvic Floor Impact Questionnaire (PFIQ) [31]. The PFDI is a 61-item measure with 3 domains. The first domain is the UDI. It contains the aforementioned UDI and 9 questions related to lower urinary tract symptoms in women with pelvic organ prolapse. Similar to the UDI, it has 3 sections: obstructive, irritative/discomfort, and stress. The second domain, the POPDI, has questions related to pelvic organ prolapse. It is divided into 3 sections: general, anterior, and posterior. The CRADI (Colorectal and Anal Distress Inventory) is the last section. This portion helps evaluate lower bowel function and is divided into 4 sections: obstructive, incontinence, pain/irritation, and rectal prolapse.

The PFIQ evaluates health-related quality of life and the affect prolapse symptoms have on a patient's daily activities relationships and emotion. It is based off of the IIQ and like the PFDI is separated into 3 scales with 31 questions each: the IIQ, the colorectal impact questionnaire (CRAIQ), and the pelvic organ prolapse impact questionnaire (POPIQ). Each scale assesses 4 areas of quality of life: travel, social, emotions, and physical activity. Though intended to be administered in entirety, each domain in the PFDI and PFIQ is scored separately. The PFDI-12 and PFIQ-7 are short forms of the PFDI and PFIQ [32].

Quality of life and bother from defecatory symptoms can be evaluated by the CRAIQ and CRADI, which are domains of the PFDI and PFIQ that address lower GI symptoms. The Fecal Incontinence Quality of Life Scale is a 29-item measure that evaluates the affect of fecal incontinence on men and women. It has 4 domains: lifestyle, coping/behavior, depression/self-perception, and embarrassment [33].

The Female Sexual Function Index (FSFI), the BFLUTS-sex, and the PISQ are three measures used to evaluate sexual function in women. The FSFI is a 19-item questionnaire with 6 domains: desire, arousal, lubrication, orgasm, satisfaction, and pain [34]. Though it can be administered to all women regardless of their sexual activity, the questionnaire is more appropriate for sexually active women.

The BFLUTS-sex is part of the BFLUTS that assesses sexual function in patients with lower urinary tract symptoms. The PISQ is a 31-item questionnaire designed to evaluate sexual function in sexually active heterosexual women with urinary incontinence or pelvic organ prolapse [35]. It has 3 domains: behavioral/emotive, physical, and partner related. The PISQ-12 is the short form of PIDQ [36].

Patient-reported outcomes are important to evaluate when performing outcomes research for pelvic organ prolapse. Two outcome measures for the medical treatment of OAB are the Benefit, Satisfaction, and Willingness questionnaire (BSW) and the Overactive Bladder Treatment Satisfaction Questionnaire (OAB-S).

The BSW is a 3 question investigator administered tool for men and women with OAB [23]. The first question measures the patient' perception of benefit from treatment, the second question measures the patient's satisfaction with treatment, and the final question measures the patient's willingness to continue treatment.

The OAB-S was developed to evaluate patient satisfaction with OAB treatment and is validated as a patient administered survey that evaluates patient satisfaction with pharmaceutical treatment for OAB [37]. There are 2 questionnaires: a 21-item pretreatment instrument and a 41 question post-treatment instrument. The pretreatment instrument has 3 domains: OAB control, impact on daily living with OAB, and interruption of day-to-day life due to OAB. The posttreatment instrument contains the aforementioned domains and 6 additional domains that evaluate medication tolerability, fulfillment of treatment expectations, overall satisfaction with treatment, willingness to continue medication, and improvement in quality of life with treatment.

The Patient Global Impression of Improvement (PGI-I) is a patient-administered single question global index validated for use in women following treatment for pelvic organ prolapse or SUI [30, 38]. The question rates the response to treatment.

From the voiding diary the physician can calculate daytime and nighttime frequency, number of incontinence episodes, number of urgency episodes, pad usage, total urine volume, maximum voided volume, and nighttime urine volume. It is a good quantitative measure of patients' urinary frequency and incontinence episodes and can be used to track treatment. A fluid diary allows the physician to evaluate a patient's fluid and caffeine intake. It also allows for measurement of polyuria and nocturnal polyuria, which are medical problems that can exacerbate lower urinary tract symptoms.

Physical Examination

A general exam should be performed that includes a patient's height, weight, and BMI. Several studies have shown that obesity is a risk factor for urinary incontinence and pelvic organ prolapse [39–43].

A patient's cognition and mental status are important to ascertain, as a direct correlation may exist in which urinary incontinence can be due to poor mental status and inability to prevent urination when it is socially appropriate. It is also important to know a patient's cognition when developing a treatment plan. Similarly a patient's functional status, mobility, and hand function are factors that can affect both urinary incontinence and treatment decisions. A patient with functional incontinence that cannot physically get to the bathroom in situations of potential incontinence may not receive adequate benefit from therapies due to these mobility issues.

A general exam usually includes abdomen and genitalia as well as a focused neurologic exam. During the abdominal exam, the patient's abdomen should be inspected for scars from prior surgeries and hernias. An attempt should be made to palpate the kidney and bladder. During palpation, the abdomen should also be evaluated for a mass or organomegaly which can increase intra-abdominal pressure. The back should be examined for costovertebral angle tenderness which could be a sign of urinary obstruction. If there is a suspicion for neurologic disease, the low back can be visualized for evidence of myelomeningocele, hairy patch, obvious scoliosis, or other spinal disease.

The lower extremities should be evaluated for lower extremity edema that can lead to nocturnal polyuria and increased nighttime lower urinary tract symptoms.

The main focus of the female incontinent or prolapsed patient is the vaginal exam which should be performed in the dorsal lithotomy position initially. If the patient's symptoms of incontinence or prolapse cannot be replicated in the dorsal lithotomy position, the exam can be repeated while the patient is standing.

The gynecological exam starts with an examination of the external genitalia: the clitoris, urethral meatus, vulva, labia, perineum, and anus. Estrogen status is evaluated. Estrogenized tissue is well perfused with thick epithelium, transverse rugae, and physiologic moisture. Atrophic tissue is pale thin and friable without rugae. During the examination of the external genitalia, evidence of irritation from urine such as excoriation, erythema, or skin breakdown should be noted. Urine within the vaginal vault should also be noted. Any discharge from the vagina or urethra should be observed and a vaginal swab for gonococcus, chlamydia, candida, bacterial vaginosis, or mycoplasma should be performed as clinically indicated. A bimanual exam can be performed to evaluate for other gynecologic pathology.

The urethral meatus is evaluated for evidence of caruncle, urethral prolapse, or uethral mass. The urethra is palpated and the position of any tenderness, mass, or discharge per urethra upon palpation should be noted for further evaluation.

While the patient is in dorsal lithotomy position with an empty bladder and the urethra exposed, the patient should be asked to strain or cough in order to elicit SUI on exam. If the patient has a history of SUI that could not be reproduced by the supine empty bladder stress test, the exam can be repeated with the patient standing.

The bladder can also be retrograde filled to around 200 cc. Resistance to filling or a rise in water level during filling can indicate detrusor overactivity. After filling the patient is asked to Valsalva or cough in supine position. The test can be repeated while the patient is standing if incontinence is not elicited.

Extra-urethral urine is suspicious for vesicovaginal fistula, urethrovaginal fistula, or ectopic urethra. Location of fistula can be evaluated with a thorough vaginal exam, cystoscopy, and vaginoscopy.

If a patient complains of leakage and the source is unknown, a pyridium pad test can be performed to determine if the fluid is urine. If the patient is leaking urine, the pad will stain orange. Similarly the bladder can be retrograde filled with methylene blue or indigo carmine. A blue stained pad indicates a bladder source of fluid. A combination of pyridium and bladder dye is given to distinguish between a ureteric and bladder source of urine. If the pad is stained orange, the patient should be evaluated for a possible ureterovesical fistula.

Urethral hypermobility can be assessed using a q-tip test. With an empty bladder, a q-tip is placed through the urethra to the area of the bladder neck. The angle of the urethra to the vertical axis at rest and with Valsalva or cough is recorded. A straining urethral angle greater than 30° above the horizontal is considered positive for urethral hypermobility. Urethral hypermobility can also be measured by cysourethrography and ultrasound.

In 1995 the International Continence Society proposed the Pelvic Organ Prolapse Quantification system (POP-Q) as the standardized measure of pelvic organ prolapse [44]. The POP-Q exam should be performed on all patients complaining of urinary incontienence and pelvic organ prolapse. When recording the results of the exam, it is important to note the patient's bladder volume, position of the patient, and whether the exam was performed during the cough or Valsalva.

Using the hymen as a fixed point of reference, the position of points Aa, Ba, C, D, Ap, and Bp are recorded (Table 1.1). The genital hiatus, perineal body, and total vaginal length are also measured and recorded (Table 1.1). Pelvic organ prolapse is then staged from stage 0 (no prolapse) to stage 4 (complete eversion) (Table 1.2).

Two modifications of the POP-Q have been introduced. A simplified version of the POP-Q was developed by Swift et al. [45]. This version measures points Aa, Ap, C, and D. Stage 0 and 1 are combined as stage 1. Stage 2 is the same as the POP-Q system. Stage 3 is defined as vaginal eversion with some mucosa not everted and stage 4 is complete vaginal eversion.

The Pelvic Organ Prolapse Quantification Index (POP-Q-I) creates a continuous variable

Table 1.1 Pelvic organ prolapse quantification system

Point	Location	Range
Aa	Midline of the anterior vaginal wall 3 cm proximal to the urethral meatus	–3 to 3 cm
Ba	Most distal portion of the upper anterior vaginal wall (from the apex to point Aa)	–3 cm to total vaginal length
C	Most distal edge of the cervix or vaginal cuff	
D	The posterior fornix in patients with an intact cervix	
Ap	Midline of the posterior vaginal wall 3 cm proximal to the hymen	–3 to 3 cm
Bp	Most distal portion of the upper posterior vaginal wall (from the apex to point Ap)	–3 cm to total vaginal length
Genital hiatus (gh)	Distance from the middle of the urethral meatus to the posterior hymen	
Perineal body (pb)	Distance from the posterior aspect of the genital hiatus to the midanal opening	
Total vaginal length (tvl)	Greatest depth of vagina when it is reduced to its normal postion	

Table 1.2 Short version of pelvic organ prolapse quantification system

Stage	Definition
0	No prolapse
1	The most distal portion of prolapse is less than –1 cm
2	The most distal portion of prolapse is –1 to 1 cm
3	The most distal portion of prolapse is more than 1 cm but less than 2 cm smaller than the total vaginal length
4	The most distal portion of prolapse is greater than total vaginal length minus 2

for the measurement of pelvic organ prolapse [46]. Two values are calculated for each POP-Q point: the actual distance of the point from its original location and an estimate of the distance of the point to where the point will be in the case of a complete eversion. Value 1 is divided by Value 2 to create the index.

Prolapse is best recorded as anterior, posterior, and apical prolapse. The terms cystocele, rectocele, and enterocele are misleading because it is difficult to determine on exam alone the organ underlying the prolapsed vaginal wall. Though digital evaluation of bowel contents in the rectovaginal septum can help diagnose enterocele, it is difficult to distinguish between rectocele and enterocele on exam alone.

In a patient with pelvic organ prolapse, it is important to test for occult SUI by asking a patient to Valsalva or cough while the prolapse is reduced. In addition, a rectal exam should be performed to evaluate for colorectal pathology such as hemorrhoids or a rectal mass. Fecal impaction, which can lead to lower urinary tract symptoms, can also be assessed.

A neurologic exam should evaluate the patient's gait, lower extremity sensation and strength, pelvic floor muscle strength, anal sphincter resting tone and contraction, perineal and posterior thigh sensation, and sacral reflexes. The sacral reflexes are the bulbocavernosus and anal reflex. In the bulbocavernosus reflex, the anus contracts after the clitoris is stimulated. In the anal reflex, the anus contracts after light stimulation of the anus with a gloved hand or Q-tip. The bulbocavernosus and anal reflex can often be absent even in neurologically normal women; however, their presence indicates an intact nerves between the conus medularis and the pudendal nerve.

A urinalysis should be performed and used as a guide for further investigation. Patients with hematuria should be evaluated for bladder cancer as a cause of their lower urinary tract symptoms. Glucosuria can indicate diabetes mellitus, and pyuria or bacteruria can indicate bladder inflammation or urinary tract infection.

A post void residual (PVR) may be performed on patient with prolapse, neurologic disease, or a possible diagnosis of urinary retention to measure the amount of residual urine in the bladder immediately following urination. The International Consultation on Incontinence states that normal sensate women with storage-specific symptoms and no risk factors for retention do not require routine PVRs [1]. PVRs can be performed by straight catheterization, a portable ultrasound bladder scanner, or transabdominal ultrasound.

Pad testing can be performed on patients with complaints of incontinence that cannot be exhibited on exam. During the test, women wear pre-weighed incontinence pads for a designated amount of time and the increase in pad weights is measured. A 1-h pad test can be performed in office. The bladder is filled with a fixed volume of fluid and the patient is asked to perform set activities to create urine loss. The 24- and 48-h tests are performed outside the office. The patient wears pre-weighed pads while performing activities of daily living. The pads are collected in a plastic pad and weighed after the test. The 24- and 48-h pad tests are more sensitive than the 1-h pad test, but can be more cumbersome to the patient [47, 48]. If clinically indicated, dynamic testing using uroflow or cystometry can be performed. This will be discussed in detail in the next chapter.

Radiologic Studies

Upper Tract and Collecting System

An ultrasound is a good initial study because it is noninvasive and less expensive than x-ray studies. The kidney can be evaluated for hydronephrosis, masses, and stones. It is not a good study to evaluate the ureters.

An IVU or CT urogram is more expensive than an ultrasound and exposes the patient to radiation and IV contrast dye. Both studies are superior to the ultrasound at showing the anatomy of the collecting system. Hydronephrosis and stones can be clearly evaluated. The anatomy of the ureter, ureteral obstruction, congenital abnormalities such as ectopic ureter and duplicated system, pathology such as ureteral injury and ureterovaginal fistulas can be seen. CT urograms are more commonly performed and have the benefit of showing the anatomy of surrounding organs and tissues. CT is superior to IVU for evaluation of kidney masses.

Lower Urinary Tract and Pelvic Organs Imaging

An ultrasound is useful for the evaluation of pelvic masses, gynecologic pathology, and bladder disease. Pelvic floor muscle structure and function can be evaluated. The degree of pelvic organ prolapse can be determined and the underlying organs can be illustrated. The ultrasound is better than physical exam alone for the detection of an enterocele. Ultrasound has also been used to evaluate urethral diverticuli and visualize slings and vaginal mesh but is clearly operator dependent.

Transabdominal ultrasound is not useful for the evaluation of pelvic organs due to shadowing from the pubic bones. However, the bladder volume can be measured with transabdominal ultrasound by measuring the height, depth, and width of the bladder. The equation is $\text{Height} \times \text{Depth} \times \text{Width} \times 0.7$.

Other methods for pelvic ultrasound include transvaginal, perineal, and introital. Perineal and introital views are used most often in the evaluation of pelvic organ prolapse and urinary incontinence.

Urethral mobility can be illustrated by an assessment of bladder neck descent and urethral rotation. These are commonly measured using perineal or introital views. Bladder neck descent is estimated by the position of the bladder neck at rest and with Valsalva, and urethral rotation is measured by the axis of the urethra at rest and with Valsalva. Transanal ultrasound can be used for imaging of suspected anal sphincter defects.

A cystogram and a CT cystogram are studies in which contrast dye is injected into the bladder. Images are obtained with a full bladder and after emptying for evaluation of a bladder injury or fistula.

During voiding cystourethrography (VCUG) the bladder is filled with contrast dye and images are obtained during filling and voiding. A VCUG evaluates bladder and urethral fistulas, urethral diverticuli, vesicoureteral reflux, and distal ureteral anomalies such as a ureterocele. Cystourethrography can also evaluate ureteral and bladder neck hypermobility similar to methods used during ultrasound. A VUCG is often combined with urodynamic studies of the bladder for a better understanding of lower urinary tract function and pathology.

In positive pressure cystourethrography a catheter with a balloon at the bladder neck and urethral meatus is used to inject dye directly into the urethra, between the balloons in order to visualize a urethral diverticulum.

A pelvic MRI has become the gold standard for the evaluation of urethral diverticuli. It gives good resolution of soft tissue in the pelvis and pelvic floor muscles and can add valuable anatomical information in the evaluation of complex pelvic organ prolapse. Though sometimes used in research for the evaluation of pelvic organ prolapse, it is an expensive test, which should not be used routinely for simple cases of prolapse.

Summary

In summary, the careful and close evaluation of a patient with urinary incontinence and prolapse usually can be done in an office visit with specific questions and a pertinent history and physical examination. The adjunctive use of questionnaires can be useful for a research setting but even in routine practice, this may be helpful to discriminate different types of incontinence, prolapse or urinary or defecatory dysfunction and its correlated impacts on quality of life. Imaging, while useful in select cases, does not need to be performed unless clinical suspicion warrants additional studies.

References

1. Abrams P, Cardoza L, Khoury S, Wein A, editors. Incontinence: 4th international consultation on incontinence. Paris: Health Publication Ltd; 2009.
2. Haylen BT, de Ridder D, Freeman RM, Swift SE, Berghmans B, Lee J, Monga A, Petri E, Rizk DE, Sand PK, et al. An International Urogynecological Association (IUGA)/International Continence Society (ICS) joint report on the terminology for female pelvic floor dysfunction. Neurourol Urodyn. 2010;29:4–20.
3. Suares NC, Ford AC. Prevalence of, and risk factors for, chronic idiopathic constipation in the community: systematic review and meta-analysis. Am J Gastroenterol. 2011;106:1582–91; quiz 1581, 1592.
4. Swift SE, Tate SB, Nicholas J. Correlation of symptoms with degree of pelvic organ support in a general population of women: what is pelvic organ prolapse? Am J Obstet Gynecol. 2003;189:372–7; discussion 377–9.
5. Ellerkmann RM, Cundiff GW, Melick CF, Nihira MA, Leffler K, Bent AE. Correlation of symptoms with location and severity of pelvic organ prolapse. Am J Obstet Gynecol. 2001;185:1332–7; discussion 1337–8.
6. Tan JS, Lukacz ES, Menefee SA, Powell CR, Nager CW. Predictive value of prolapse symptoms: a large database study. Int Urogynecol J Pelvic Floor Dysfunct. 2005;16:203–9; discussion 209.
7. Bradley CS, Zimmerman MB, Wang Q, Nygaard IE. Vaginal descent and pelvic floor symptoms in postmenopausal women: a longitudinal study. Obstet Gynecol. 2008;111:1148–53.
8. Ghetti C, Gregory WT, Edwards SR, Otto LN, Clark AL. Pelvic organ descent and symptoms of pelvic floor disorders. Am J Obstet Gynecol. 2005;193:53–7.
9. Miedel A, Tegerstedt G, Maehle-Schmidt M, Nyren O, Hammarstrom M. Symptoms and pelvic support defects in specific compartments. Obstet Gynecol. 2008;112:851–8.
10. Reddy J, Barber MD, Walters MD, Paraiso MF, Jelovsek JE. Lower abdominal and pelvic pain with advanced pelvic organ prolapse: a case–control study. Am J Obstet Gynecol. 2011;204:537 e1–5.
11. Heit M, Culligan P, Rosenquist C, Shott S. Is pelvic organ prolapse a cause of pelvic or low back pain? Obstet Gynecol. 2002;99:23–8.
12. Serati M, Salvatore S, Uccella S, Nappi RE, Bolis P. Female urinary incontinence during intercourse: a review on an understudied problem for women's sexuality. J Sex Med. 2009;6:40–8.
13. Coyne KS, Zyczynski T, Margolis MK, Elinoff V, Roberts RG. Validation of an overactive bladder awareness tool for use in primary care settings. Adv Ther. 2005;22:381–94.
14. Blaivas JG, Panagopoulos G, Weiss JP, Somaroo C. Validation of the overactive bladder symptom score. J Urol. 2007;178:543–7; discussion 547.
15. Bradley CS, Rovner ES, Morgan MA, Berlin M, Novi JM, Shea JA, Arya LA. A new questionnaire for urinary incontinence diagnosis in women: development and testing. Am J Obstet Gynecol. 2005;192:66–73.
16. Jackson S, Donovan J, Brookes S, Eckford S, Swithinbank L, Abrams P. The Bristol Female Lower Urinary Tract Symptoms questionnaire: development and psychometric testing. Br J Urol. 1996;77:805–12.
17. Brookes ST, Donovan JL, Wright M, Jackson S, Abrams P. A scored form of the Bristol Female Lower Urinary Tract Symptoms questionnaire: data from a randomized controlled trial of surgery for women with stress incontinence. Am J Obstet Gynecol. 2004;191:73–82.
18. Corcos J, Behlouli H, Beaulieu S. Identifying cut-off scores with neural networks for interpretation of the

incontinence impact questionnaire. Neurourol Urodyn. 2002;21:198–203.
19. Hagen S, Hanley J, Capewell A. Test-retest reliability, validity, and sensitivity to change of the urogenital distress inventory and the incontinence impact questionnaire. Neurourol Urodyn. 2002;21:534–9.
20. Shumaker SA, Wyman JF, Uebersax JS, McClish D, Fantl JA. Health-related quality of life measures for women with urinary incontinence: the Incontinence Impact Questionnaire and the Urogenital Distress Inventory. Continence Program in Women (CPW) Research Group. Qual Life Res. 1994;3:291–306.
21. FitzGerald MP, Kenton K, Shott S, Brubaker L. Responsiveness of quality of life measurements to change after reconstructive pelvic surgery. Am J Obstet Gynecol. 2001;185:20–4.
22. Woodman PJ, Misko CA, Fischer JR. The use of short-form quality of life questionnaires to measure the impact of imipramine on women with urge incontinence. Int Urogynecol J Pelvic Floor Dysfunct. 2001;12:312–5; discussion 315–6.
23. Kelleher CJ, Cardozo LD, Khullar V, Salvatore S. A new questionnaire to assess the quality of life of urinary incontinent women. Br J Obstet Gynaecol. 1997;104:1374–9.
24. Coyne K, Revicki D, Hunt T, Corey R, Stewart W, Bentkover J, Kurth H, Abrams P. Psychometric validation of an overactive bladder symptom and health-related quality of life questionnaire: the OAB-q. Qual Life Res. 2002;11:563–74.
25. Matza LS, Thompson CL, Krasnow J, Brewster-Jordan J, Zyczynski T, Coyne KS. Test-retest reliability of four questionnaires for patients with overactive bladder: the overactive bladder questionnaire (OAB-q), patient perception of bladder condition (PPBC), urgency questionnaire (UQ), and the primary OAB symptom questionnaire (POSQ). Neurourol Urodyn. 2005;24:215–25.
26. Coyne K, Lai J, Zyczynski HM, Kopp Z, Avery K, Abrams P. An overactive bladder symptom and quality-of-life short form: development of the overactive bladder questionnaire short form (OAB-q SF). In: Thirty fourth Joint Meeting of the International Continence Society and the International UroGynecological Association, Paris, France; 2004.
27. Avery K, Donovan J, Peters TJ, Shaw C, Gotoh M, Abrams P. ICIQ: a brief and robust measure for evaluating the symptoms and impact of urinary incontinence. Neurourol Urodyn. 2004;23:322–30.
28. Lee PS, Reid DW, Saltmarche A, Linton L. Measuring the psychosocial impact of urinary incontinence: the York Incontinence Perceptions Scale (YIPS). J Am Geriatr Soc. 1995;43:1275–8.
29. Coyne KS, Matza LS, Kopp Z, Abrams P. The validation of the patient perception of bladder condition (PPBC): a single-item global measure for patients with overactive bladder. Eur Urol. 2006;49:1079–86.
30. Yalcin I, Bump RC. Validation of two global impression questionnaires for incontinence. Am J Obstet Gynecol. 2003;189:98–101.
31. Barber MD, Kuchibhatla MN, Pieper CF, Bump RC. Psychometric evaluation of 2 comprehensive condition-specific quality of life instruments for women with pelvic floor disorders. Am J Obstet Gynecol. 2001;185:1388–95.
32. Barber MD, Walters MD, Bump RC. Short forms of two condition-specific quality-of-life questionnaires for women with pelvic floor disorders (PFDI-20 and PFIQ-7). Am J Obstet Gynecol. 2005;193:103–13.
33. Rockwood TH, Church JM, Fleshman JW, Kane RL, Mavrantonis C, Thorson AG, Wexner SD, Bliss D, Lowry AC. Fecal Incontinence Quality of Life Scale: quality of life instrument for patients with fecal incontinence. Dis Colon Rectum. 2000;43:9–16; discussion 16–7.
34. Rosen R, Brown C, Heiman J, Leiblum S, Meston C, Shabsigh R, Ferguson D, D'Agostino Jr R. The Female Sexual Function Index (FSFI): a multidimensional self-report instrument for the assessment of female sexual function. J Sex Marital Ther. 2000;26:191–208.
35. Rogers GR, Villarreal A, Kammerer-Doak D, Qualls C. Sexual function in women with and without urinary incontinence and/or pelvic organ prolapse. Int Urogynecol J Pelvic Floor Dysfunct. 2001;12:361–5.
36. Rogers RG, Coates KW, Kammerer-Doak D, Khalsa S, Qualls C. A short form of the Pelvic Organ Prolapse/Urinary Incontinence Sexual Questionnaire (PISQ-12). Int Urogynecol J Pelvic Floor Dysfunct. 2003;14:164–8; discussion 168.
37. Piault E, Evans CJ, Espindle D, Kopp Z, Brubaker L, Abrams P. Development and validation of the Overactive Bladder Satisfaction (OAB-S) Questionnaire. Neurourol Urodyn. 2008;27:179–90.
38. Srikrishna S, Robinson D, Cardozo L. Validation of the Patient Global Impression of Improvement (PGI-I) for urogenital prolapse. Int Urogynecol J. 2010;21:523–8.
39. Danforth KN, Townsend MK, Lifford K, Curhan GC, Resnick NM, Grodstein F. Risk factors for urinary incontinence among middle-aged women. Am J Obstet Gynecol. 2006;194:339–45.
40. Hannestad YS, Rortveit G, Daltveit AK, Hunskaar S. Are smoking and other lifestyle factors associated with female urinary incontinence? The Norwegian EPINCONT Study. BJOG. 2003;110:247–54.
41. Kudish BI, Iglesia CB, Sokol RJ, Cochrane B, Richter HE, Larson J, Hendrix SL, Howard BV. Effect of weight change on natural history of pelvic organ prolapse. Obstet Gynecol. 2009;113:81–8.
42. Melville JL, Katon W, Delaney K, Newton K. Urinary incontinence in US women: a population-based study. Arch Intern Med. 2005;165:537–42.
43. Waetjen LE, Liao S, Johnson WO, Sampselle CM, Sternfield B, Harlow SD, Gold EB. Factors associated with prevalent and incident urinary incontinence in a cohort of midlife women: a longitudinal analysis of data: study of women's health across the nation. Am J Epidemiol. 2007;165:309–18.
44. Bump RC, Mattiasson A, Bo K, Brubaker LP, DeLancey JO, Klarskov P, Shull BL, Smith AR. The

standardization of terminology of female pelvic organ prolapse and pelvic floor dysfunction. Am J Obstet Gynecol. 1996;175:10–7.
45. Swift S, Woodman P, O'Boyle A, Kahn M, Valley M, Bland D, Wang W, Schaffer J. Pelvic Organ Support Study (POSST): the distribution, clinical definition, and epidemiologic condition of pelvic organ support defects. Am J Obstet Gynecol. 2005;192:795–806.
46. Lemos NL, Auge AP, Lunardelli JL, Carramao Sda S, Faria AL, Aoki T. Validation of the Pelvic Organ Prolapse Quantification Index (POP-Q-I): a novel interpretation of the POP-Q system for optimization of POP research. Int Urogynecol J Pelvic Floor Dysfunct. 2008;19:995–7.
47. Lose G, Jorgensen L, Thunedborg P. 24-hour home pad weighing test versus 1-hour ward test in the assessment of mild stress incontinence. Acta Obstet Gynecol Scand. 1989;68:211–5.
48. Victor A, Larsson G, Asbrink AS. A simple patient-administered test for objective quantitation of the symptom of urinary incontinence. Scand J Urol Nephrol. 1987;21:277–9.

Urodynamics: Indications, Technique, and Fluoroscopy

2

Mayank Mohan Agarwal and Yogesh R. Barapatre

Women with pelvic floor disorders present with a myriad of symptomatology. It may range from stress urinary incontinence and pelvic organ prolapse (POP), urgency with or without incontinence, to voiding/defecatory dysfunction or pelvic pain/dyspareunia. Initial evaluation is almost entirely clinical, i.e. a detailed history and thorough clinical examination; an ultrasound of kidney–ureter–bladder–pelvis may be added (in my clinical practice, rather liberally) considering it an 'extension of clinical examination'. Urodynamic assessment starts at this stage only in the form of bladder diary or *the urolog*.

It must be understood at this point that urodynamic study (UDS) must not be performed for every patient with the goal of achieving a definitive diagnosis in one test. Initial treatment for any incontinence in women is behavioural, physical, and medical after non-invasive evaluation as described above. Invasive urodynamic evaluation, in other words a definitive urodynamic diagnosis, is needed only when it would make a difference in the management.

M.M. Agarwal, M.S., D.N.B., M.R.C.S.(Ed.), M.Ch. (✉)
• Y.R. Barapatre, M.S., M.Ch.
Department of Urology, Postgraduate Institute
of Medical Education and Research, Level II,
B Block, Nehru Hospital, PGIMER, Sector 12,
Chandigarh 160012, India
e-mail: drmayank.22@gmail.com

Urolog

The *Urolog*, is an extremely helpful, non-invasive tool to document the patient's drinking habits and voiding patterns over a finite period of time. Often, it is the sole metric to initiate treatment. At the most basic level, a voiding diary is just what it sounds like: a schedule for going to the bathroom. For a 24- to 48-h period the patient records all fluid intakes, and measures and records all urine output, including frequency and episodes of leakage. These data are beneficial to the physician because they clarify home voiding patterns, particularly in the elderly. They are often useful to patients as well because they provide a focus on the problem (feedback) and can serve as a baseline for treatment interventions such as behavioural training, bladder training, and pharmacologic management. This type of diary answers a lot of questions about bladder health and patterns, and creates a baseline picture of bladder control. A prototype of bladder diary used at our institute is given in Fig. 2.1.

The following information can be readily interpreted from a comprehensive urolog:

(a) Amount of urine passed in 24 h (polyuria); amount passed in nighttime (nocturnal polyuria). It can be correlated with the pattern and timing of liquid intake.
(b) Functional bladder capacity (normal/high/low); whether passing relatively fixed volumes (hypersensate bladder) or highly variable

G.H. Badlani (ed.), *Minimally Invasive Therapy for Urinary Incontinence and Pelvic Organ Prolapse*, Current Clinical Urology, DOI 10.1007/978-1-4939-0008-4_2,

BLADDER DIARY, Department of Urology, Postgraduate Institute of Medical Education and Research, Chandigarh, India

INSTRUCTIONS:

Date	Day 1			Day 2			Day 3		
	Drinks		Urine	Drinks		Urine	Drinks		Urine
	What?	How much?	How much	What?	How much?	How much? (ml)	What?	How much?	How much? (ml)
Sample	Tea	1 cup	<u>200</u> 300 S						
6-7 AM									
7-8 AM									
8-9 AM									
9-10 AM									
10-11 AM									
11-12 PM									
12-1 PM									
1-2 PM									
2-3 PM									
3-4 PM									
4-5 PM									
5-6 PM									
6-7 PM									
7-8 PM									
8-9 PM									
9-10 PM									
10-11 PM									
11-12 MN									
12-1 AM									
1-2 AM									
2-3 AM									
3-4 AM									
4-5 AM									
5-6 AM									

- Choose a 3 days period to keep this record when you can conveniently measure your voids.
- If you are unable to keep the diary for a 24 hour period, try to keep it for as many hours as possible.
- Include all voids, even if they occur in the middle of the night
- **Underline** each void accompanied by abnormal urgency (a sudden compelling desire to void which is difficult to postpone).
- If you leak urine, please wear pad all the time during the days of bladder diary. Record the number of soaked pads you had to change during each day. Note your activity at the time of any leakage
- Enter the following marks in the box when have an accidental leak of urine (even the slightest amount) –
  - "U": because you could not make it to toilet.
  - "S": during cough, sneeze, laugh, physical exertion, straining or activity.
  - "W": without knowing.
- Enter "P" in the box when you feel pain which you think is related to your bladder (pain in lower belly, urinary passage, and pain on filling of bladder).
- Mark the box you went to bed at night and you woke up in the morning finally.

The information you provide on this diary will help us better understand your urinary symptoms.

Fig. 2.1 Bladder diary prototype. (Courtesy of Postgraduate Institute of Medical Education and Research, Chandigarh, India.)

(overactive bladder). This would also help to determine appropriate fill rate during multichannel UDS if required.

(c) Quantification of urgency/incontinence/pain; the patient is asked to keep pads during the observation period.

(d) The diary would act as visual feedback for the patient for behavioural modification, scheduled/timed voiding, and judging response to therapy.

The problem of a comprehensive bladder diary is patient-compliance. The following simpler modifications are often clinically used:

(a) **Frequency-volume chart**—no record of fluid intake.

(b) **Micturition chart**—no record of fluid intake or measurement of urine volume.

Diary duration may be an important factor in terms of the reliability/representativeness of symptoms; longer diary duration is known to provide less variable diary data. Thus, a 7-day diary would be more reliable than a 3-day. The most appropriate duration of the test has not been established. Whatever the duration, it would be preferable to have diary of a weekday and a weekend to evaluate for a 'psychogenic voiding pattern'. Further details on various patterns on the urolog would be redundant here and can be found in appropriate text books.

Uroflowmetry

Uroflowmetry is defined as a measurement of rate of urine flow over time. It is easy to perform, non-invasive and requires little time and preparation. It is reflection of the final result of the act of voiding and therefore influenced by a number of variables. These include effectiveness of detrusor contractions, completeness of sphincteric relaxation, patency of urethra and, in females, adequate support of pelvic organs. It is very useful in selecting patients presenting with voiding dysfunction for more complex urodynamic testing. It also provides an objective way of determining response to treatment of certain diseases, e.g. flow after sling surgery. Since women are poor historians as far as LUTS are concerned, it is prudent to screen with uroflowmetry before undertaking invasive procedure for any pelvic floor dysfunction, whether incontinence or prolapse.

Various types of uroflowmeters are available for measurement of uroflow, viz gravimetric, rotating disc, electronic dipstick, and integral trap magnetic type. Whatever type, it is important to conform to certain standardization requirements. The International Continence Society (ICS) technical report [1] recommends a range of at least 0–50 mL/s for Qmax, 0–1,000 mL for voided volume, maximum time constant of 0.75 s, and an accuracy of +5 % relative to full scale. Uroflowmeter can be, rather preferably, set up in a toilet where tension-free, conducive environment with adequate privacy can be arranged for a hassle-free void.

Normal Uroflow Curve

The flow curve is characteristically a bell-shaped curve (Fig. 2.2) whose Qmax is achieved within initial 1/3rd of total voiding time. The relevant quantitative parameters obtained from the free flow curve are Qmax, Qave (= voided volume/ flow time), flow time, voided volume, and post-void residual urine (ultrasound).

Flow rate is affected by many factors, including volume, psychological inhibition, age, race, and

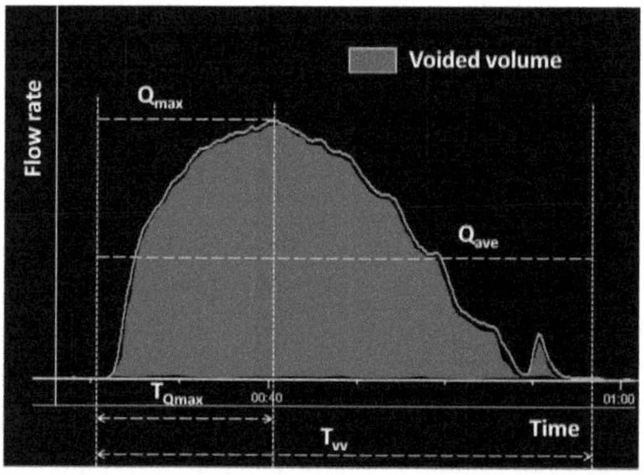

Fig. 2.2 A typical normal flow curve showing various measurements

abdominal straining. Volume is the single most important determinant of flow rates; therefore, it is imperative to mention volume with Qmax for correct interpretation. Flow–volume nomograms (Fig. 2.3) and volume normalized flow rates (cQ) are two ways to aid in interpretation [2, 3]. Since flow and volume share a quadratic relation, cQ=Q (max or average)/√bladder volume (voided volume+postvoid residue). This value is considered to be a constant for a given individual for a given condition of outlet over wide range of volumes. We found the following values [median (interquartile range)] in Indian population.

cQmax = 1.39 (1.14 – 1.66)

cQave = 0.79 (0.62 – 0.96)

We found this concept to be useful in our clinical practice akin to body mass index.

Uroflow Curve Patterns

Various abnormal flow patterns have been described (Fig. 2.4):

- Supervoid/hypervoid: a peaked curve, high Qmax with short voiding time. Often seen in patients with bladder overactivity
- Compressive obstruction: Qmax is reached early in the flow and then a prolonged tail continues
- Constrictive obstruction: a box-shaped plateau curve
- Intermittent curve: straining pattern

In the presence of abnormal flow pattern with normal urethral calibration, usually invasive UDS will be the next logical step.

Multichannel Urodynamics (UDS)

Uroflowmetry is the final outcome of function of bladder and status of urethral resistance. Therefore, it cannot differentiate between detrusor underactivity and bladder outlet obstruction. If further information is needed for management, invasive multichannel UDS would be required. It comprises pressure-flow analysis and urethral pressure profilometry (UPP) with or without fluoroscopic surveillance (video-urodynamics

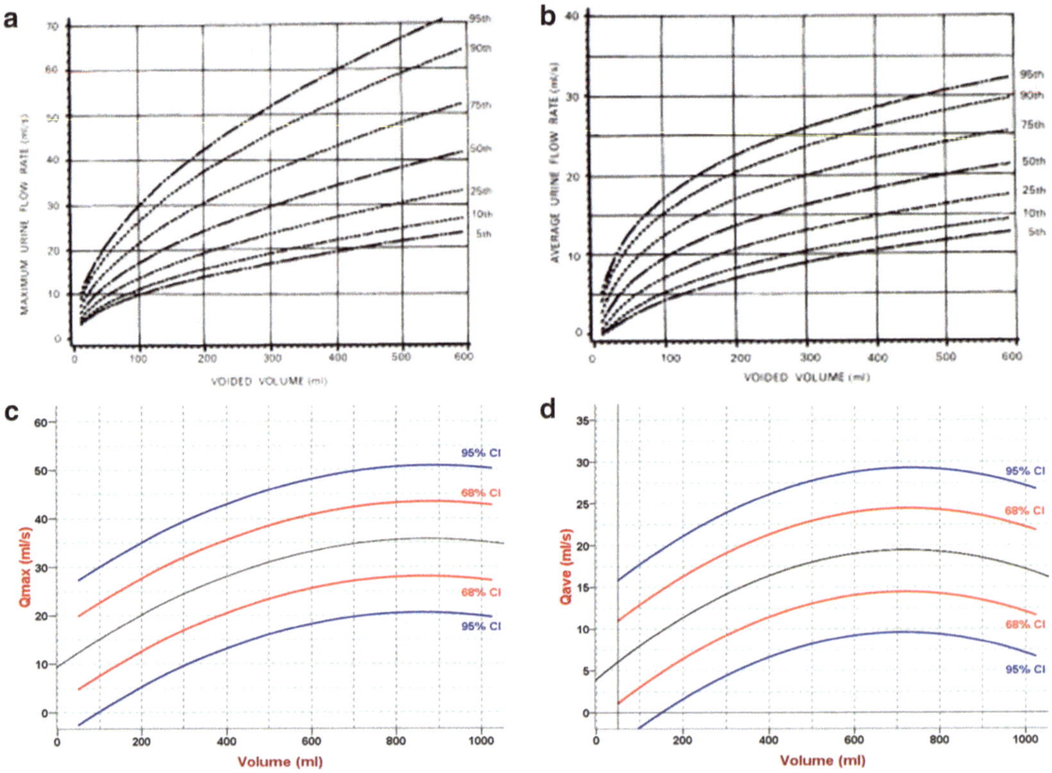

Fig. 2.3 Flow–volume nomograms for women: (**a**, **b**) liverpool nomograms for Caucasian women, and (**c**, **d**) PGIMER nomograms for Indian women. (From Barapatre Y, Agarwal MM, Singh SK, et al. Uroflowmetry in healthy women: development and validation of flow–volume and corrected flow–age nomograms. Neurourol Urodyanm 2009; 28(8): 1003–9, with permission.)

[VUDS]). The key component for pressure-measurement is a pressure transducer which converts mechanical energy into electrical signals.

For urodynamic apparatus, technical recommendations of the Working Party of Urodynamic Equipment of the ICS have been published [1] and are available on its website (www.icsoffice.org). Briefly, the transducer requirements are as follows:

- Pressure range—0–300 cmH_2O
- A sensitivity drift with temperature—less than 0.1 %/°C
- Linearity and hysteresis deviation—equal or less than ±1 % over pressure range 0–100 cmH_2O
- Should be able to sustain an overload pressure of 1,500–5,000 cmH_2O. The calibration should not change >1 % once overload pressure is removed
- A zero offset signal (a small electrical output from transducer in the presence of zero pressure) should not change >0.1 cmH_2O/°C with temperature

Multichannel UDS is always an embarrassing investigation for patients, since the woman's private parts are exposed and touched. Therefore, no stone should be left unturned to put the woman at ease, so that she will tolerate the investigator 'staring' at her introitus. Privacy should be respected at all times.

As discussed above, UDS is required for further classification and quantification of cause of LUTS in patients presenting with incontinence and POP when it would make a difference in the management. A UDS is generally not warranted when presentation is purely prolapse symptoms, i.e. 'something coming out' with or without

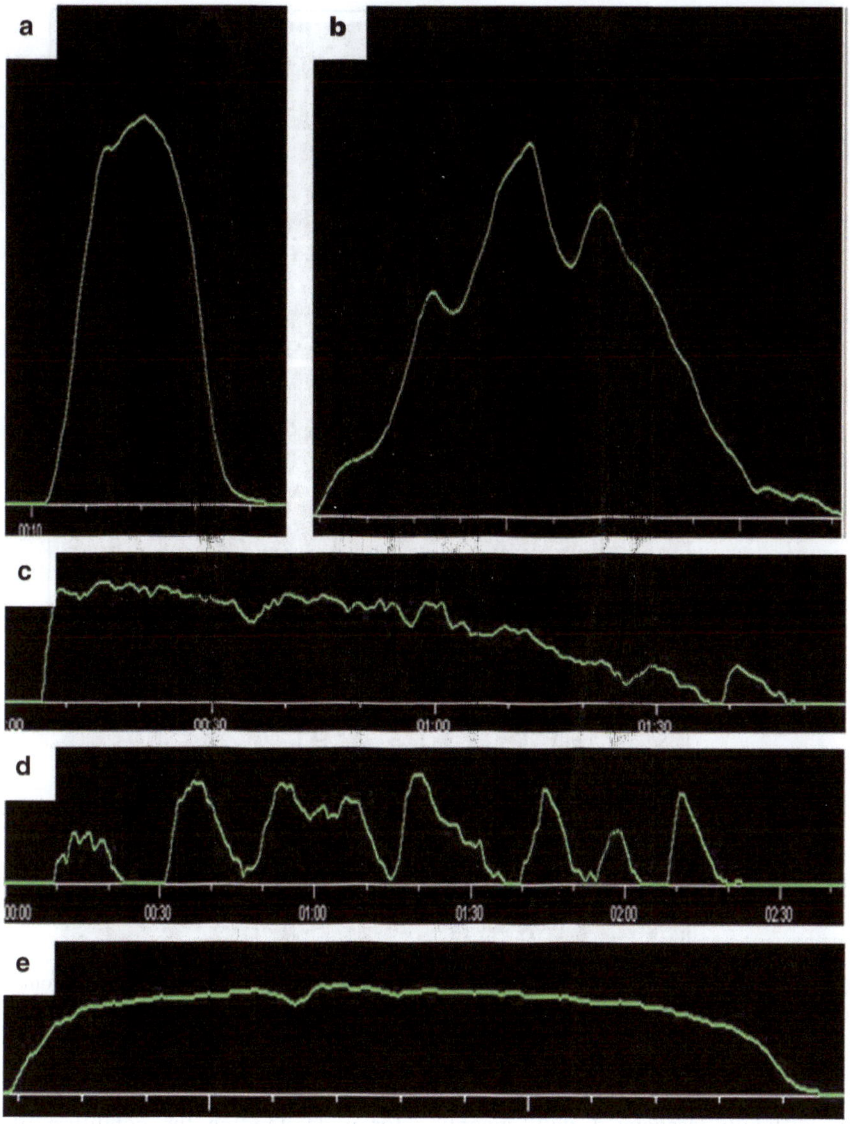

Fig. 2.4 (**a**) A peaked pattern of hypervoider; (**b**) a stattaco pattern; (**c**) compressive obstruction; (**d**) straining pattern; (**e**) constrictive obstruction

dragging in pelvis getting relieved on repositioning the prolapse. Similarly, it may possibly be omitted before midurethral sling surgery in a woman in menstrual age group presenting with pure stress urinary incontinence of moderate degree, and urethral hypermobility is demonstrable on clinical examination. However, scientific societies lack consensus on this aspect.

Nevertheless, it would be preferable to undertake a UDS before surgical intervention in the following circumstances in women:

- Severe stress incontinence, previous pelvic radiation, previous anti-incontinence surgery.
- Overactive bladder symptoms, with or without incontinence, with or without stress incontinence symptoms.

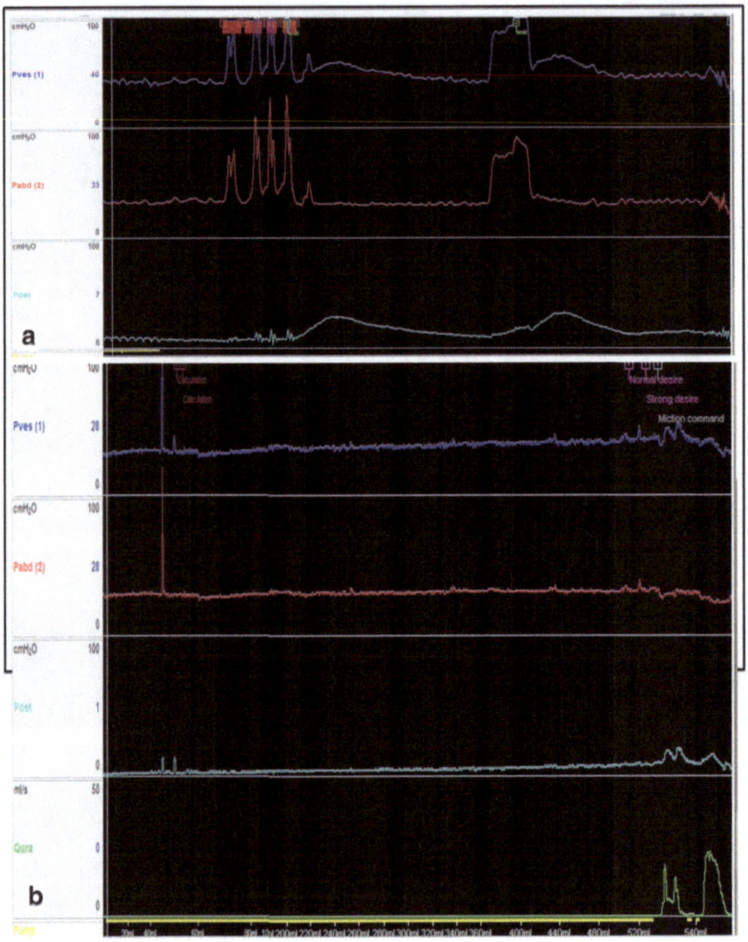

Fig. 2.5 (**a**) Stress-induced detrusor overactivity in a woman presenting with pure SUI symptoms; (**b**) urethral relaxation type voiding pattern without significant rise in detrusor pressure during voiding in a woman with severe SUI without urethral hypermobility

- Voiding difficulty associated with incontinence or POP.
- POP associated with LUTS, including in-continence.
- Poorly definable or variable symptoms.
- Associated with diseases which can affect the function of LUT/pelvic floor, e.g. diabetes mellitus, Parkinson's disease, cerebrovascular accident, and prolapsed intervertebral disc.

Various experts have suggested routine use of UDS before any anti-incontinence surgery, be it sling surgery for SUI or onabotulinum toxin A/sacral neuromodulation for urge incontinence. It not only provides useful information for understanding the condition of LUT and planning of treatment, but also helps in more informed counselling and prognostication. A significant minority of women presenting with 'pure SUI' actually have detrusor overactivity and urethral relaxation type voiding pattern (without significant detectable detrusor contraction) which may become unmasked after surgery (Fig. 2.5). Similarly, performing UDS in case of POP, both before and after reduction of POP before surgery may provide clue to occult stress incontinence and provide functional correlate to improvement (or not) in clinical symptomatology.

Table 2.1 Urodynamic description based on International Continence Society classification

Storage phase	Voiding phase
1. Bladder function	1. Bladder function
(a) Detrusor activity: normal/overactive (neurogenic/non-neurogenic)	(a) Detrusor activity: normal/underactive/acontractile
	2. Urethral function
	(a) Normal/abnormal
(b) Bladder sensation: normal/hypersensitive/ hyposensitive/absent	(b) Location of obstruction—from bladder neck
(c) Bladder capacity: normal/high/low	(c) Degree of obstruction—Blaivas' criteria, AG no. (?), DAMPF (?), Pura—Pves (max)
(d) Bladder compliance: normal/high/low	
2. Urethral function	
(a) Closure mechanism: normal/incompetent	
(b) Maximum urethral closure pressure	
(c) Urethral profile length	
(d) Leak point pressures (ALPP/DLPP)	

Advantages of UDS evaluation in women with incontinence:

- Description of detrusor activity during filling.
- Determination of bladder compliance.
- Confirmation of incontinence and its cause.
- Assessment of detrusor voiding function.
- Assessment of degree of sphincter weakness.
- Assessment of pelvic floor function.
- Assessment of urethral function.

Various classification systems exist for LUT dysfunction. Out of these, the ICS and expanded functional classifications provide the most reasonable platforms for understanding the pathophysiology of LUT dysfunction in a given patient and planning/prognosticating its treatment-outcome. A classification scheme used at our institute adopted from the ICS is presented in Table 2.1.

Cystometry: Filling and Voiding (Pressure-Flow Analysis)

A free uroflowmetry should be done before UDS as described above since it would be required for a combined interpretation. Patient should be seated comfortably on the urodynamic chair. Multipurpose UDS chairs are available some of which are also radiolucent and can be electromechanically made into various positions/heights (Fig. 2.6). The patient is placed in reclining position which helps placement of catheters and electrodes. Alternatively, if a sophisticated chair is not available, placement of catheters and filling cystometry can be performed in supine position on a couch. Subsequently, she can be shifted to the micturitional chair for a voiding phase. Of course, this method is more cumbersome. During voiding the patient may be asked to be in sitting or squatting position (whichever is her preferred voiding position), the urethral meatus should be clearly visible and a light source like torch should be available for assessment of urinary leak. The latter is very important and we believe that it is more sensitive than a fluoroscopic contrast assessment of leakage. Three types of measurement systems (catheter-transducer) are available, i.e. fluid infusion system, air-charged system and catheter-mounted microtip-transducer. Of these, the former is most widely available system.

A 6Fr double-lumen cystometry catheter is placed in the bladder and taped to the skin. Balloon rectal catheter (5–8Fr) is then placed; care is taken to place the balloon above anorectal junction without any kink in the tubing (Fig. 2.7a, b). The catheters are then attached to respective pressure transducers kept at the level of superior border of the pubic symphysis. After flushing out air from the catheter-transducer system, the transducers are zeroed to the atmosphere before starting the study. Surface Electromyography (EMG) electrodes (preferably button electrodes) are placed in the perianal region.

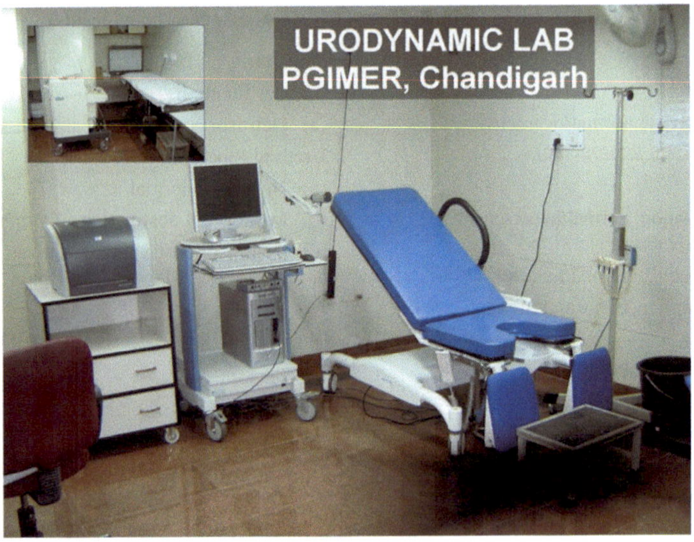

Fig. 2.6 Urodynamic suite at our institution showing the Sonesta Stille radiolucent urodynamic chair, the Solar Silver® urodynamic apparatus (MMS International, the Netherlands) and (inset) ultrasound machine

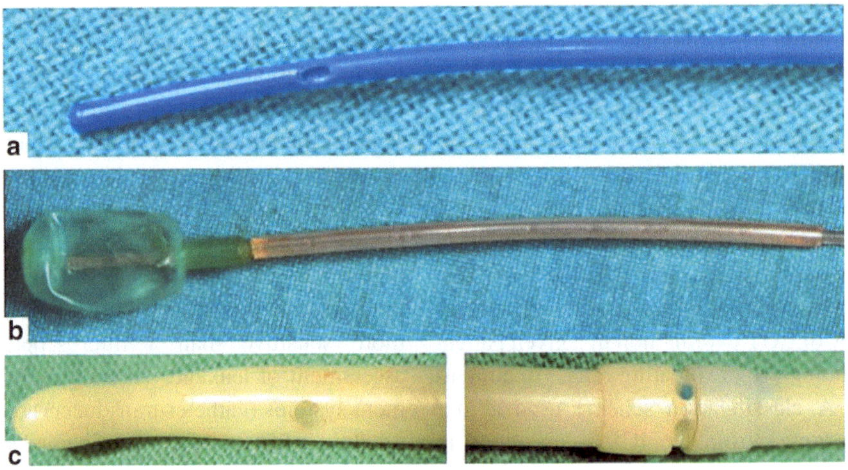

Fig. 2.7 Fluid perfusion urodynamic catheters, (**a**) a 6Fr double lumen cystometry catheter; (**b**) an 8Fr single lumen perforated balloon rectal catheter with inserter; (**c**) a 7Fr triple lumen urethral pressure profilometry (UPP) catheter

The common filling medium is sterile normal saline (0.9 % w/v). Alternatively, a diluted iodinated contrast medium is used if video-fluoroscopic surveillance is needed. It is important to calibrate the uroflowmeter to the density of the fluid used. Ideally, the fluid should be warmed to body temperature to avoid artefacts due to bladder irritation at cold temperature. The filling is started at physiological rate which has been defined as 1/4th of the body weight or less. Alternatively, a moderate fill rate (~50 mL/min) or ~10 % of functional bladder capacity (from bladder diary) can be used. Often, the first filling cycle may show artefacts due to rapid filling; therefore, it is prudent to repeat a filling-voiding cycle at the same sitting. To further allay anxiety and to develop a repo with the patient a light conversation should continue throughout the procedure

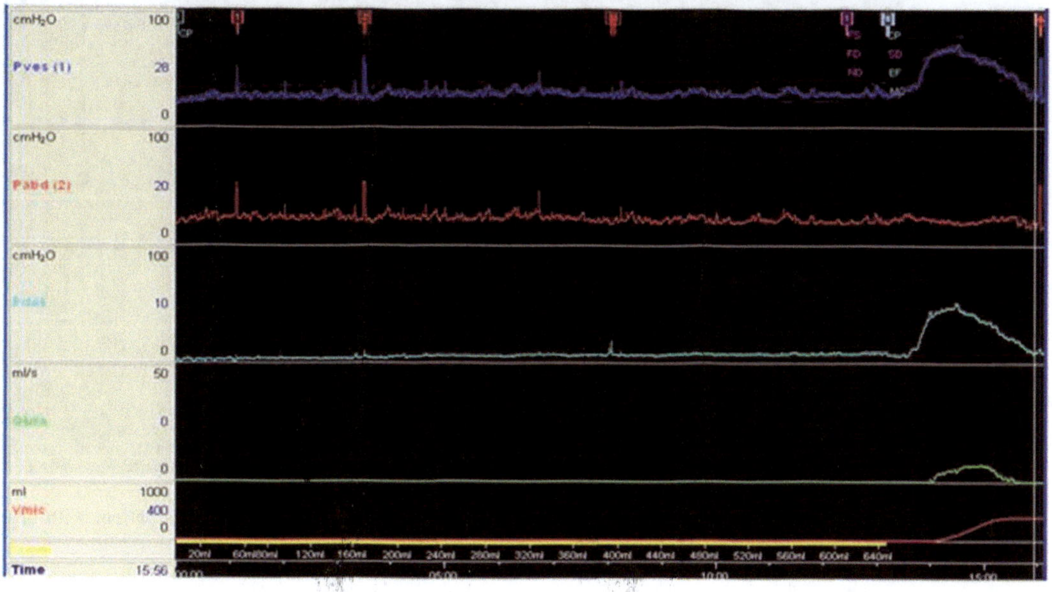

Fig. 2.8 Irregular baseline of Pves and Pabd indicates continuous conversation between doctor and patient during the study. Cough response during filling and at the end of the study suggests good equivalence between Pabd/Pves

and the following sensations are marked—first sensation, first desire, normal desire, strong desire, urgency (if felt), and maximum cystometric capacity (Fig. 2.8). Any leakage associated with urgency/detrusor overactivity is marked.

The following measurements are relevant in cystometry from the point of view of urinary incontinence:

Detrusor Overactivity

It is a urodynamic observation characterized by involuntary detrusor contractions of any amplitude during the filling phase which may be spontaneous or provoked. It can be provoked by rapid filling, use of cooled or acidic filling medium and hand wash. The term 'detrusor overactivity' replaces the previous term 'detrusor instability' as well as its definition of at least 15 cmH_2O amplitude. Detrusor overactivity is of two types as follows (Fig. 2.9):

1. **Phasic**: with or without incontinence
2. **Terminal**: single, involuntary detrusor contraction, occurring at cystometric capacity, which cannot be suppressed and results in incontinence usually resulting in bladder emptying.

It is not only important to be able to diagnose DO but also to quantify it. There have been efforts to develop indices of severity taking into account summation of all DO amplitudes or area under curve as a function of cystometric capacity (e.g. $\sum Pdet/MCC$ or $Pdet_{AUC}/MCC$). However, unfortunately, none of these concepts have been standardized.

Abdominal Leak Point Pressure

Similar to maximum urethral closure pressure (MUCP), abdominal leak point pressure (ALPP) is a measure of obstructive quality of urethra in storage phase. It is defined as the intravesical pressure at which urine leakage occurs due to increased abdominal pressure in the absence of a detrusor contraction. A value <60 cmH_2O is considered indicative of intrinsic sphincteric deficiency. It is measured at bladder volumes 150–250 mL, preferably in upright position. It can be measured by either graded cough or progressive Valsalva manoeuvre (Fig. 2.10).

The latter is considered more representative for a couple of reasons, firstly there is no significant reflex pelvic floor contraction during this manoeuvre (unlike cough) and secondly the pressure rise is

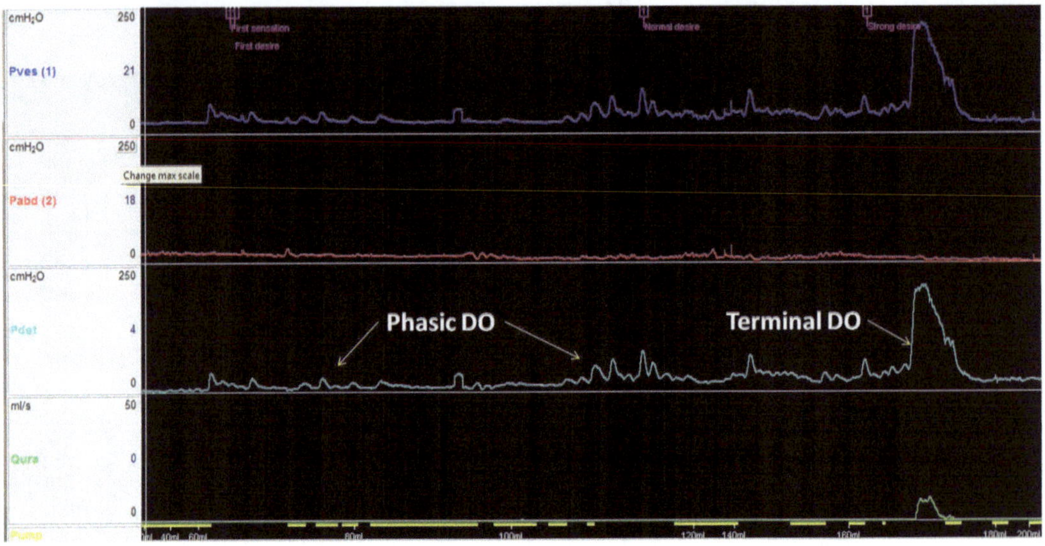

Fig. 2.9 A filling phase multichannel UDS graph showing phasic as well as terminal DO in a patient with urge incontinence and obstructive voiding

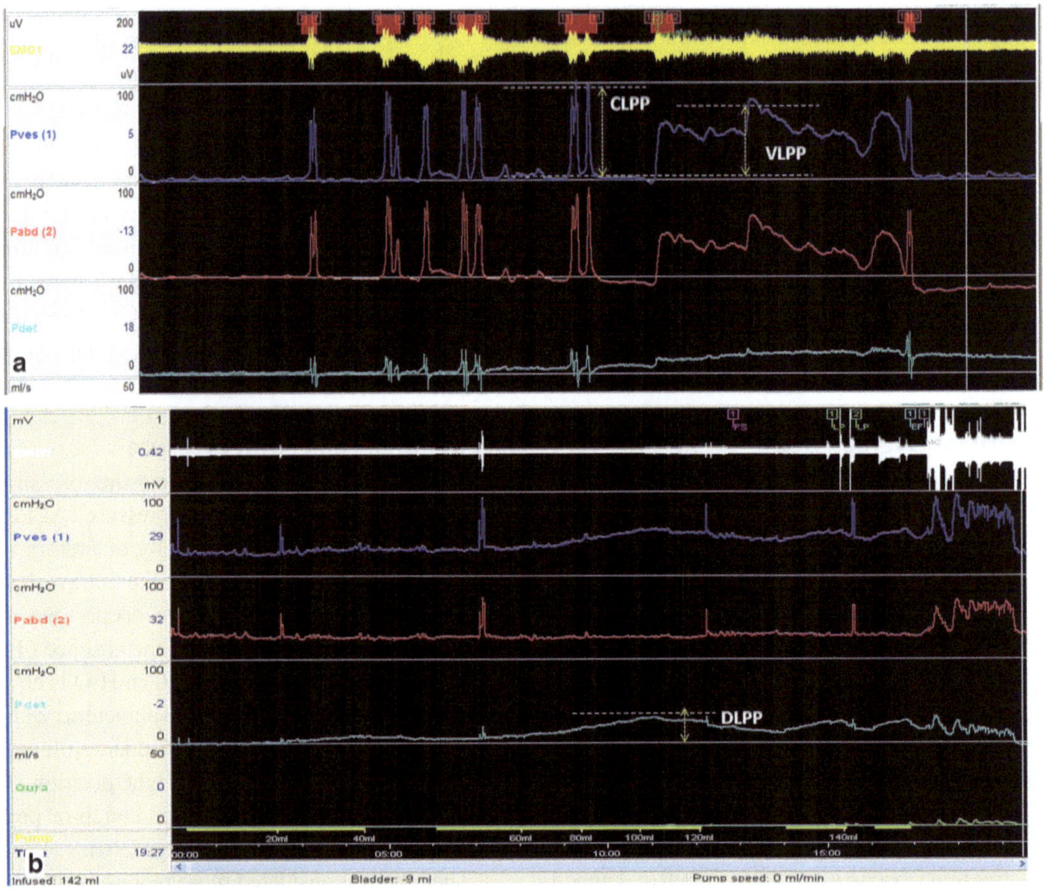

Fig. 2.10 Leak point pressure measurement. (**a**) Abdominal leak point pressures in a patient with stress urinary incontinence—difference in CLPP and VLPP is notable; (**b**) Detrusor leak point pressure in a patient with voiding dysfunction after repair of complex vesicovaginal fistula—this patient presented with bilateral hydroureteronephrosis with thick-walled bladder, which can be explained by high DLPP. Compliance in this patient had an active component suggested by a drop in Pdet on stopping flow

more controlled and graded and therefore more accurately measurable. It is based on the assumption that the 6–8Fr catheter present in the urethra does not change the measurements significantly or change the urethral disposition during stress. Although the technical aspects of measurements of ALPP have not been evaluated comprehensively, the ALPP value correlate reasonably with MUCP and in fact correlate more closely to the presence of ISD compared to the latter. During measurement, the leak is observed either directly at the meatus or using fluoroscopy; we prefer the former method. It has been found that ALPP and MUCP when considered together are more predictive of ISD from the perspective of surgical results [4].

In case the investigator is not able to demonstrate the leakage with stress manoeuvre (the urodynamic stress incontinence; USI), there are various ways to demonstrate the same.

(a) Remove the urethral catheter and ask to cough/strain. Making urethra catheter-free removes however small obstructive effect of catheter (either mechanical or sphincteric spasm)
(b) Spread the legs widely in standing position, one on the floor and another on a short stool. Spreading the legs tends to weaken the pelvic floor support to the sphincter mechanism and therefore unmask the USI
(c) Ambulatory UDS (*vide infra*)

Bladder Compliance

It indicates the status of accommodation function of the bladder. Normally the bladder should 'accommodate' the urine/filling fluid without much rise in Pdet (<10 cmH_2O) over filling volume 300–500 mL. Therefore, the compliance, defined as maximal cystometry capacity/end fill Pdet (considering it zero at zero volume) normally ranges from 30 to 50 mL/cmH_2O. A compliance less than 12.5 mL/cmH_2O is considered risk factor for damage to upper urinary tracts. Sphincteric urinary incontinence in women having poor compliance (e.g. pelvic radiation, neurogenic bladder) is a kind of 'safety valve' and therefore, it is of paramount importance to improve compliance before any anti-incontinence procedure. Compliance has two components, passive (interstitial tissue and collagen) and active (detrusor); only the latter component is sensitive to pharmacological interventions. Urodynamically, the two components of the compliance can be differentiated by stopping the filling for about 2 min and watching for decrease in Pdet (and hence improvement in compliance) (Fig. 2.10b).

Detrusor leak point pressure (DLPP) is a measure of implication of poor compliance on upper tract drainage into bladder. Pioneered by Dr J McGuire in children with meningomyelocoele, it is defined as detrusor pressure in the absence of an active detrusor contraction at which urinary leakage occurs (Fig. 2.10b). DLPP >40 cmH_2O is associated with upper tract damage.

Voiding Phase

After completion of filling and stress phases as described above, the patient is asked to void into uroflowmeter with the catheter in situ. Some women would be habitual to void with variable amount of abdominal straining; however, the patient is encouraged to relax during voiding and avoid straining at all cost. This is to avoid artefacts during the study and correctly measure the contribution of active detrusor contraction for voiding. This is important since a low Pdet during voiding (PdetQmax <12 cmH_2O) has been associated with increased incidence of voiding dysfunction after midurethral sling procedures for incontinence (Fig. 2.5b).

Diagnosis of bladder outlet obstruction in women is not as straightforward as in men since definitions lack standardization. Concept of bladder outlet obstruction index and Abrams-Griffiths nomogram are not applicable in women. Various criteria have been laid down, as follows:

(a) Massey and Abrams [5] defined BOO as the presence of two or more of the following:
   i. PdetQmax – >50 cmH_2O
   ii. Qmax – <12 mL/s
   iii. Urethral resistance factor (PdetQmax/Qmax^2) – >0.2
   iv. Significant postvoid residual urine in the presence of i or iii
(b) Defreitas et al. [6] defined BOO as the presence of Qmax <10 cmH_2O in the presence of PdetQmax > 25 cmH_2O (odds ratio 28.62)

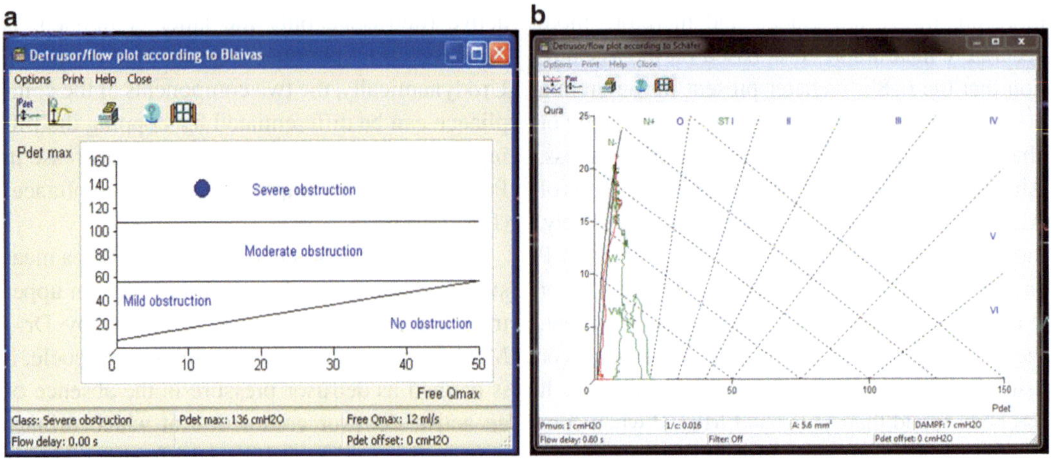

Fig. 2.11 Pressure flow nomograms. (**a**) Blaivas-Groutz nomogram, (**b**) Schaefer nomogram

(c) Blaivas and Groutz [7] developed detrusor pressure and free uroflow nomogram to predict the presence and severity of BOO and found a good correlation between subjective severity of symptoms and nomogram grading (Fig. 2.11a).

(d) Schaefer et al. conceptualized obstruction coefficient [OCO = PdetQmax/(40 + 2XQmax)] and developed pressure flow nomograms grading for BOO as well as detrusor strength simultaneously (Fig. 2.11b). This nomogram was initially validated for men. They recently suggested that the concept of OCO and the nomogram are valid for women as well [8]. Normal values for OCO are in range of 0.35 for women and 0.56 for men.

Urethral Pressure Profilometry

This UDS is indicated when the clinician is interested in knowing the function of urethra. Similar to cystometry, urethrometry, or the UPP is performed both during storage and voiding phase. During storage, it is performed during rest as well as stress manoeuvres.

A triple lumen 7Fr UPP catheter is placed in bladder, connected to appropriate transducers and fixed to an automated motor-driven puller. The catheter has three apertures, the one close to the tip for cystometry, one of the two proximal ones for urethrometry and third for fluid infusion (Fig. 2.7c).

Resting UPP

After 50–100 mL filling, the filling rate is decreased to 2–6 mL/min and puller is started to pull the UPP catheter at a predefined fixed rate (we typically keep at 2 mm/s). Once the urethral pressure aperture reaches functional bladder neck, the Pura graph shows an uprising pattern whereas the Pves continues to be at the baseline. In this way the pressure along the whole of the urethra is recorded.

Maximum Urethral Closure Pressure

Urethral closure pressure (Pclo) is defined as the urethral pressure over and above vesical pressure (Pclo = Pura − Pves) (Fig. 2.12). Understandably, it indicates the urethral resistance during storage and its maximum value (i.e. MUCP) indicates the occlusive quality of the urethra. Normally, it ranges from 40 to 60 cmH_2O; a value of less than 20–30 cmH_2O is often defined as intrinsic sphincter deficiency and is associated with poorer surgical outcomes, particularly with suspension procedures.

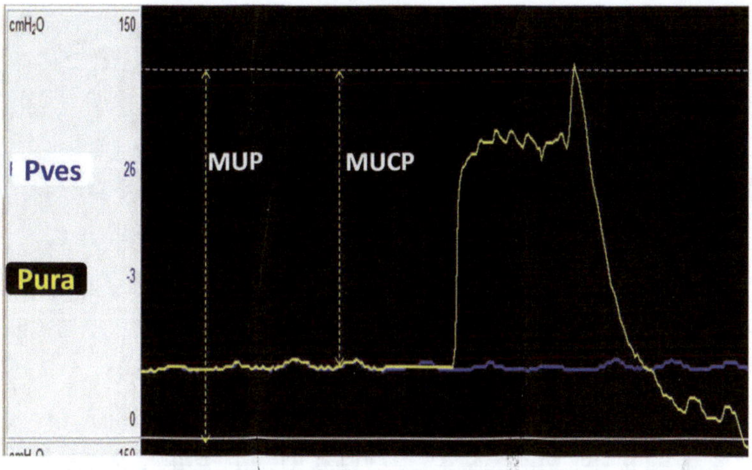

Fig. 2.12 A resting urethral pressure profilometry of a woman showing calculation of maximum urethral closure pressure

Urethral Relaxation Incontinence

This is measured during resting UPP cycle. Previously known as 'urethral instability' it is an uncommon phenomenon, sometimes detected in women presenting with large volume urinary leakage without prior warning/urgency. It is defined as a fall of Pura >15 cmH_2O during filling without concomitant rise in abdominal pressure or detrusor overactivity. Alternatively, maximum urethral pressure variation ratio of 33 % or more (ΔMUPX100/highest MUP) is considered indicative of this condition. It is not clear whether or not it is a variant of a prematurely activated micturition reflex, in which the rise in detrusor pressure due to an involuntary contraction is too small to see. According to the ICS, it is better to give a full description if symptoms are seen in association with a decrease in urethral pressure during cystometry.

Stress UPP

Once the static profile is taken, at approximately 150–250 mL of filling the catheter is pulled just below the midurethra detected by a point just past the MUCP (*vide infra*). Stress manoeuvre is performed by cough or Valsalva (blowing in a balloon is simple technique) for calculation of pressure transmission ratio and ALPP.

Pressure Transmission Ratio

This is measured in stress UPP cycle. In a normally continent woman with supported urethra, transmission of abdominal pressure to urethra is equal or greater than that to bladder in order to maintain continence. The PTR is defined as ratio of rise in Pura to rise in Pves during cough (PTR = ΔPuraX100/ΔPves). Care should be taken that during this measurement, the patient should not leak, since a fluid-bridge thus formed would transmit Pves directly giving false negative result. As discussed above, normally it should be ≥100 %. A value less than 100 % in an incontinent woman is indicative of urethral hypermobility (Fig. 2.13).

Bump et al. [9] found a PTR cut-off of 90 % to have a sensitivity and normal predictive value to be 97 %. Unfortunately, it has remained an orphan concept and its clinical relevance has not been evaluated in details.

ALPP

Another, possibly more accurate method is employing the 'fluid bridge' principle of UPP (*vide infra*). In this, the urethral aperture of the UPP catheter is placed just distal to midurethra. The patient performs Valsalva manoeuvre or graded cough and deflections are observed in the Pves, Pabd as well as Pura graphs.

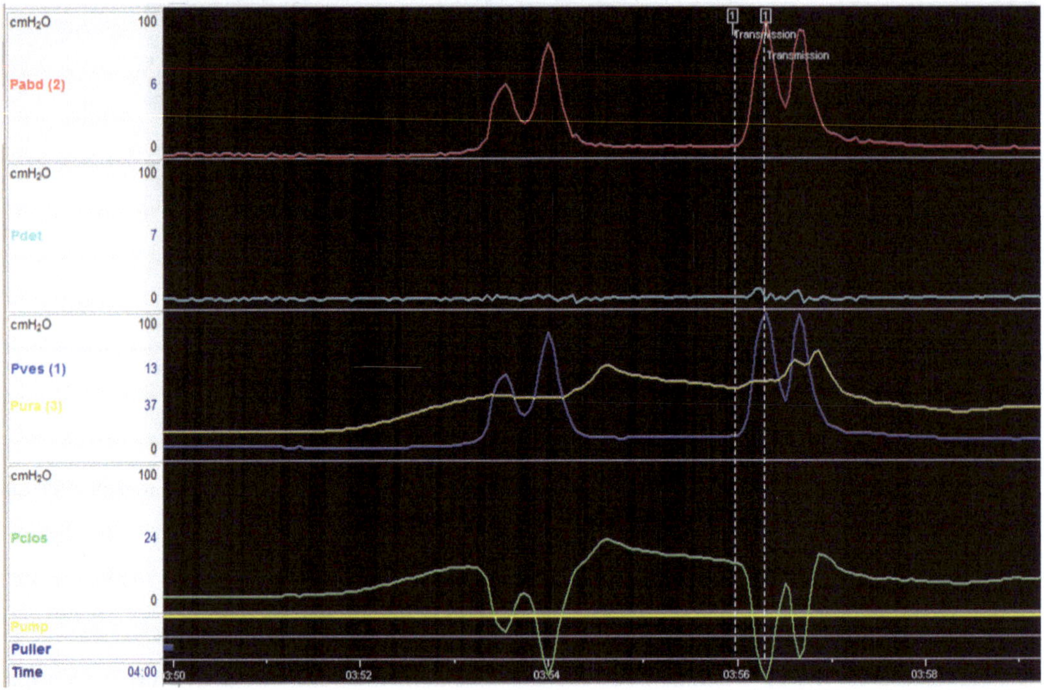

Fig. 2.13 Stress UPP graph showing measurement of pressure transmission ratio (PTR). Two points are taken, one at the start of cough and another at the peak (*broken white lines*). Difference in Pura as a percentage of Pves is PTR

As soon as there is leakage, a fluid bridge is formed and the vesical pressures are transmitted to the urethral aperture. This point is recorded and corresponding Pves is marked as ALPP (Fig. 2.14).

Voiding UPP

In the absence of standard criteria for diagnosis of bladder outlet obstruction, we have found micturitional UPP with or without fluoroscopic surveillance are quite helpful in diagnosis and localization of BOO. MUPP is performed as follows:

Once the static and stress (if indicated) have been performed, the UPP catheter is pulled back to the bladder neck, marked by elevation of Pura over Pves and kept there. The filling CMG is resumed in standard fashion. Once voiding phase is started and micturition is initiated, the puller is given command to pull at a fixed rate (2 mm/s) so that the urethral pressure orifice negotiates the urethra recording the urethral pressures all along, in real time. Normally, there should be no pressure gradient in any part of urethra (i.e. Pclo → 0) except for a minor dip in Pura at the level of urethral meatus. Any pressure gradient >5 cmH_2O is diagnostic of BOO and the point at which this happens marks the most proximal level of obstruction (Fig. 2.15).

Electromyography

The measurement of electrical activity of pelvic floor muscles is performed to study the behaviour of the muscles during micturitional cycle (storage + voiding). In the evaluation of incontinence and voiding dysfunction in women, EMG activity is helpful in indicating neurological intactness of the LUT and pelvic floor. It can be measured using needle, luminal or surface electrodes. Needle electrodes are inserted directly into the muscle in question (external urethral sphincter) and hence most accurate. However, in non-neurological conditions, this would be too invasive and painful for the information sought. Most

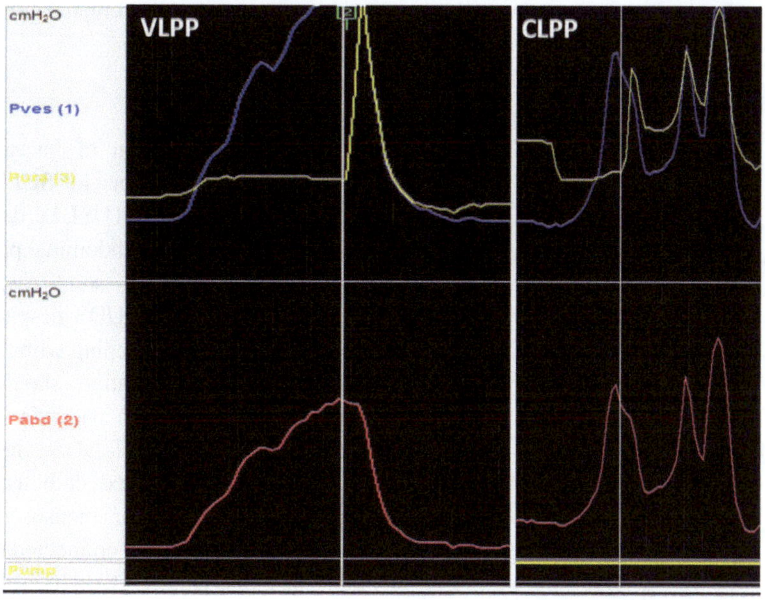

Fig. 2.14 Stress UPP graph showing measurement of abdominal leak point pressures. ALPP (CLPP and VLPP) is defined as Pves at a point (*solid vertical white line*) where Pura shows a sudden rise indicative of formation of fluid-bridge (i.e. leakage)

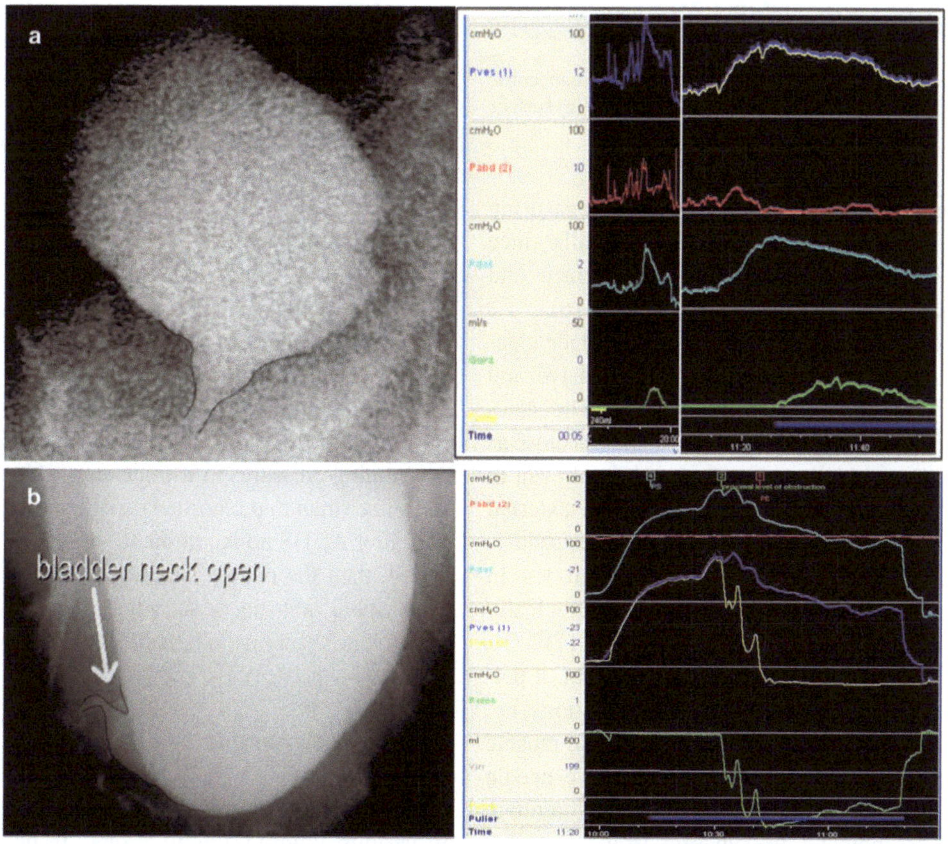

Fig. 2.15 Micturitional UPP (**a**) patient with obstructive nephropathy with incontinence—high pressure-low flow voiding pattern indicative of BOO; however, MUPP did not show any obstruction (no Pura-Pves gradient) confirmed on fluoroscopy; (**b**) patient with stage II cystocoele with voiding dysfunction showing high pressure-low flow voiding pattern indicative of BOO. It was localized by the MUPP (Pura-Pves gradient starting at midurethra) confirmed on fluoroscopy

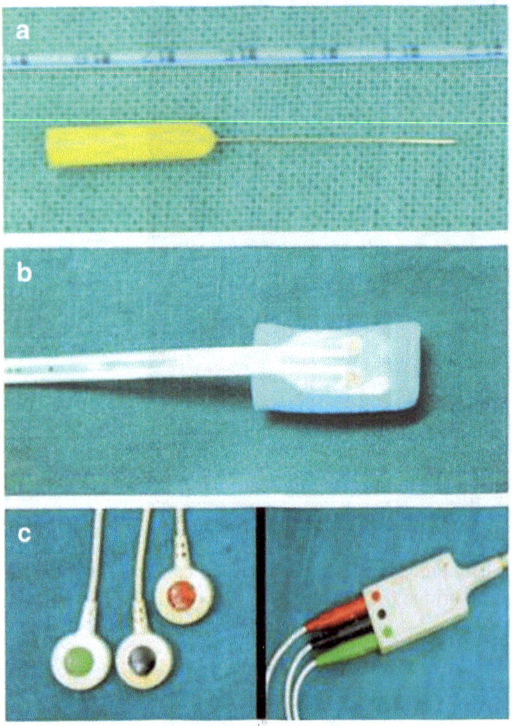

Fig. 2.16 Electromyography electrodes: (**a**) concentric needle electrode, (**b**) vaginal sponge electrode, (**c**) surface electrodes

of the information can be gathered by measuring activity of anal sphincter or puborectalis since these are easily accessible using surface and luminal electrodes, respectively (Fig. 2.16).

We most frequently use perineal surface electrodes since these are totally non-invasive and offer maximum patient-compliance. The electrodes are placed on either side of anus as close as possible. At this location, fat is minimal even in obese patients and superficial part of external anal sphincter is adjacent. Neutral electrode is placed close to the other two electrodes in perineum. The EMG patterns in neurologically intact individuals are detailed in (Fig. 2.17).

Since, surface electrodes measure sum of pelvic floor activity, there are certain limitations, i.e. noise is more and amplitude of change in muscle activity is less, compared to an invasive needle electrode. It may be difficult to differentiate detrusor sphincter dyssynergia from increased pelvic floor activity from straining.

Ambulatory UDS

The foremost indication of invasive UDS in a patient undergoing surgery for SUI is to be able to demonstrate the so-called USI, i.e. demonstration of leakage with increased abdominal pressure without any detrusor activity. In some cases, USI is not demonstrable in office UDS despite a suggestive history. Therefore, in keeping with the urodynamic principle 'the investigation should be able to explain/corroborate with patient's symptoms', an ambulatory, or natural fill, UDS is indicated.

It utilizes air-charged catheters or microtip transducer-catheters for measurement of pressures. The catheters are connected to a small portable machine (Fig. 2.18) which the patient can hang conveniently. Three cycles are recorded:

(a) Resting: patient comfortably sits in a chair or lies down
(b) Stress: patient is asked to perform stress manoeuvres
(c) Voiding: patient voids in natural voiding position in the regular toilet with/without uroflowmeter in complete privacy.

Patient is asked to mark events or accidents during recording phase (e.g. leak, urgency, or pain). The recorded data is downloaded on a desktop for interpretation.

Ambulatory UDS has revealed various surprises:

(a) DO will be detected in almost every individual if recorded long enough
(b) Poor compliance recorded on office UDS often turns out to be phasic DO
(c) Voiding pressures in women are significantly higher than that recorded on office UDS.

If after AUDS no incontinence can be demonstrated, then the patient should be told that surgery would not be wise when the cause of incontinence remains to be defined.

Video-Urodynamics

VUDS is considered gold standard for diagnosis of various voiding dysfunctions. It helps in delineating bladder outline and capacity, vesico-

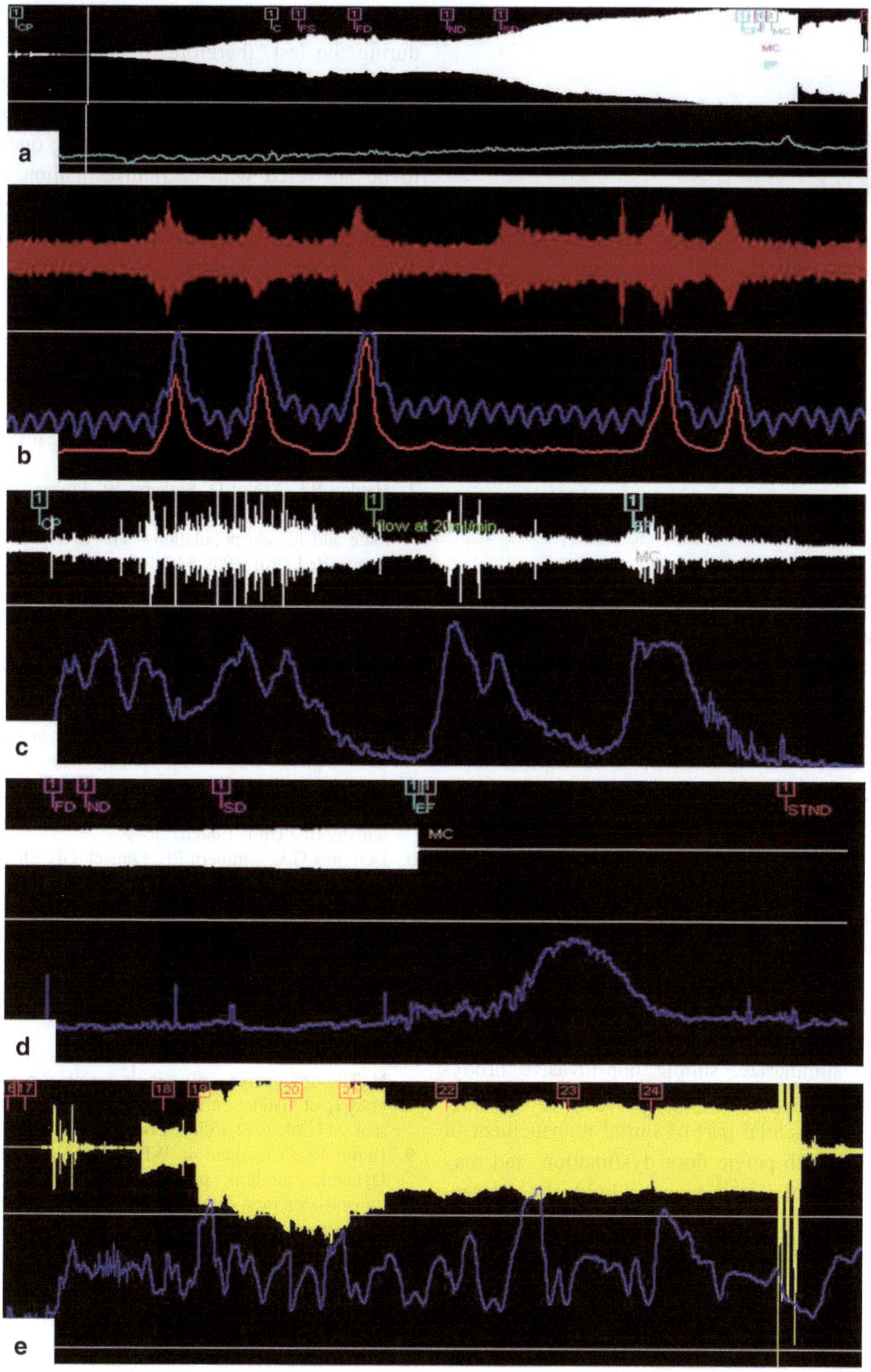

Fig. 2.17 (**a**) Progressively increasing EMG activity during storage phase; (**b**) cough response of pelvic floor activity; (**c**) reflex increase in EMG activity with detrusor overactivity; (**d**) EMG activity becomes silent just before detrusor contraction during voiding phase; (**e**) increased EMG activity of pelvic floor with abdominal straining during attempt to void. *Blue lines* represent Pves

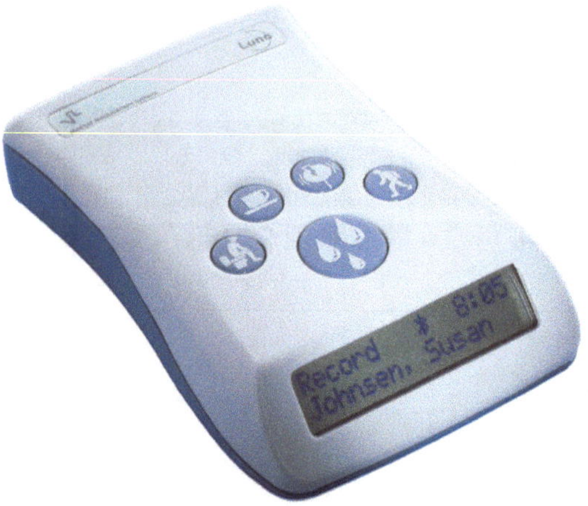

Fig. 2.18 LUNA ambulatory urodynamics apparatus. (Courtesy of MMS International, the Netherlands.)

ureteral reflux, position of bladder neck at rest, stress and during voiding, inspection of leakage during stress manoeuvre, the presence and location of BOO as well as status of anterior vaginal wall support.

Despite the benefit, there are certain disadvantages and limitations. It involves an expensive and elaborate setup which may not be practicable everywhere and it is associated with radiation hazard. Moreover, delineation of bladder outlet may not be clear at times due to positioning. In our setup, we perform UPP as described earlier which is conclusive in most circumstances. Whenever fluoroscopic surveillance is required, we perform a cystourethrogram separately in our high power fluoroscopy and radiography suite.

To summarize, simple non-invasive urodynamic investigations, e.g. urolog and uroflowmetry are essential part of initial management of patients with pelvic floor dysfunction, and may even be sufficient in many individuals undergoing invasive treatment. Multichannel UDS should be used judiciously for its invasiveness, cost, and inconvenience. It is best interpreted in real-time during the test; therefore, it is preferably performed in front of the treating team member. Whatever UDS investigation, it is of paramount importance to have clear urodynamic questions to be answered with each investigation and it must always be interpreted in clinical perspective; ultimately, it is the patients who need treatment and not the investigation!

References

1. Rowan D, James ED, Kramer AEJL, Sterling AM, Suhel PF. Urodynamic equipment: technical aspects. J Med Eng Technol. 1987;11:57–64.
2. Haylen BT, Ashby D, Sutherst JR, Frazer MI, West CR. Maximum and average urine flow rates in normal male and female populations- The Liverpool nomograms. Br J Urol. 1989;64:30–8.
3. Barapatre Y, Agarwal MM, Singh SK, Sharma SK, Mavuduru RM, Mete UK, et al. Uroflowmetry in healthy women: development and validation of flow—volume and corrected flow—age nomograms. Neurourol Urodyanm. 2009;28(8):1003–9.
4. Kilicarslan H, Gokce G, Ayan S, Guvenal T, Kaya K, Gultekin EY. Predictors of outcome after in situ anterior vaginal wall sling surgery. Int Urogynol J. 2003;14:339–41.
5. Massey JA, Abrams PH. Obstructed voiding in the female. Br J Urol. 1988;61:36–9.
6. Defreitas GA, Zimmern PE, Lemack GE, Shariat SF. Refining diagnosis of anatomic female bladder outlet obstruction: comparison of pressure-flow study parameters in clinically obstructed women with those of normal controls. Urology. 2004;64:675–9.
7. Blaivas JG, Groutz A. Bladder Outlet obstruction nomogram for women with lower urinary tract symptomatology. Neurourol Urodyn. 2000;19(5):554–64.
8. Schaefer W, Clarkson B, Griffiths D, Tadic S, Resnick N. The urodynamics of voiding function in females: grading of bladder outflow conditions on a continuous scale. J Urol. 2011;185(4S):e682–3.
9. Bump RC, Copeland Jr WE, Hurt WG, Fantl JA. Dynamic urethral pressure/profilometry pressure transmission ratio determinations in stress incontinent and stress-continent subjects. Am J Obs Gyn. 1988;159:749–55.

Part II

Female Stress Urinary Incontinence

3 Retropubic Midurethral Synthetic Slings for Female Stress Urinary Incontinence

Oussama El Yazami Adli and Jacques Corcos

Female stress urinary incontinence (SUI), defined as involuntary leakage on effort, exertion, sneezing, or coughing [1], is a prevalent condition with significant impact on patient quality of life (QoL). About 18.3 million American women suffered from urinary incontinence in 2010, and almost 50 % of them reported SUI as the primary or sole symptom, with a financial burden of over US $12 billion a year [2, 3]. This number is expected to increase substantially as the population ages. Worldwide, the prevalence of female SUI ranges from 5 to 61 %, and its incidence is estimated to be 4–11 % per year [4, 5].

Tension-free vaginal tape (TVT®; Gynecare, Ethicon, Somerville, NJ, USA) was the first retropubic midurethral synthetic sling (MUSS) [6] proposed to address defective suburethral support, hypothesized to be responsible for the development of stress incontinence. Since then, the procedure has changed the perspective of SUI treatment and has become standard of care. It has several advantages, including a mini-invasive vaginal approach, short operation time, and hospital stay, combined with excellent short- and long-term results.

O.E.Y. Adli, M.D. • J. Corcos, M.D., F.R.C.S.(S). (✉)
Department of Urology, McGill University, Jewish General Hospital, 3755 Côte Sainte-Catherine Road, Montreal, QC, Canada H3T 1E2
e-mail: jcorcos@uro.jgh.mcgill.ca

Development of the TVT Procedure

The retropubic MUSS procedure was first based on the work of Petros and Ulmsten [7] describing the "integral theory" as the basis of female urinary continence during sudden increases in intra-abdominal pressure through the vaginal connective tissue and/or pelvic ligamentous support. In 1994, the "hammock theory" of DeLancey postulated the role of two elements, the sphincter and urethral support [8]. The supportive hammock under the urethra provides a firm backstop against which it is compressed during heightened abdominal pressure, preventing urine leakage.

Retropubic MUSSs (Fig. 3.1) reinforce urethral support at the level of the pubourethral ligaments. Sling placement at the midurethra enables dynamic urethral kinking when abdominal pressure is amplified and provides continence without affecting the bladder neck. This has been well-demonstrated in sonographic and dynamic magnetic resonance imaging studies [9, 10].

In its original description, the procedure involved sling positioning in a retrograde manner (bottom-to-top). Since then, several modifications have been made regarding trocar passage and sling composition.

Based on animal and clinical studies [11–14], most commercially available MUSSs nowadays are made from type I, macroporous, monofilament, uncoated mesh that is believed to be resistant to infection and inflammation (Table 3.1).

G.H. Badlani (ed.), *Minimally Invasive Therapy for Urinary Incontinence and Pelvic Organ Prolapse*, Current Clinical Urology, DOI 10.1007/978-1-4939-0008-4_3,

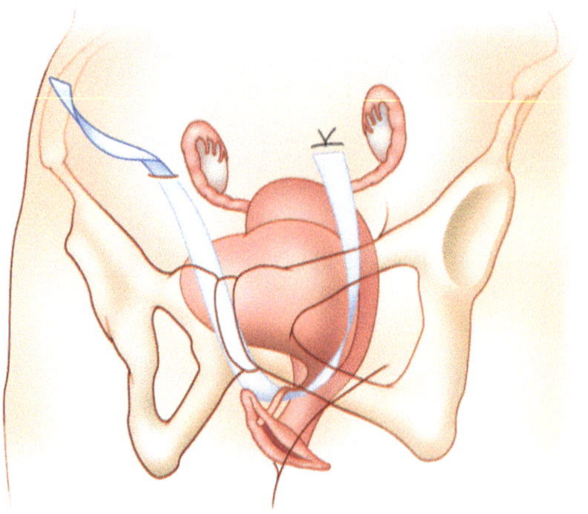

Fig. 3.1 Position of the retropubic tension-free vaginal tape

Table 3.1 Commercially available retropubic slings

Brand	Approach	Material
TVT® (Gynecare, Ethicon, Somerville, NJ, USA)	Retrograde	Monofilament
Advantage® (Boston Scientific Corporation, Natick, MA, USA)	Retrograde	Monofilament
SPARC® (American Medical Systems, Minnetonka, MN, USA)	Antegrade	Monofilament
Lynx® (Boston Scientific)	Antegrade	Monofilament
Anterior intravaginal slingplasty (Tyco Healthcare LP, Norwalk, CT, USA)	Retrograde	Multifilament

Interestingly, in a randomized controlled trial (RCT) on 100 female SUI patients, Rechberger et al. [15] reported similar cure and complication rates with both monofilament and multifilament meshes up to 18 months, but published no long-term data.

Surgical Procedure

We first describe a surgical technique inspired by the original bottom-to-top procedure, with some minor changes. The top-to-bottom approach is addressed thereafter.

The TVT® kit consists of two curved needles attached to a 1.1×40 cm polypropylene mesh sling sheathed in plastic, with a detachable handle to facilitate retropubic passage of the needles and a guide to rigidify the Foley catheter.

Although the original method emphasized the use of local anesthesia, most procedures are now performed under spinal or general anesthesia. Patients are placed in the dorsal supine lithotomy position, prepped and draped in a sterile manner. Perioperative broad spectrum antibiotics are administered, and appropriate anti-embolism precautions are taken, depending on hospital policy. An 18-Fr Foley catheter is placed in the urethra.

Local anesthetics are infiltrated vaginally (10 cc on the side of the urethra up to the urogenital diaphragm and 5 cc under the vaginal mucosa) prior to incision if the procedure is to be performed under local anesthesia. Anesthetics (20 cc) are injected in the suprapubic area as well as on each side of the planned skin incision site.

A 1.5-cm midline vaginal incision is made, starting 0.5 cm from the external meatus of the urethra. Blunt dissection with Metzembaum scissors is undertaken in the paraurethral area between the vaginal mucosa and the pubocervical, orienting towards the symphysis pubis. Special care must be taken to coagulate or compress any bleeding. Dissection is advanced as far as the subsymphysial space with scissors or finger through the incision.

The guide is placed in the Foley catheter which is tented towards the ipsilateral side of trocar passage to mobilize the bladder neck and proximal urethra away from the trocar path. The needle is secured to the handle, then placed within the paraurethral tunnel with the needle tip between the surgeon's index finger in the vagina and the lower rim of the pubic ramus. Slow, controlled pressure is needed to bring the needle, oriented along the previously dissected path, through the urogenital diaphragm, the space of retzius and the rectus abdominal fascia, in close contact with the pubic bone, targeting the skin mark about 1 cm from midline above the pubis (Fig. 3.2a, b). The skin is then breached with a scalpel, and the needle is externalized. The same procedure is

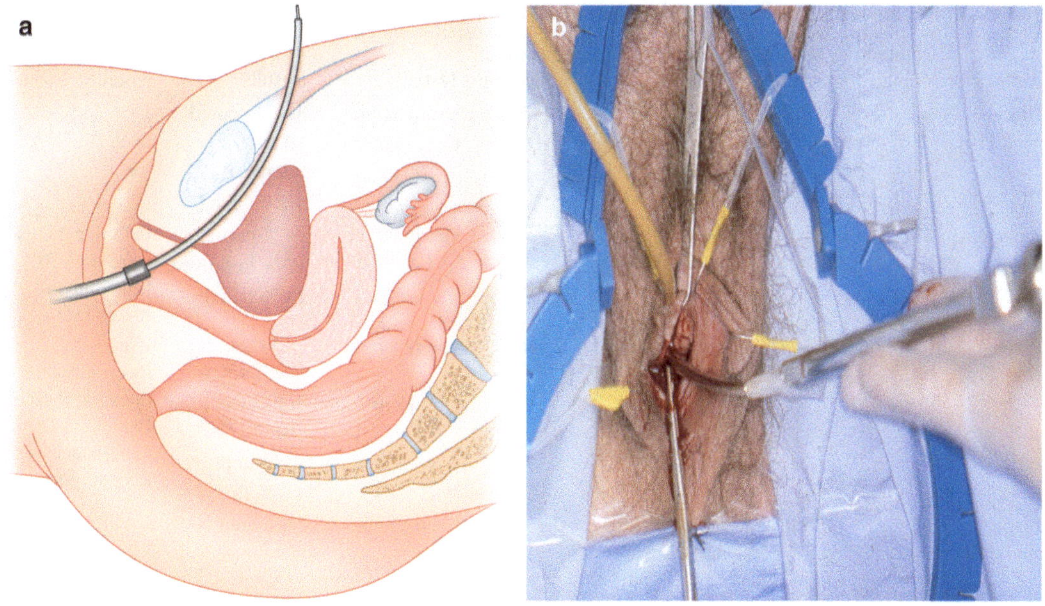

Fig. 3.2 Passage of the trocar in bottom-to-top fashion. (**a**) Schematic view of the path of passage from the vaginal incision through the urogenital diaphragm, the space of retzius, and the rectus abdominal fascia in close contact with the pubic bone and (**b**) perioperative view

followed on the other side. At this point, cystoscopy is undertaken to ensure bladder integrity.

The sling is positioned suburethrally by pulling on the threads and adjusted. The bladder is filled with 250–300 cc of saline, and a cough test is performed. The tape is tightened accordingly, until only a drop of saline is at the meatus. The Metzembaum scissors are then placed between the urethra and the tape to avoid over-adjustment, and the plastic sheet is removed. The tips of the sling are sectioned at the level of the skin and retracted from the cutaneous plane. Hemostasis is verified, and the vaginal incision is sutured. A vaginal gauze pad is left in the vagina for 24 h.

In the top-to-bottom approach, the suprapubic arc sling kit (SPARC® American Medical Systems, Minnetonka, MN, USA) contains two needles that are smaller than TVT® trocars. Prepubic incisions are first made 1 cm from midline on each side above the pubis, and the needles are passed from there onto the surgeon's finger placed within the periurethral dissection. The mesh is attached to the needles by sliding dilating connectors and withdrawn from the prepubic incisions. It is tensioned similar to the bottom-to-top approach.

Results

Efficacy

TVT is the best studied and documented procedure among MUSSs. Table 3.2 summarizes the long-term outcome data. Cure rates up to 11.5 years are reported to be up to 90 % and are in the same order as those reported in initial, early trials [6], indicating effective maintenance over the years.

Comparison Between Retropubic MUSSs According to the Tape Placement Approach

Few RCTs comparing TVT® with other retropubic MUSSs have been published. Comparison of different bottom-to-top slings has revealed no significant differences [26]. Andonian et al. [27]

Table 3.2 Results of retropubic midurethral slings in the literature

Authors	Number of patients	Mean age at surgery	Recruitment criteria	Length of follow-up	Testing	Results	Notes
Nilsson et al. [16]	85	57	Primary SUI	5 years	Urodynamics QoL evaluation	84.7 % cured 10.6 % improved 4.7 % failed	
Rezapour and Ulmsten [17]	49	66	Stress incontinence and ISD	4 years	Urodynamics QoL evaluation	74 % cured 12 % improved 14 % failed	Failing patients were over 70 years old with severe ISD
Reich et al. [18]	108	63	Unselected group	7 years	Urodynamics QoL evaluation	Objective cure rate: 89.8 % Subjective cure rate: 82 % 13 % improved 4.6 % failed	Urge incontinence is the main reason for dissatisfaction after surgery
Liapis et al. [19]	65	58.1	SUI with stage 1 cystocele	7 years	Urodynamics	Cure rate: 80 % Failure rate: 13.5 %	
Song et al. [20]	306	50.7	SUI	7 years	Urodynamics QoL evaluation	Cure rate: 84.6 %	23.2 % had complications at 1-month follow-up after surgery
Groutz et al. [21]	52	62.4	Urodynamically confirmed SUI	10 years	Questionnaire	Subjective cure rate: 65 % Improvement: 12 % Failure rate: 23 %	54 % of patients had concomitant UUI
Serati et al. [22]	58	58	SUI without ISD or POP	10 years	Urodynamics	Objective cure rate: 93.1 % Subjective cure rate: 89.7 %	
Abdul-Rahman et al. [23]	12	53.3	Neuropathic bladder dysfunction and SUI	10 years	Urodynamics (incontinence impact questionnaire)	7 patients cured 2 patients improved 1 failed	2 patients lost to follow-up at 10 years were continent at 5 years
Olsson et al. [24]	128	54.4	SUI	11.5 years	Stress test, 23-h pad test, questionnaire	Objective cure rate: 84 % Subjective cure rate: 77 % 18 % improved	
Nilsson et al. [25]	–	69	SUI	11 years	Urodynamics QoL evaluation	Objective cure rate: 90 % Subjective cure rate: 77 %	

randomized 41 patients with SUI to either SPARC® or TVT® but did not find statistically significant differences in terms of cure rates and complications at 1-year follow-up. Lord et al. [28] and Tseng et al. [29] reported a higher cure rate and fewer short-term complications with the bottom-to-top compared to the top-to-bottom approach. Meta-analysis by Novara et al. [30] led

Table 3.3 Complication rates with the TVT procedure

Authors	Number of patients	Bladder injury	Bleeding	Voiding difficulties	De novo urgency	Hematoma	Urinary tract infections	Sling erosion/ extrusion	Notes
Tamussino et al. [37]	2,795	2.70 %	2.30 %	Not reported	Not reported	0.67 %	17.0 %	Not reported	41 % of patients had concomitant surgery
Kuuva and Nilsson [38]	1,455	3.80 %	1.90 %	7.60 %	0.20 %	1.90 %	4.1 %	Not reported	
Olsson et al. [24]	124	2.7	2.7	12.1 %	21.2	–	7.2 %	0	
Kristensen et al. [39]	788	6.6 %	0.6 %	56 %	Not reported	0.8 %	3.1 %	Not reported	
Pushkar et al. [40]	207	5.4 %	Not reported	5.9 %	8 %	9.1 %	Not reported	0.5 %	
Tincello et al. [41]	437	2.1 %	1 %	2.1 %	3 %	2 %	1.9 %	1.5 %	1-year data
Lleberia-Juanos et al. [42]	243	6.2 %	1.6 %	13.2 %	24.7 %	Not reported	4.5 %	4.1 %	
Serati et al. [22]	63	2 cases	0	0	18.9 %	Not reported	Not reported	Not reported	10-year data

to the conclusion that the bottom-to-top procedure was more efficacious than the top-to-bottom mode, and similar results were published recently by Ogah et al. [31]. The long-term follow-up data of Heidler et al. [32] seem to endorse this conclusion.

TVT Versus Other Procedures for the Treatment of Incontinence

Meta-analyses of available RCTs suggest that retropubic MUSSs outperform Bursh colposuspension in terms of postoperative cure rates, but colposuspension is associated with fewer perioperative complications, shorter indwelling catheter duration and less long-term voiding dysfunction [30, 33, 34]. Similar success rates have been reported for both TVT® and fascial pubovaginal slings.

Comparison of retropubic and transobturator approaches reveals that both have globally similar postoperative outcomes. Sung et al. [35] and Long et al. [36] did not discern statistically significant differences in subjective cure or improvement rates, but the objective cure rate seemed to favor retropubic MUSS (88 % vs. 84 % for the transobturator approach) [31]. On the other hand, the transobturator route is linked with lower peri- and postoperative complication rates as well as shorter surgery time but with more frequent postoperative groin pain.

Minimally invasive, synthetic suburethral slings appear to be as effective as retropubic MUSSs in the short-term but with fewer postoperative complications (shorter operation time, less postoperative voiding dysfunction, and *de novo* urgency). However, quality of the evidence is insufficient because available trials and long-term data are lacking [31].

Complications

Perioperative and postoperative complications after retropubic MUSSs are rare. Table 3.3 summarizes the complication rate with the TVT® procedure. The risk of intraoperative complications is not related to patient age, body mass index (BMI), or parity, but may be due to surgeon experience and previous prolapse or incontinence surgery [39, 40]. Long-term follow-up data do not disclose any signs of rejection or adverse tissue reactions to the polypropylene tape.

Perioperative Complications

The **bladder injury** rate seems to be consistent in different series. Insufficient surgeon experience, previous incontinence, and pelvic surgery are independent risk factors for trocar injury [39], which should be promptly recognized on perioperative cystoscopy for correct application needle reinsertion. There is no need for primary closure or longer than usual bladder drainage, so that healing can take place without sequelae. Urethral injury is rare (less than 1 %) and should be repaired immediately [43].

Bowel injury is a rare complication that may occur during trocar passage in patients with a previous history of abdominal or pelvic surgery [44].

The incidence of **vascular injury**, estimated to be 2.7–6 % with the TVT® procedure, is due to lack of direct pelvic vascular structure visualization during trocar passage. The risk can be minimized (but not entirely eliminated) by a good operating technique. **Bleeding** can be managed by vaginal packing or compression of the anterior vaginal wall directly against the symphysis pubis. Persistent bleeding indicates major vessel injury and warrants retropubic exploration.

Postoperative Complications

Voiding dysfunction may present as complete urinary retention, persistently elevated post-void residual (PVR) or bothersome and poorly characterized lower urinary tract symptoms with variable incidence, depending on its definition [45]. It may occur despite standard perioperative use of scissors contact to provide a space between the tape and the urethra. Preoperative voiding difficulties and concomitant prolapse surgery are independent risk factors for postoperative voiding problems [46]. In case of complete, immediate postoperative urinary retention, re-intervention within 48 h is strongly advocated to release tension. This procedure is easily performed under local anesthesia compared to delayed sling mobilization (after 3–4 days) which can prove to be extremely difficult. The options for patients with initially high PVR include long-term clean intermittent catheterization, suprapubic catheterization, and alpha-blocker pharmacotherapy. Insufficient improvement after 1 month should prompt transvaginal sling excision or urethrolysis, acknowledging the significant risk of recurrent SUI symptoms [45].

***De novo* urgency**, with or without incontinence episodes, is a significant problem after all types of incontinence surgery. The incidence rate after retropubic MUSSs ranges from 4 to 33 % [34, 47–49], and the symptoms are reported to be as bothersome as preoperative SUI [50]. The origin of *de novo* urgency and its mechanism are unclear. Risk factors include old age, parity, history of cesarean section and recurrent urinary tract infections (UTI), elevated detrusor pressure over 15 cmH_2O during the filling phase, and maximal detrusor pressure (P_{detmax}) of less than 28 cmH_2O during the voiding phase on preoperative cystometry [51]. Antimuscarinics in this particular type of symptomatic DO seem to be less efficient in this than in idiopathic overactive bladder syndrome [34]. Urethrolysis with sling resection remains an option in the presence of obstruction.

The incidence of **vaginal extrusion** and **urinary tract erosion** is reported to be around 2 %. Interestingly, Nilsson et al. [25] did not encounter any cases of tape extrusion/erosion on 11-year patient follow-up. Extrusion may be related to poor surgical technique, infection, or physical properties of the implanted material [45]. Large extrusions should be managed by excision and removal of the extruded sling segment, but simple observation could be an option for nonsexually active patients with small extrusions. On the other hand, urinary tract erosion is confirmed by endoscopy and must be managed operatively by scissors or laser transection of the intraluminal portion of the sling or by an open technique.

The incidence of **other complications**, such as dyspareunia, is poorly documented, but must warn of possible sling extrusion. Surgical site infections are rare and occur mostly with multifilament meshes.

Special Considerations

Mixed Urinary Incontinence

Mixed urinary incontinence is defined as the involuntary loss of urine associated with the sensation of urgency and also with exertion, sneezing, or coughing [1]. Up to 80 % of patients diagnosed with SUI report mixed symptoms [49], and these women may be difficult to manage with conservative measures alone.

Several studies have described retropubic MUSS outcomes in patients, showing overall improvement of both stress and urge components [52–54]. Paick et al. [55] reported an overall cure rate of 81.9 % at mean follow-up of 10.9 months, and multivariate analysis disclosed that failure to cure urgency urinary incontinence was related to low maximum urethral closure pressure (MUCP) and the presence of uninhibited DO. Resolution of urodynamic DO after the retropubic MUSS procedure has been noted in 23–40 % of patients [56, 57]. Objective and subjective cure rates are encouraging in women with a predominant stress component and in those with equal urgency and stress incontinence than in subjects with predominant urgency [58]. In a systemic review of the published data, Jain et al. [59] found good cure rates of the stress component (85–97 %) and lower (30–85 %) and declining cure rates of urgency incontinence over time.

Intrinsic Sphincter Deficiency

Intrinsic sphincter deficiency (ISD), defined by objective urodynamic measurements of urethral function as MUCP of 20 cmH_2O or less, or Valsalva leak point pressure (VLPP) lower than 60 cmH_2O [60, 61], is associated with poor surgical outcome after urethral suspension procedures [62]. We strongly support the statement that, to a certain degree, ISD is always coupled with SUI.

Most studies of retropubic MUSSs excluded or contained small numbers of patients with ISD. Thus, fewer series are available for analysis. Overall, the retropubic approach is effective in treating SUI and ISD, although the cure rates are slightly lower than those of SUI without ISD. Rodriguez et al. [63] did not detect a significant impact of various VLPP values on TVT outcomes. Rezapour et al. [64], who reported 4-year follow-up of TVT in ISD patients, obtained objective and subjective cure rates of 74 % and improvement in 12 % of patients, which are lower than the cure rates of SUI without ISD. Multivariate analysis of several observational studies failed to demonstrate ISD as an independent risk factor for surgical failure. Some authors suggested that the coexistence of poor urethral mobility and ISD may be associated with a higher surgical failure rate [65]. The failure rate with retropubic MUSSs remains lower than with transobturator slings, as seen in two large, comparative, retrospective, and randomized controlled studies [66, 67]. Proper explanations remain unclear.

Recurrent SUI

Recurrent SUI may be related to the underlying mechanism in SUI (ISD) or inappropriate intraoperative tape adjustment. Management of these situations can be difficult. Clinical guidelines from the Society of Obstetricians and Gynaecologists of Canada call for conservative measures as the first-line modality in recurrent SUI [68]. However, such conclusions are mainly extrapolated from studies of primary SUI. Surgical options include bulking agents, abdominal urethropexy, artificial urinary sphincter (AUS), and repeat MUSSs. The success rate with bulking agents tends to decrease over time. The failure rate of Bursh colposuspension is 55 % in patients with recurrent ISD without urethral hypermobility. The cure rates of AUS in properly selected patients are reported to be 76–89 % [69–72].

Secondary retropubic MUSSs are associated with significant cure rates after retropubic or transobturator synthetic sling placement. Objective and subjective cure rates in retrospective and prospective studies varied between 77.4 % and 62 % after median follow-up of 19 and 40 months, respectively [73–75]. It is noteworthy that all these studies exclusively or predominantly recruited patients with ISD. The repeat retropubic approach is significantly more successful than the repeat transobturator procedure (71 % vs. 48 %) with no increase in the incidence of complications compared to primary surgery, except for *de novo* urgency (30 % vs. 14 %, $p<0.001$).

Concomitant Pelvic Organ Orolapse Surgery

The TVT procedure is more easily undertaken with a vaginal Pelvic Organ Orolapse (POP) approach than with abdominal surgery. The sequence of MUSS placement depends on POP procedure, but the tape should be adjusted after its completion [76].

Despite limited follow-up in most published studies, the objective cure rate of urinary incontinence is between 84 and 94 % [77–80]. The question of whether or not to perform a TVT procedure for occult SUI at the time of prolapse surgery was addressed by Liang et al. [81] who reported a significantly higher rate of postoperative stress incontinence in women who did not undergo TVT® vs. those who did (64 % vs. 10 %). In a Cochrane database review, Maher et al. [82] concluded that the addition of TVT to prolapse repair may reduce the incidence of postoperative urinary incontinence (relative risk 5.5, 95 % confidence interval 1.32–22.32), but needs to be balanced against possible differences in adverse effects.

Retropubic MUSS in Obese (BMI >30) and Elderly (>65-Year-Old) Women

Several small studies have evaluated the outcomes of retropubic MUSS procedures in overweight and obese patients. Killingsworth et al. [83] reported no differences in improvement or complication rates between normal, overweight (BMI 25–29.9), and obese patients at 12-month follow-up. In another retrospective investigation, obesity did not appear to influence the rate of bladder injury or urinary retention after TVT® procedure [84]. On the other hand, in a study with median 5.7-year follow-up, Hellberg et al. [85] noted a decrease in the subjective cure rate between women with BMI less than 25 and those above 35 (81.2 % vs. 52.1 %). However, these obese patients were significantly older and more often suffered from diabetes mellitus and chronic bronchitis. There was no increase in the complication rate between patient groups, depending on the BMI.

As for age, older women are more prone to ISD and mixed urinary incontinence than younger women [86]. The retropubic MUSS procedure is associated with decreased cure rates in elderly patients. Jun et al. [87] observed a decline of cure and improvement rates in elderly patients (over 65 years old) vs. younger patients at median 48.8-month follow-up (66.7 % vs. 80.2 % and 3.3 % vs. 4.7 %). Hellberg et al. [85] compared patients older than 75 years with younger subjects. Older women more frequently had mixed urinary incontinence with inferior subjective cure rates than their younger counterparts (55.7 % vs. 79.7 %), and a higher failure rate for the stress component over urgency symptoms. Adjustment for previous vaginal repair, incontinence surgery, and history of recurrent UTI did not alter the lower odds ratios for cure in these women.

Conclusion

Retropubic MUSSs represent standard care in female SUI. The procedure has the advantage of minimally invasive surgery (short operation time, ambulatory surgery) with excellent objective and subjective cure rates in all groups of patients on long-term follow-up. The complication rate is low, provided the procedure is performed in a standardized manner.

References

1. Abrams P, Cardozo L, Fall M, Griffiths D, Rosier P, Ulmsten U, Van Kerrebroeck P, Victor A, Wein A, Standardisation Sub-committee of the International Continence Society. The standardisation of terminology in lower urinary tract function: report from the Standardisation Sub-committee of the International Continence Society. Urology. 2003;61(1):37–49.
2. Reynolds WS, Dmochowski RR, Penson DF. Epidemiology of stress urinary incontinence in women. Curr Urol Rep. 2011;12(5):370–6.
3. Wu JM, Hundley AF, Fulton RG, Myers ER. Forecasting the prevalence of pelvic floor disorders in U.S. women: 2010 to 2050. Obstet Gynecol. 2009;114(6):1278–83.
4. Walker GJ, Gunasekera P. Pelvic organ prolapse and incontinence in developing countries: review of prevalence and risk factors. Int Urogynecol J. 2011;22(2): 127–35. Epub 2010 Jul 9.

5. Milsom I, Altman D, Lapitan MC, Nelson R, Sillen U, Thom DH. Epidemiology of urinary (UI) and faecal (FI) incontinence and pelvic organ prolapse (POP). In: Abrams P, Cardozo L, Khoury S, Wein AJ, editors. Incontinence: 4th international consultation on incontinence. Paris, France: Health Publications Ltd.; 2009. p. 35–112.
6. Ulmsten U, Henriksson L, Johnson P, Varhos G. An ambulatory surgical procedure under local anesthesia for treatment of female urinary incontinence. Int Urogynecol J. 1996;7(2):81–6; discussion 85–6.
7. Petros PE, Ulmsten UI. An integral theory of female urinary incontinence. Experimental and clinical considerations. Acta Obstet Gynecol Scand Suppl. 1990; 153:7–31.
8. DeLancey JO. Structural support of the urethra as it relates to stress urinary incontinence: the hammock hypothesis. Am J Obstet Gynecol. 1994;170(6): 1713–20; discussion 1720–3.
9. Atherton MJ, Stanton SL. A comparison of bladder neck movement and elevation after tension-free vaginal tape and colposuspension. BJOG. 2000;107(11): 1366–70.
10. Rinne K, Kainulainen S, Aukee S, Heinonen S, Nilsson CG. Dynamic MRI confirms support of the mid-urethra by TVT and TVT-O surgery for stress incontinence. Acta Obstet Gynecol Scand. 2011; 90(6):629–35.
11. Slack M, Sandhu JS, Staskin DR, Grant RC. In vivo comparison of suburethral sling materials. Int Urogynecol J Pelvic Floor Dysfunct. 2006;17(2):106–10. Epub 2005 Jul 2.
12. Meschia M, Pifarotti P, Bernasconi F, Magatti F, Viganò R, Bertozzi R, Barbacini P. Tension-free vaginal tape (TVT) and intravaginal slingplasty (IVS) for stress urinary incontinence: a multicenter randomized trial. Am J Obstet Gynecol. 2006;195(5):1338–42.
13. Domingo S, Alamá P, Ruiz N, Perales A, Pellicer A. Diagnosis, management and prognosis of vaginal erosion after transobturator suburethral tape procedure using a nonwoven thermally bonded polypropylene mesh. J Urol. 2005;173(5):1627–30.
14. Prien-Larsen JC, Hemmingsen L. Long-term outcomes of TVT and IVS operations for treatment of female stress urinary incontinence: monofilament vs. multifilament polypropylene tape. Int Urogynecol J Pelvic Floor Dysfunct. 2009;20(6):703–9.
15. Rechberger T, Rzeźniczuk K, Skorupski P, Adamiak A, Tomaszewski J, Baranowski W, Jakowicki JA. A randomized comparison between monofilament and multifilament tapes for stress incontinence surgery. Int Urogynecol J Pelvic Floor Dysfunct. 2003; 14(6):432–6.
16. Nilsson CG, Kuuva N, Falconer C. Long-term results of the tension-free vaginal tape (TVT) procedure for surgical treatment of female stress urinary incontinence. Int Urogynecol J Pelvic Floor Dysfunct. 2001;12 Suppl 2:S5–8.
17. Rezapour M, Ulmsten U. Tension-free vaginal tape (TVT) in women with recurrent stress urinary incontinence—a long-term follow up. Int Urogynecol J Pelvic Floor Dysfunct. 2001;12 Suppl 2:S9–11.
18. Reich A, Kohorst F, Kreienberg R, Flock F. Long-term results of the tension-free vaginal tape procedure in an unselected group: a 7-year follow-up study. Urology. 2011;78(4):774–7.
19. Liapis A, Bakas P, Creatsas G. Long-term efficacy of tension-free vaginal tape in the management of stress urinary incontinence in women: efficacy at 5- and 7-year follow-up. Int Urogynecol J Pelvic Floor Dysfunct. 2008;19(11):1509–12.
20. Song PH, Kim YD, Kim HT, Lim HS, Hyun CH, Seo JH, Yoo ES, Park CH, Jung HC, Gomelsky A. The 7-year outcome of the tension-free vaginal tape procedure for treating female stress urinary incontinence. BJU Int. 2009;104(8):1113–7.
21. Groutz A, Rosen G, Cohen A, Gold R, Lessing JB, Gordon D. Ten-year subjective outcome results of the retropubic tension-free vaginal tape for treatment of stress urinary incontinence. J Minim Invasive Gynecol. 2011;18(6):726–9.
22. Serati M, Ghezzi F, Cattoni E, Braga A, Siesto G, Torella M, Cromi A, Vitobello D, Salvatore S. Tension-free vaginal tape for the treatment of urodynamic stress incontinence: efficacy and adverse effects at 10-year follow-up. Eur Urol. 2012;61(5): 939–46.
23. Abdul-Rahman A, Attar KH, Hamid R, Shah PJ. Long-term outcome of tension-free vaginal tape for treating stress incontinence in women with neuropathic bladders. BJU Int. 2010;106(6):827–30.
24. Olsson I, Abrahamsson AK, Kroon UB. Long-term efficacy of the tension-free vaginal tape procedure for the treatment of urinary incontinence: a retrospective follow-up 11.5 years post-operatively. Int Urogynecol J. 2010;21(6):679–83.
25. Nilsson CG, Palva K, Rezapour M, Falconer C. Eleven years prospective follow-up of the tension-free vaginal tape procedure for treatment of stress urinary incontinence. Int Urogynecol J Pelvic Floor Dysfunct. 2008;19(8):1043–7.
26. Lim YN, Dwyer P, Muller R, Rosamilia A, Lee J, Stav K. Do the Advantage slings work as well as the tension-free vaginal tapes? Int Urogynecol J. 2010; 21(9):1157–62.
27. Andonian S, Chen T, St-Denis B, Corcos J. Randomized clinical trial comparing suprapubic arch sling (SPARC) and tension-free vaginal tape (TVT): one-year results. Eur Urol. 2005;47(4): 537–41.
28. Lord HE, Taylor JD, Finn JC, Tsokos N, Jeffery JT, Atherton MJ, Evans SF, Bremner AP, Elder GO, Holman CD. A randomized controlled equivalence trial of short-term complications and efficacy of tension-free vaginal tape and suprapubic urethral support sling for treating stress incontinence. BJU Int. 2006;98(2):367–76.
29. Tseng LH, Wang AC, Lin YH, Li SJ, Ko YJ. Randomized comparison of the suprapubic arc sling procedure vs tension-free vaginal taping for stress

incontinent women. Int Urogynecol J Pelvic Floor Dysfunct. 2005;16(3):230–5.
30. Novara G, Ficarra V, Boscolo-Berto R, Secco S, Cavalleri S, Artibani W. Tension-free midurethral slings in the treatment of female stress urinary incontinence: a systematic review and meta-analysis of randomized controlled trials of effectiveness. Eur Urol. 2007;52(3):663–78.
31. Ogah J, Cody DJ, Rogerson L. Minimally invasive synthetic suburethral sling operations for stress urinary incontinence in women: a short version Cochrane review. Neurourol Urodyn. 2011;30(3):284–91.
32. Heidler S, Ofner-Kopeinig P, Puchwein E, Pummer K, Primus G. The suprapubic arch sling procedure for treatment of stress urinary incontinence: a 5-year retrospective study. Eur Urol. 2010;57(5):897–901.
33. Rehman H, Bezerra CC, Bruschini H, Cody JD. Traditional suburethral sling operations for urinary incontinence in women. Cochrane Database Syst Rev. 2011;(1):CD001754.
34. Novara G, Galfano A, Boscolo-Berto R, Secco S, Cavalleri S, Ficarra V, Artibani W. Complication rates of tension-free midurethral slings in the treatment of female stress urinary incontinence: a systematic review and meta-analysis of randomized controlled trials comparing tension-free midurethral tapes to other surgical procedures and different devices. Eur Urol. 2008;53(2):288–308.
35. Sung VW, Schleinitz MD, Rardin CR, Ward RM, Myers DL. Comparison of retropubic vs transobturator approach to midurethral slings: a systematic review and meta-analysis. Am J Obstet Gynecol. 2007;197(1):3–11.
36. Long CY, Hsu CS, Wu MP, Liu CM, Wang TN, Tsai EM. Comparison of tension-free vaginal tape and transobturator tape procedure for the treatment of stress urinary incontinence. Curr Opin Obstet Gynecol. 2009;21(4):342–7.
37. Tamussino KF, Hanzal E, Kölle D, Ralph G, Riss PA, Austrian Urogynecology Working Group. Tension-free vaginal tape operation: results of the Austrian registry. Obstet Gynecol. 2001;98(5 Pt 1):732–6.
38. Kuuva N, Nilsson CG. A nationwide analysis of complications associated with the tension-free vaginal tape (TVT) procedure. Acta Obstet Gynecol Scand. 2002;81(1):72–7.
39. Kristensen I, Eldoma M, Williamson T, Wood S, Mainprize T, Ross S. Complications of the tension-free vaginal tape procedure for stress urinary incontinence. Int Urogynecol J. 2010;21(11):1353–7.
40. Pushkar DY, Godunov BN, Gvozdev M, Kasyan GR. Complications of mid-urethral slings for treatment of stress urinary incontinence. Int J Gynaecol Obstet. 2011;113(1):54–7.
41. Tincello DG, Botha T, Grier D, Jones P, Subramanian D, Urquhart C, Kirkemo A, Khandwala S, TVT Worldwide Registry Investigators. The TVT Worldwide Observational Registry for Long-Term Data: safety and efficacy of suburethral sling insertion approaches for stress urinary incontinence in women. J Urol. 2011;186(6):2310–5.
42. Lleberia-Juanós J, Bataller-Sánchez E, Pubill-Soler J, Mestre-Costa M, Ribot-Luna L, Vizcaíno MA. De novo urgency after tension-free vaginal tape versus transobturator tape procedure for stress urinary incontinence. Eur J Obstet Gynecol Reprod Biol. 2011; 155(2):229–32.
43. Morton HC, Hilton P. Urethral injury associated with minimally invasive mid-urethral sling procedures for the treatment of stress urinary incontinence: a case series and systematic literature search. BJOG. 2009;116(8):1120–6.
44. Rooney KE, Cholhan HJ. Bowel perforation during retropubic sling procedure. Obstet Gynecol. 2010; 115(2 Pt 2):429–31.
45. Gilchrist AS, Rovner ES. Managing complications of slings. Curr Opin Urol. 2011;21(4):291–6.
46. Vervest HA, Bisseling TM, Heintz AP, Schraffordt Koops SE. The prevalence of voiding difficulty after TVT, its impact on quality of life, and related risk factors. Int Urogynecol J Pelvic Floor Dysfunct. 2007;18(2):173–82.
47. Debodinance P, Delporte P, Engrand JB, Boulogne M. Tension-free vaginal tape (TVT) in the treatment of urinary stress incontinence: 3 years experience involving 256 operations. Eur J Obstet Gynecol Reprod Biol. 2002;105(1):49–58.
48. Ustün Y, Engin-Ustün Y, Güngör M, Tezcan S. Tension-free vaginal tape compared with laparoscopic Burch urethropexy. J Am Assoc Gynecol Laparosc. 2003;10(3):386–9.
49. Ward KL, Hilton P, UK and Ireland TVT Trial Group. A prospective multicenter randomized trial of tension-free vaginal tape and colposuspension for primary urodynamic stress incontinence: two-year follow-up. Am J Obstet Gynecol. 2004;190(2):324–31.
50. Holmgren C, Nilsson S, Lanner L, Hellberg D. Frequency of de novo urgency in 463 women who had undergone the tension-free vaginal tape (TVT) procedure for genuine stress urinary incontinence—a long-term follow-up. Eur J Obstet Gynecol Reprod Biol. 2007;132(1):121–5.
51. Alperin M, Abrahams-Gessel S, Wakamatsu MM. Development of de novo urge incontinence in women post sling: the role of preoperative urodynamics in assessing the risk. Neurourol Urodyn. 2008;27(5): 407–11.
52. Athanasiou S, et al. Mixed urinary incontinence/TVT or TVT-O. Oral presentation at the 34th Annual IUGA Meeting. Int Uroynecol J. 2009;20 Suppl 2:S218.
53. Sinha D, Blackwell A, Moran PA. Outcome measures after TVT for mixed urinary incontinence. Int Urogynecol J Pelvic Floor Dysfunct. 2008;19(7): 927–31.
54. Duckett JR, Basu M. The predictive value of preoperative pressure-flow studies in the resolution of detrusor overactivity and overactive bladder after tension-free vaginal tape insertion. BJU Int. 2007; 99(6):1439–42.
55. Paick JS, Oh SJ, Kim SW, Ku JH. Tension-free vaginal tape, suprapubic arc sling, and transobturator tape in the treatment of mixed urinary incontinence in

women. Int Urogynecol J Pelvic Floor Dysfunct. 2008;19(1):123–9.
56. Botros SM, Miller JJ, Goldberg RP, Gandhi S, Akl M, Beaumont JL, Sand PK. Detrusor overactivity and urge urinary incontinence following transobturator versus midurethral slings. Neurourol Urodyn. 2007; 26(1):42–5.
57. Choe JH, Choo MS, Lee KS. The impact of tension-free vaginal tape on overactive bladder symptoms in women with stress urinary incontinence: significance of detrusor overactivity. J Urol. 2008;179(1):214–9.
58. Kulseng-Hanssen S, Husby H, Schiøtz HA. Follow-up of TVT operations in 1,113 women with mixed urinary incontinence at 7 and 38 months. Int Urogynecol J Pelvic Floor Dysfunct. 2008;19(3):391–6.
59. Jain P, Jirschele K, Botros SM, Latthe PM. Effectiveness of midurethral slings in mixed urinary incontinence: a systematic review and meta-analysis. Int Urogynecol J. 2011;22(8):923–32.
60. Sand PK, Bowen LW, Panganiban R, Ostergard DR. The low pressure urethra as a factor in failed retropubic urethropexy. Obstet Gynecol. 1987;69(3 Pt 1): 399–402.
61. McGuire EJ, Fitzpatrick CC, Wan J, Bloom D, Sanvordenker J, Ritchey M, Gormley EA. Clinical assessment of urethral sphincter function. J Urol. 1993;150(5 Pt 1):1452–4.
62. Lim YN, Dwyer PL. Effectiveness of midurethral slings in intrinsic sphincteric-related stress urinary incontinence. Curr Opin Obstet Gynecol. 2009; 21(5):428–33.
63. Rodríguez LV, de Almeida F, Dorey F, Raz S. Does Valsalva leak point pressure predict outcome after the distal urethral polypropylene sling? Role of urodynamics in the sling era. J Urol. 2004;172(1):210–4.
64. Rezapour M, Falconer C, Ulmsten U. Tension-Free vaginal tape (TVT) in stress incontinent women with intrinsic sphincter deficiency (ISD)—a long-term follow-up. Int Urogynecol J Pelvic Floor Dysfunct. 2001;12 Suppl 2:S12–4.
65. Liapis A, Bakas P, Salamalekis E, Botsis D, Creatsas G. Tension-free vaginal tape (TVT) in women with low urethral closure pressure. Eur J Obstet Gynecol Reprod Biol. 2004;116(1):67–70.
66. Jeon MJ, Jung HJ, Chung SM, Kim SK, Bai SW. Comparison of the treatment outcome of pubovaginal sling, tension-free vaginal tape, and transobturator tape for stress urinary incontinence with intrinsic sphincter deficiency. Am J Obstet Gynecol. 2008; 199(1):76.e1–4.
67. Schierlitz L, Dwyer PL, Rosamilia A, Murray C, Thomas E, De Souza A, Lim YN, Hiscock R. Effectiveness of tension-free vaginal tape compared with transobturator tape in women with stress urinary incontinence and intrinsic sphincter deficiency: a randomized controlled trial. Obstet Gynecol. 2008; 112(6):1253–61.
68. Lovatsis D, Easton W, Wilkie D, Society of Obstetricians and Gynaecologists of Canada Urogynaecology Committee. Guidelines for the evaluation and treatment of recurrent urinary incontinence following pelvic floor surgery. J Obstet Gynaecol Can. 2010;32(9):893–904.
69. Walsh CA. Recurrent stress urinary incontinence after synthetic mid-urethral sling procedures. Curr Opin Obstet Gynecol. 2011;23(5):355–61.
70. Gorton E, Stanton S, Monga A, Wiskind AK, Lentz GM, Bland DR. Periurethral collagen injection: a long-term follow-up study. BJU Int. 1999;84(9):966–71.
71. Amaye-Obu FA, Drutz HP. Surgical management of recurrent stress urinary incontinence: a 12-year experience. Am J Obstet Gynecol. 1999;181(6):1296–307.
72. Costa P, Mottet N, Rabut B, Thuret R, Ben Naoum K, Wagner L. The use of an artificial urinary sphincter in women with type III incontinence and a negative Marshall test. J Urol. 2001;165(4):1172–6.
73. Lee KS, Doo CK, Han DH, Jung BJ, Han JY, Choo MS. Outcomes following repeat mid urethral synthetic sling after failure of the initial sling procedure: rediscovery of the tension-free vaginal tape procedure. J Urol. 2007;178(4 Pt 1):1370–4; discussion 1374.
74. Moore RD, Gamble K, Miklos JR. Tension-free vaginal tape sling for recurrent stress incontinence after transobturator tape sling failure. Int Urogynecol J Pelvic Floor Dysfunct. 2007;18(3):309–13.
75. Stav K, Dwyer PL, Rosamilia A, Schierlitz L, Lim YN, Chao F, De Souza A, Thomas E, Murray C, Conway C, Lee J. Repeat synthetic mid urethral sling procedure for women with recurrent stress urinary incontinence. J Urol. 2010;183(1):241–6.
76. Lo TS. Tension-free vaginal tape procedures in women with stress urinary incontinence with and without co-existing genital prolapse. Curr Opin Obstet Gynecol. 2004;16(5):399–404.
77. Jomaa M. Combined tension-free vaginal tape and prolapse repair under local anaesthesia in patients with symptoms of both urinary incontinence and prolapse. Gynecol Obstet Invest. 2001;51(3):184–6.
78. Partoll LM. Efficacy of tension-free vaginal tape with other pelvic reconstructive surgery. Am J Obstet Gynecol. 2002;186(6):1292–5; discussion 1295–8.
79. Lo TS, Chang TC, Chao AS, Chou HH, Tseng LH, Liang CC. Tension-free vaginal tape procedure on genuine stress incontinent women with coexisting genital prolapse. Acta Obstet Gynecol Scand. 2003;82(11):1049–53.
80. Groutz A, Gold R, Pauzner D, Lessing JB, Gordon D. Tension-free vaginal tape (TVT) for the treatment of occult stress urinary incontinence in women undergoing prolapse repair: a prospective study of 100 consecutive cases. Neurourol Urodyn. 2004;23(7):632–5.
81. Liang CC, Chang YL, Chang SD, Lo TS, Soong YK. Pessary test to predict postoperative urinary incontinence in women undergoing hysterectomy for prolapse. Obstet Gynecol. 2004;104(4):795–800.
82. Maher C, Baessler K, Glazener CM, Adams EJ, Hagen S. Surgical management of pelvic organ prolapse in women: a short version Cochrane review. Neurourol Urodyn. 2008;27(1):3–12.
83. Killingsworth LB, Wheeler 2nd TL, Burgio KL, Martirosian TE, Redden DT, Richter HE. One-year

outcomes of tension-free vaginal tape (TVT) mid-urethral slings in overweight and obese women. Int Urogynecol J Pelvic Floor Dysfunct. 2009;20(9): 1103–8.
84. Revicky V, Mukhopadhyay S, de Boer F, Morris EP. Obesity and the incidence of bladder injury and urinary retention following tension-free vaginal tape procedure: retrospective cohort study. Obstet Gynecol Int. 2011;2011:746393.
85. Hellberg D, Holmgren C, Lanner L, Nilsson S. The very obese woman and the very old woman: tension-free vaginal tape for the treatment of stress urinary incontinence. Int Urogynecol J Pelvic Floor Dysfunct. 2007;18(4):423–9.
86. Milsom I, Ekelund P, Molander U, Arvidsson L, Areskoug B. The influence of age, parity, oral contraception, hysterectomy and menopause on the prevalence of urinary incontinence in women. J Urol. 1993;149(6):1459–62.
87. Jun KK, Oh SM, Choo GY, Park HK, Paick SH, Lho YS, Kim HG. Long-term clinical outcomes of the tension-free vaginal tape procedure for the treatment of stress urinary incontinence in elderly women over 65. Korean J Urol. 2012;53(3):184–8.

Transobturator Tape

4

Saad Juma

Stress urinary incontinence (SUI) is the most common form of urinary incontinence and is estimated to affect more than 13 million adult women in the United States [1]. Burch colposuspension and pubovaginal sling have been the most popular surgical treatments for female SUI. The cure rate for the retropubic open suspension (including Burch colposuspension) at 12–23 months is 82 %, and at 24 months and beyond is 73–76 %. For slings at the midurethra (transvaginal/retropubic technique), the estimated cure/dry rate is 81–84 % [2].

The tension-free vaginal tape (TVT) procedure was introduced by Ulmsten in 1996 [3]. In an attempt to minimize the complications associated with the TVT technique, Delorme in 2001 devised and first described the Transobturator tape (TOT) technique [4, 5]. In the original description of the TOT by Delorme the tunneler needle is advanced through the skin overlying the obturator fossa towards the vaginal incision (outside-in). In 2003 de Leval described an inside-out (TVT-O) technique where the tunneler needle is advanced through the vaginal incision towards the skin overlying the obturator fossa (inside-out) [6].

The TOT is a *midurethral sling*. It reproduces the natural suspension of the urethra while preserving the retropubic space. It replaces the pubourethral ligament, providing continence by creating functional kinking of the midurethra during increase intra-abdominal pressure and the associated rotational descent of the bladder neck and proximal urethra [7]. The TOT is a *tension-free sling* as the resting urethral angle is not changed by the procedure, nor is it necessary to correct urethral hypermobility [8]. This approach is more anatomically correct and poses *no significant impact on voiding function* [9]. Patients who undergo the TOT procedure have significantly *lower rates of de novo urgency/urge incontinence* than those who undergo other midurethral sling procedures as demonstrated by Botros and Juma in 2007 [10, 11].

In 2005 Delmas demonstrated that the anatomical course of the TOT avoids major neurovascular structures, and the anatomical structures crossed by the tape are muscles and fascia. It avoids femoral and obturator vessels in the thigh and pudendal vessels in the perineum [12]. Because of the nature of the procedure, *major hemorrhage and bowel perforation are not reported* in the TOT procedure [13, 14].

In 2006, Achtari demonstrated the course of the dorsal nerve of the clitoris (DNC) and the obturator canal in cadavers relative to the path of the tape in transobturator inside-out (TVT-O) and transobturator outside-in (TOT) procedures. The DNC passes beneath the pubic bone at a distance of 14.3 ± 4.7 mm of the midline. Given the course of the DNC along the medial aspect of the

S. Juma, M.D., F.A.C.S. (✉)
Incontinence Research Institute,
320 Santa Fe Dr., Suite 300,
Encinitas, CA 92024, USA
e-mail: urodawk@gmail.com

G.H. Badlani (ed.), *Minimally Invasive Therapy for Urinary Incontinence and Pelvic Organ Prolapse*, Current Clinical Urology, DOI 10.1007/978-1-4939-0008-4_4,

ischiopubic ramus, he concluded the outside-in (TOT) technique may be safer [15]. Further, Hinoul in 2007 concluded that the inside-out (TVT-O) tape trajectory is subject to wider variability than was originally postulated based on a study of the trajectory of the tape study in six fresh cadavers [16]. In 2007 Zahn demonstrated in cadavers that TOTs placed by the inside-out (TVT-O) technique were significantly closer to the obturator canal than with the outside-in (TOT) method, and the greater proximity of the inside-out method was noted in all dissections. This leads the authors to conclude the outside-in (TOT) technique results in the mesh being placed farther from the obturator canal and closer to the ischiopubic ramus, theoretically *reducing the risk of neurovascular injury* [17].

This minimally invasive midurethral sling technique (TOT) has become *the standard procedure for the surgical treatment of SUI*. Several studies in the literature have confirmed the feasibility, safety, and efficacy of this operation, [5, 11, 18–20].

Indications and Contraindications

This minimally invasive midurethral sling technique has become the most commonly performed surgical procedure for the management of female SUI. The TOT is indicated in the treatment of patients with SUI due to urethral hypermobility or mixed urinary incontinence with predominant stress component. The TOT may be performed in conjunction with pelvic organ prolapse (POP) repair and/or hysterectomy. The role of TOT in SUI due to intrinsic sphincter deficiency (ISD) is controversial. It may be used in the majority of patient with ISD and urethral hypermobility [11]. However, patients with stem pipe urethra (ISD and fixed urethra) are better served with a midurethral retropubic sling or pubovaginal sling.

The TOT is not indicated for patients with urge urinary incontinence (UUI) or mixed incontinence with predominant urge component. Patients, who undergo urethral diverticulectomy, urethral reconstruction, or repair of urethrovaginal fistula, should not have a mesh sling placed during the same procedure though a later sling may be considered once the repair has healed. Great caution should be exercised in patient with Parkinson's disease, Multiple Sclerosis, and Myasthenia Gravis because of the increased functional urethral resistance due to detrusor sphincter dyssynergia or pseudo-dyssynergia.

Transobturator Tape

In evaluating the efficacy of a surgical procedure in the treatment of patients with SUI, dry rates are the ideal outcome and a precise end point. However, dry rates do not equate with, nor are they necessary for patient satisfaction. Patient satisfaction rate is as important outcome measure as it encompasses patient overall perception of outcome and not merely dry rates. The *functional efficacy and patient satisfaction with the outcome of TOT in the treatment of patient with SUI* have been demonstrated in several retrospective as well as prospective randomized controlled trials. In 2007, Juma reported 90 % subjective resolution of SUI in 130 women who underwent the TOT procedure at a mean follow-up of 16.85 ± 4.68 months [11]. Several series have reported similar success rates for the TOT procedure in the treatment of SUI [18, 19, 21, 22]. de Tayrac reported a 1-year cure rate of 84 % with the TOT procedure, and in a series of 117 patients with a median follow-up of 16.3 months, Spinosa reported subjective complete and partial satisfaction rates of 92.3 % and 4.2 %, respectively [18]. Abdel-Fattah in 2011, demonstrated that TOTs have good patient-reported and objective success rates at 1 year of follow-up in women with previous failed incontinence surgery [23].

Several studies have demonstrated the *subjective and objective cure rate of TOT is similar to pubovaginal and midurethral retropubic slings*. In a study of 104 women with SUI, the condition was "cured" in 81.8 % of cases in the TVT group and 83.7 % in the TOT group, and improvement occurred in 10.9 % and 10.2 % of cases, respectively [24]. In a study comparing the retropubic and the TOT slings, a total of 597 women were randomly assigned to a study group; 565 (94.6 %) completed the 12-month assessment. The rates of objectively assessed treatment success were

80.8 % in the retropubic-sling group and 77.7 % in the transobturator-sling group. The rates of subjectively assessed success were 62.2 % and 55.8 %, respectively [25]. In a review and meta-analysis of 12 randomized controlled trials that compared TOT with TVT, and 15 that compared TVT-O vs. TVT for treating SUI; the subjective and objective cure of TOT was similar to TVT. For TVT-O, the subjective and objective cure was also similar to TVT [26]. Another study demonstrated that the cure rate for TVT, TVT-O, and TOT in three groups of women were 90.9 %, 92.3 %, and 91.1 %, respectively [27]. In a study comparing the TOT and TVT-O techniques and involving 341 women who completed 1-year follow-up, the patient-reported success rate was 80 % with no statistically significant differences between the groups. The objective cure rate was 91 % with no statistically significant difference between the groups [28].

In the author's opinion, the *TOT is effective in the majority of patients with ISD*. The reason for success of the TOT in patients with low VLPP is due to the fact that not all these patients have a fixed urethra. In fact most of these patients have some degree of urethral mobility albeit less than that seen in patients with higher VLPP. The placement of a transobturator midurethral sling will correct the problem in the majority of these patients. Such a benefit cannot be achieved with similar success in patients with fixed urethra. In a series of 130 patients, we demonstrated the functional results and patient satisfaction of the TOT procedure in patients with VLPP ≤ 60 cmH_2O are comparable to the results of the procedure in patients with VLPP > 60 cmH_2O [11]. In another study, Valsalva leak point pressure, maximum urethral closure pressure, and urodynamic stress incontinence were the only urodynamic variables consistently associated with objective failure on multivariate analysis. It is the author's opinion that patients with low Valsalva leak point pressure, and low maximum urethral closure pressure have a higher failure rate irrespective of the technique used. This was demonstrated in a study by Nager of the value of these urodynamic parameters, where no specific cut point was determined for predicting failure for Valsalva leak point pressure or maximum urethral closure pressure. The lowest quartile (Valsalva leak point pressure less than 86 cmH_2O, maximum urethral closure pressure less than 45 cmH_2O) conferred an almost twofold increased odds of objective failure 1 year after transobturator or retropubic midurethral sling [29]. In yet another study, multivariate analysis demonstrated a low maximal urethral closure pressure of <30 cmH_2O was the only independent predictor of failure in patients who had previously failed incontinence surgery [23]. In a study of 145 subjects to compare TOT with TVT in patients with low maximum urethral closure pressure. A cut-off point of 42 cmH_2O for preoperative maximum urethral closure pressure was identified as predictor of success in the entire cohort. In this study though, subjects with maximum urethral closure pressure of 42 cm or less H_2O, the TOT subjects were nearly six times more likely to fail than TVT subjects [30].

One of the important and not well-recognized advantages of the TOT as compared to other midurethral sling procedures is the *lower rate of de novo urgency/urge incontinence*. The low incidence of de novo urgency/urge incontinence observed in our series [11] is consistent with what has been reported by others including a review and meta-analysis of 12 randomized controlled trials [18, 26, 31, 32]. Roumeguere reported only 2.5 % de novo urgency [30], and Spinosa reported 0.85 % de novo urge incontinence [18]. Morey reported lower incidence of de novo urgency after TOT (1.3 %) compared to retropubic midurethral slings (6 %) [31]. In another study of 276 subjects with urodynamic stress or mixed urinary incontinence who underwent retropubic midurethral slings or transobturator slings, de novo subjective urge incontinence differed significantly between the TOT and the other two retropubic midurethral slings. Fourteen to sixteen percent of patients with preoperative urge incontinence who underwent TVT or other retropubic midurethral slings had worsening of their urge incontinence symptoms while only 6 % of the TOT group did ($P=0.02$). There was no difference in rates of resolution of detrusor overactivity among the groups (40 % vs. 48 % vs. 32 %, $P=0.39$) or de novo detrusor overactivity (32 % vs. 22 % vs. 22 %, $P=0.64$) at 3 months. The authors concluded patients who undergo transobturator procedures have significantly lower rates of de novo urge incontinence than those who undergo midurethral sling procedures. Rates of resolution of detrusor overactivity, urge incontinence, and de novo detrusor overactivity do not differ between groups [10]. The lower incidence of de novo urgency/urge incontinence may be explained by two factors. In the transobturator approach, the path of the tape, crossing the obturator foramen, muscle, and fascia, reproduces the natural suburethral suspension by reinforcing the rotational pivot point, restoring continence while sparing the retropubic space. Sparing the retropubic space may preserve any periurethral nerve fibers that may be associated with urethral function and stability. Second, the TOT is associated with a lower risk of urethral obstruction as compared to other midurethral sling procedures [11].

The TOT and the transabdominal midurethral slings appear equally efficacious in eliminating the need for incontinence pad use. However, *signs of obstructive voiding are reported less often after TOT than TVT procedures* whether done as the only procedure or combined with pelvic prolapse repair procedures [26, 31]. Obstructive voiding dysfunction is the most commonly reported complication of TVT midurethral sling placement. Because the TOT is positioned horizontally across the urethra, it provides less chance for static urethral kinking and the associated urethral obstruction that may follow. In a series of 104 women, urinary obstruction rates (temporary and permanent) in the TVT group were approximately twice those in the TOT group [24]. In yet another series of 597 women, the rates of voiding dysfunction requiring surgery were 2.7 % in those who received retropubic slings and 0 % in those who received transobturator slings ($P=0.004$) [25].

The TVT midurethral sling is associated with serious though rare complications including intestinal perforation, vascular injury, and obturator nerve injury, and even death [26, 27, 33–35]. The transobturator sling procedure spares the retropubic space and thus *eliminates the risk of major bowel, neural and vascular complications* which have been reported with the TVT. Several series and meta-analysis that compared TOT with TVT, demonstrated that adverse events such as bladder injuries and hematoma were less with TOT than TVT [26, 27, 36]. Bladder perforation is uncommon and resolves spontaneously with catheter drainage. We believe the presence of a distended bladder in the presence of a moderate to large cystocele increases the likelihood of this adverse event. Ensuring an empty bladder during needle passage particularly in the presence of a moderate to large cystocele will eliminate this adverse event [11]. In one study, two cases of retropubic hematoma have been reported with the TOT [37]. The authors suggest a technical error in passing the needle through the obturator internus muscle and into the retropubic space as the potential etiology.

The rate of vaginal extrusion of the tape in our series [11] is consistent with the rate of vaginal extrusion reported by other large series [18] and lower than reported with smaller series [38, 39]. This difference between large and small series may be related to differences in technique and patient selection and will need further evaluation. All extrusions in our series occurred in otherwise healthy women. There was no difference in the vaginal estrogen status in patients with and without extrusion. Management with estrogen vaginal cream did not result in resolution of extrusion and delayed the treatment of what is otherwise a simple to manage adverse outcome. Based on these results, we recommend early and limited excision of the extruded portion of the tape with primary closure of the incision in the majority of patients. The patient continence status in our series was not adversely affected by this approach [11].

In conclusion, the TOT has equal efficacy to other midurethral sling procedures in the treatment of patients with urodynamic demonstrated SUI. No significant difference was demonstrated in the functional outcome and patient satisfaction rates in the majority of patients with low VLPP. The incidence of de novo urgency/urge incontinence and obstructive voiding dysfunction is lower than other midurethral sling procedures. Serious adverse events are rare with this technique. The earlier report by Juma is supported by recent meta-analysis and prospective studies [26, 29, 40, 41].

Technique

The procedure may be performed as the sole procedure or in combination with pelvic prolapse repair (cystocele repair, enterocele repair, rectocele repair, sacrospinous suspension) and/or hysterectomy. Hysterectomy, apical repair (enterocele repair and sacrospinous suspension), and cystocele repair should be performed prior to the TOT procedure to allow for proper adjustment of tension of the sling without further manipulation of the tissue once the sling is in position. If the patient is to undergo POP repair, an enema the night before surgery and liquid diet is advised to minimize the risk of postoperative constipation which may jeopardize the repair. Cephalosporin or Quinilone antibiotic prophylaxis (within the first 24 h of surgery) is given starting within 1 h of surgery.

The procedure can be performed under general, spinal, or local anesthesia with intravenous sedation. In one study comparing local vs. general anesthesia, the operative times were identical in the two groups, but the time spent in the recovery room was significantly longer in the general anesthesia group. Patients undergoing local anesthesia experienced less pain than did those undergoing general anesthesia. No significant differences were observed for the rates of complications [42]. Our experience in over 200 cases done under local anesthesia is consistent with the results of this study. The patient is positioned in the modified lithotomy position. In patients with artificial hip prosthesis, the rotation of the pelvis may be different on the side of the prosthesis even though the leg position is similar on both sides. This may result in the wider portion of the ischiopubic ramus being in the path of the tunneler needle on the side of the hip prosthesis. The lower abdomen, external genitalia, vaginal canal, and the proximal thighs should be prepped and draped in the usual sterile manner. The pubic hair should be clipped below the level of the clitoris to avoid entrapment of hair by the advancing tape. When intravenous sedation with local anesthesia is used, the anterior vaginal wall is infiltrated with 0.25 % Bupivacaine (Marcaine) from the midurethra to the bladder neck proximally, and from the urethra in the midline to the endopelvic fascia bilaterally. The anticipated path of the transobturator needle is likewise infiltrated with Bupivacaine (Marcaine).

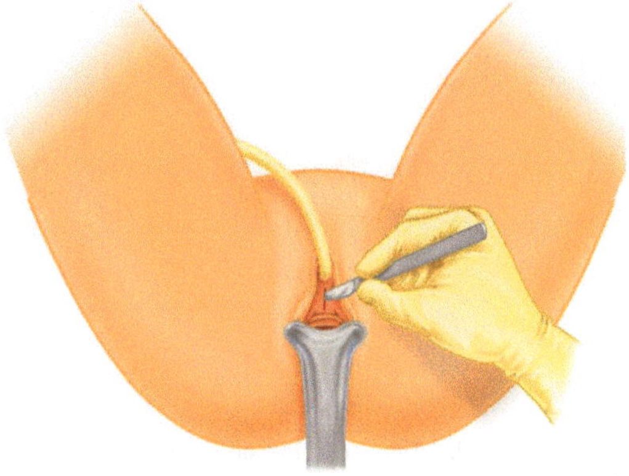

Fig. 4.1 An Allis clamp is applied to the anterior vaginal wall over the midurethra, and a short incision (1–2 cm) is made in the anterior vaginal wall over the midurethra

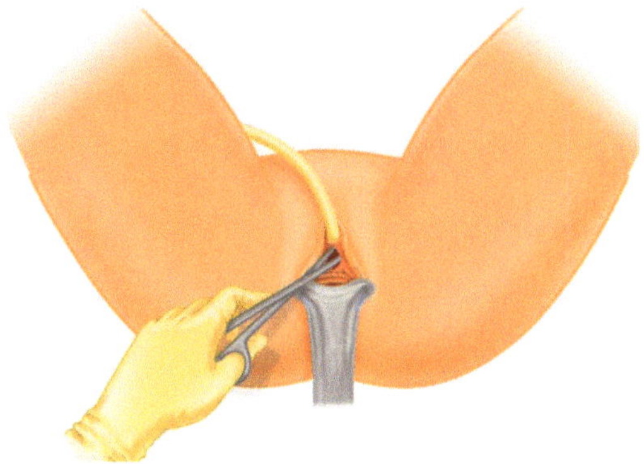

Fig. 4.2 The vaginal wall is dissected in the submucosal plane on both sides of the midline and extended laterally to the ischiopubic rami

A Foley catheter placed in the bladder and a weighted vaginal speculum on the posterior vaginal wall facilitate the vaginal dissection. An Allis clamp or two are applied to the anterior vaginal wall over the midurethra, and a short incision (1–2 cm) is made in the anterior vaginal wall over the midurethra (Fig. 4.1). The vaginal wall is then dissected in the submucosal plane on both sides of the midline. The dissection is extended laterally to the ischiopubic rami (Fig. 4.2). Two stab

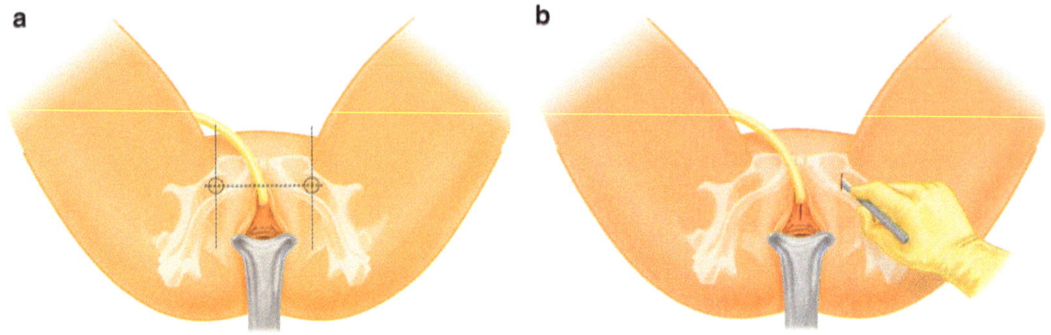

Fig. 4.3 (**a**, **b**) Two stab incisions are made in the Genitofemoral folds, one on either side of the midline at the level of the clitoris and overlying the superior medial aspect of the obturator fossa just below the insertion of Adductor Longus tendon

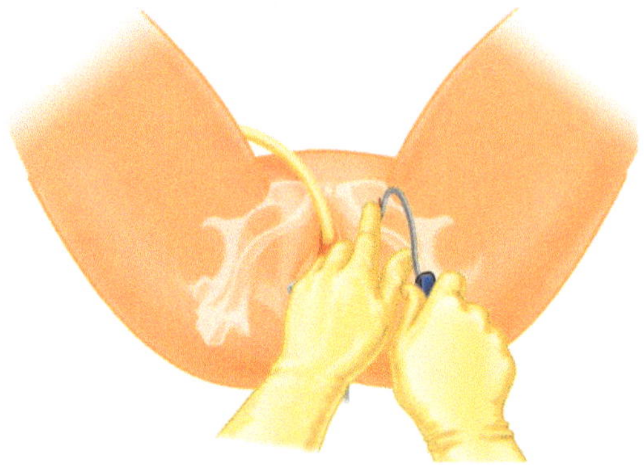

Fig. 4.4 The tunneler needle is advanced through the skin incision, subcutaneous tissue, the adductor muscles (below the Adductor Longus tendon), the obturator externus, obturator internus muscle, and the obturator fascia

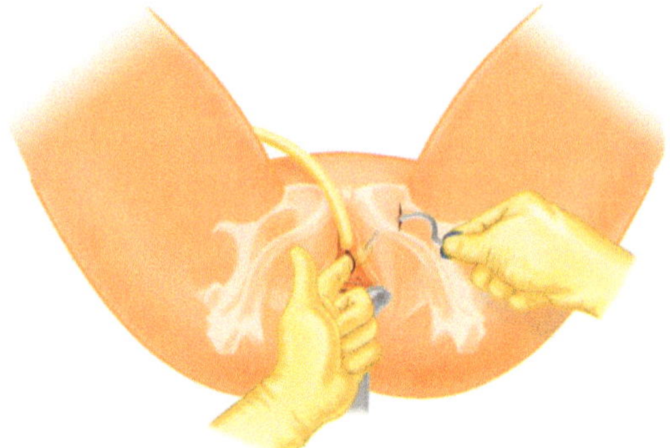

Fig. 4.5 The needle is rotated medially below the Levator Ani and around the posterior edge of the ischiopubic ramus towards the midurethra while a finger in the vaginal incision guides the needle into the vaginal incision and protects the urethra from the advancing needle

incisions are made in the Genitofemoral folds, one on either side of the midline. These stab incisions should be at the level of the clitoris and overlying the superior medial aspect of the obturator fossa just below the insertion of Adductor Longus tendon (Fig. 4.3a, b). The lateral and the inferior portions of the obturator fossa should be avoided to minimize the risk of nerve and/or vascular injuries. The tunneler needle is then advanced through the skin incision, subcutaneous tissue, the adductor muscles (below the Adductor Longus tendon), the obturator externus, obturator internus muscle, and the obturator fascia (Fig. 4.4). The needle is then rotated medially below the Levator Ani and around the posterior edge of the ischiopubic ramus towards the midurethra while a finger in the vaginal incision guides the needle into the vaginal incision and protects the urethra from the advancing needle (Fig. 4.5). Caution should be exercised as the needle is passed over the lateral fold in the vaginal wall (sulcus) to avoid a button hole in the vaginal wall. A woven polypropylene tape is used for the sling. Once the needle is in the vaginal incision, one free end of the tape is threaded or attached to the end of the needle, and the needle is pulled back until the free end of the tape exits through the skin incision over the Genitofemoral fold (Fig. 4.6). The procedure is repeated on the opposite side in a similar fashion

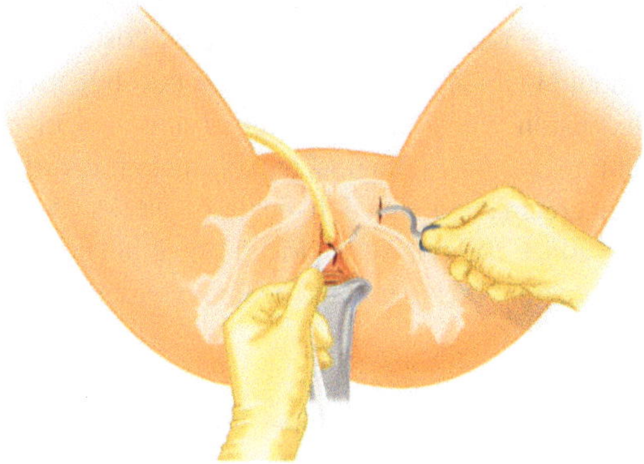

Fig. 4.6 Once the needle is in the vaginal incision, one free end of the tape is threaded or attached to the end of the needle, and the needle is pulled back until the free end of the tape exits through the skin incision over the Genitofemoral fold

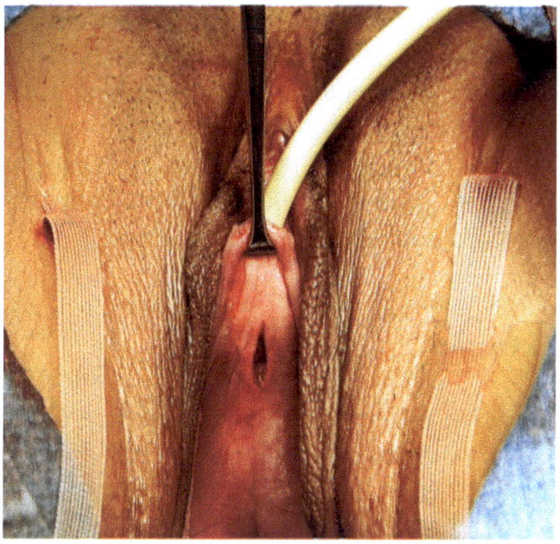

Fig. 4.7 The procedure is repeated on the opposite side in a similar fashion so that the tape is positioned over the midurethra and its free ends exit through the incisions in the Genitofemoral folds

so that the tape is positioned over the midurethra and its free ends exit through the incisions in the Genitofemoral folds (Fig. 4.7). The tape tension is adjusted to provide passive support to the urethra during Valsalva. We prefer to tension the sling mesh with the Foley catheter in the urethra and a spacer is placed between the urethra and the sling mesh (Fig. 4.8). Alternatively, the sling is adjusted so as to leave a visual separation (1 mm) between the tape and the urethral wall. A right angle clamp may be placed between the mesh and the urethral wall to adjust the tension as well (Fig. 4.9). Excessive tension is avoided to minimize the risk of postoperative urethral obstruction and prolonged need for catheterization. The excess tape is excised just below the level of the skin incision (Fig. 4.10), the vaginal incision and the two skin incisions are irrigated with antibiotic solution, and the vaginal incision is closed with 2-0 Polyglycolic suture while the skin incisions are closed with 2-Octyl Cyanoacrylate (Dermabond) topical skin adhesive.

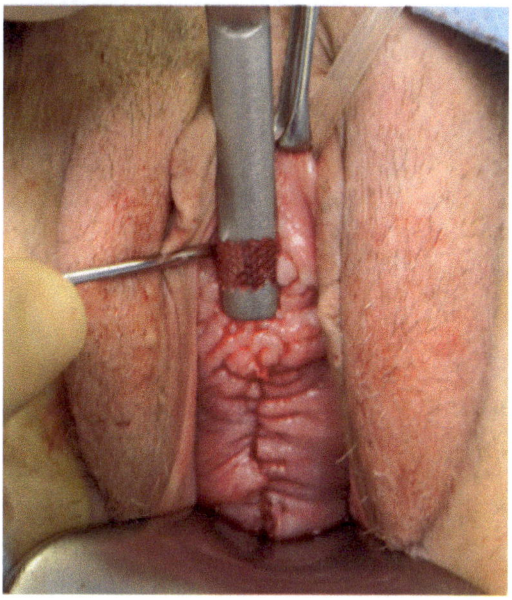

Fig. 4.8 Tension is placed on the sling mesh with the Foley catheter in the urethra, and a spacer is placed between the urethra and the sling mesh

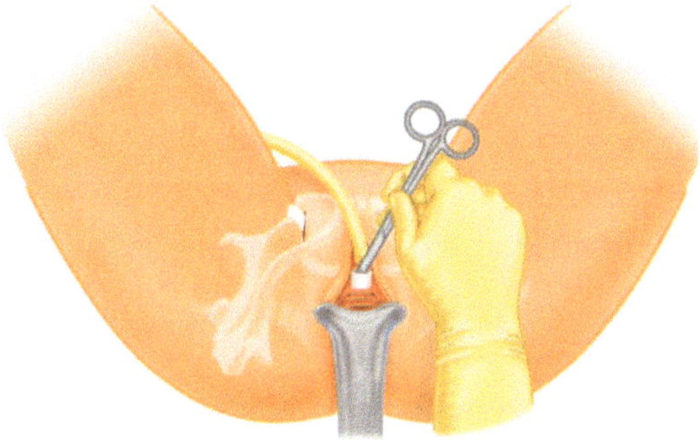

Fig. 4.9 A right angle clamp may be placed between the mesh and the urethral wall to adjust the tension

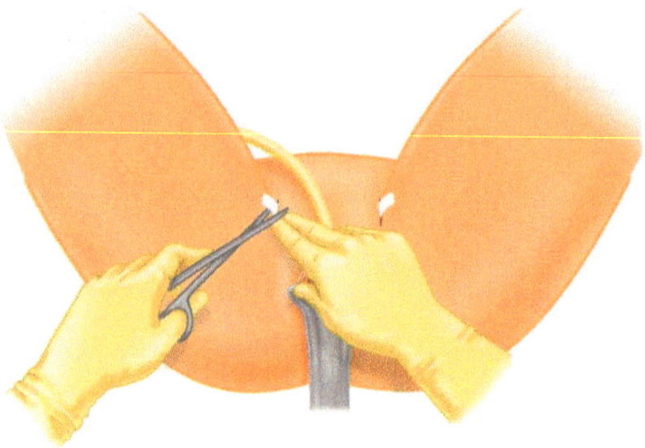

Fig. 4.10 The excess tape is excised just below the level of the skin incision

Following technical landmarks are mandatory to ensure successful procedure: the vaginal incision must include all the thickness of the vaginal wall; the transobturator end point must be located at the level of the midurethra; the tunneling needle must have a close contact with the ischiopubic bone; the finger inside the vaginal incision protects the urethra [43]. The tape has a transverse course; it crosses the adductor muscles close to their pubic insertion and passes through the obturator foramen by crossing the obturator membrane, before reaching the middle plane of the perineum after having crossed the obturator internus muscle. The tape passes above the internal pudendal pedicle and then under the Levator Ani muscle, under the tendinous arch of the pelvic fascia and continues in the middle third of the urethrovaginal septum [12]. At the end of the procedure, cystoscopy is done to ensure patency of the ureters and to exclude bladder or urethral injuries [9, 44]. Removal of the Foley catheter concludes the procedure.

In the recovery room, a voiding trial is done when the bladder is full. Patients who void successfully can be discharged without a catheter while those who don't will require an indwelling catheter usually for 1–2 days. Self-catheterization can also be used as an alternate to indwelling catheter. The patient is discharged home with oral analgesics and antibiotic prophylaxis. The patient is instructed to remove the vaginal pack within 24 h. They can resume ambulation the same day, resume driving within 1 week, and may return to work after 2 weeks; however, they should avoid straining for 6 weeks. Postop care should include pelvic exam to rule out sling mesh extrusion which can be minimal and very difficult to recognize. Vaginal creams including estrogen cream are avoided in the first 6 weeks postop to reduce the risk of accidental manipulation of the vaginal incision in the healing phase.

Postoperative Adverse Outcome

Urinary Retention and Obstruction

Voiding dysfunction after midurethral sling procedures is uncommon. If a patient is unable to void 48 h postoperatively, and there is a concern that excessive tension may be the cause, early tape release is advisable before any tissue in growth has occurred. Ozel et al. reported on a method to adjust the transobturator midurethral sling under local anesthesia in the early postoperative period for postoperative voiding difficulty. Both patients had immediate resolution of their symptoms while maintaining urinary continence [45].

Extrusion

Extrusion refers to the vaginal exposure of the tape mesh through the vaginal mucosa. It could be at the incision site (central) or at the sulcus (lateral). Several theories regarding the tape extrusion has been proposed. It's the author's belief that the etiology may vary depending upon host (patient), technique (surgeon), device (tape) factors, or any combination thereof. Although several reports suggest that estrogen should be used as the primary method of treatment for all tape extrusion, we believe tape excision and primary closure in the office under local anesthesia is more effective in most cases.

Urethral and Vesical Erosion

Erosion of the tape into the urethra may result if the dissection in the vaginal incision is carried deep and close to the urethral wall. Erosion into the bladder may occur due to in advert passage of the introducer needle into the bladder during passage. The presence of cystocele may increase this risk. If the patient presents with history of recurrent UTI or irritative voiding symptoms, erosion should be suspected, and cystoscopy should be done. Urethral erosions may be repaired transvaginal with mesh removal, urethral repair with/without Martius flap. Placing another sling at the same time should be avoided because the risk of recurrent erosion is high. If erosion occurs in the bladder, a transvaginal repair with/without Martius flap may be done; however, a transvesical approach may be needed if the mesh is embedded in the bladder wall and there is excessive tissue ingrowth or stone formation. In an assessment of factors increasing risk of injury, and comparison of the "outside-in" and "inside-out" techniques, 241 women underwent TOT technique and 148 of them underwent TVT-O technique. Four injuries occurred (1 %): two urethral injuries (0.5 %) and two bladder injuries (0.5 %). All injuries occurred in the outside-in group, although this difference did not reach significance ($P=0.146$). Bladder injuries occurred in women who underwent concomitant vaginal surgery, while urethral injuries occurred in women undergoing secondary procedures. They concluded that lower urinary tract injury is an uncommon complication of the TOT procedures and in their hands only occurred with the outside-in technique. Intraoperative cystoscopy should be considered only in selected cases [44].

Urinary Tract Infection

If a patient presents with recurrent UTI, it should raise the suspicion of urethral or bladder erosion, and cystoscopy should be considered once the acute infection is treated. A single episode of UTI should be treated with antibiotics in the usual fashion.

Dyspareunia

If a patient reports Dyspareunia postoperatively, proper evaluation to rule out mesh extrusion or granuloma formation should be sought and addressed accordingly. However, in the absence of specific reversible physical findings, proper evaluation of the potential etiology of female sexual dysfunction should be conducted and the necessary treatment recommended accordingly.

Urinary incontinence is a common condition that negatively impacts female sexuality. In one study, at 60-month follow-up, 52 patients (72 %) were objectively cured of SUI but only 44 patients (61 %) were satisfied. The mean cause of dissatisfaction was the development of sexual dysfunction resulting from Dyspareunia or incontinence during intercourse, which was found in 37.5 % [40]. Another study of 46 women who completed 12-month follow-up, 71 % of sexually active women showed an improvement in the total 12-item POP/Incontinence Sexual Function Questionnaire scores [23].

In yet another study of 133 patients who underwent TOT procedure, or a retropubic procedure, and who completed 12-month follow-up, data showed that after a midurethral sling procedure, female sexual function improves. The authors also found that a very relevant percentage of nonsexually active women reported renewed sexual activity after midurethral sling [46].

Recurrent Incontinence

If urinary incontinence persists beyond 3 months of surgery, complete evaluation including urodynamics should be done to elicit the etiology of persistent or recurrent incontinence. In the majority of cases, persistent detrusor overactivity/urge incontinence, or de novo urge incontinence is the etiology and conservative management should be considered first. In those who demonstrate urethral obstruction on urodynamic studies, initial trial at urethral dilation and if it fails, tape release should be considered. In those who have recurrent SUI, consideration should be given to proximal tape placement or migration as the possible etiology, and tape removal and replacement should be considered. If this is done, tape fixation will increase the likelihood of success. Alternatively, bulking agents may be used or otherwise in a lead pipe urethra consideration for midurethral retropubic sling should be given.

In one study done in 463 patients with SUI who were randomly allocated to treatment with a standard TOT procedure or to a TOT procedure with additional 2-point tape fixation. Two absorbable sutures parallel to the urethra were added to fix the tape and prevent displacement during tape tensioning. Objective clinical efficacy of the procedure at 12 months with fixation was significantly higher with 95.12 % cured or improved compared to 88.73 % cured or improved with the standard sling ($P=0.0169$). Also, among patients with ISD they noted a significantly better outcome in the fixation group than in the control group, 95.1 % cured or improved vs. 73.8 % ($P=0.0011$). The authors concluded tape fixation significantly increases the clinical efficacy of the transobturator sling, especially in patients with ISD [47].

De novo Urgency

In patients who develop de novo urgency/urge incontinence, obstruction should be ruled out. In the absence of obstruction, the majority of cases will resolve spontaneously. In those in whom it persists, it should be treated with behavioral modification with or without pharmacotherapy. If obstruction is suspected, urodynamic studies should be done, and urethrolysis should be considered if obstruction is diagnosed.

Leg pain

Based on cadaver studies, the outside-in (TOT) technique results in the mesh being placed farther from the obturator canal and closer to the ischiopubic ramus, theoretically *reducing the risk of neurovascular injury* [16]. In a study of TOT vs. TVT-O, severe postoperative thigh pain was twice as common in the inside-out group but this was not statistically significant [48]. In another study of 127 women, the TVT-O caused more transient leg pain than the TVT (26.4 % vs. 1.7 %, $P=0.0001$) [49]. In the author's experience, thigh pain is mild and transient, and responds well to nonsteroidal anti-inflammatory agents.

References

1. Fultz NH, Burgo K, Diokno AC, et al. Burden of stress urinary incontinence for community-dwelling women. Am J Obstet Gynecol. 2003;189:1275–82.
2. Dmochowski RR, Blaivas JM, Juma S, et al. Update of AUA guideline on the surgical management of female stress urinary incontinence. J Urol. 2010;183(5):1906–14.
3. Ulmsten U, Henriksson L, Johnson P, et al. An ambulatory surgical procedure under local anesthesia for treatment of female urinary incontinence. Int Urogynecol J. 1996;7:81–6.
4. Delorme E. Transobturator urethral suspension: mini-invasive procedure in the treatment of stress urinary incontinence in women. Prog Urol. 2001;11(6): 1306–13.
5. Delorme E, Droupy S, de Tayrac R, et al. Transobturator tape (Uratape). A new minimally invasive method in the treatment of urinary incontinence in women. Prog Urol. 2003;13(4):656–9.
6. de Leval J. Novel surgical technique for the treatment of female stress urinary Incontinence: transobturator vaginal tape inside-out. Eur Urol. 2003;44(6): 724–30.
7. Petros PF, Ulmsten UI. An integral theory and its method for the diagnosis and management of female urinary incontinence. Scand Urol Nephrol Suppl. 1993;153:193.
8. Minaglia S, Ozel B, Hurtado E, et al. Effect of transobturator tape procedure on proximal urethral mobility. Urology. 2005;65(1):55–9.
9. Wang AC, Lin YH, Tseng LH, et al. Prospective randomized comparison of transobturator suburethral sling (Monarc) vs. suprapubic arc (Sparc) sling procedures for female urodynamic stress incontinence. Int Urogynecol J Pelvic Floor Dysfunct. 2006;17(5): 439–43.
10. Botros SM, Miller JJ, Goldberg RP, et al. Detrusor overactivity and urge urinary incontinence following trans obturator versus midurethral slings. Neurourol Urodyn. 2007;26(1):42–5.
11. Juma S, Brito CG. Transobturator tape (TOT): two years follow-up. Neurourol Urodyn. 2007;26(1):37–41.
12. Delmas V. Anatomical risks of transobturator sub urethral tape in the treatment of female stress urinary incontinence. Eur Urol. 2005;48(5):793–8.
13. Gunnemann A, Heleis W, Pohl J, et al. The transobturator tape (TOT). A minimally-invasive procedure for the treatment of female urinary stress incontinence. Urologe A. 2004;43(9):1106–10.
14. Mellier G, Benayed B, Bretones S, et al. Suburethral tape via the obturator route: is the TOT a simplification of the TVT? Int Urogynecol J Pelvic Floor Dysfunct. 2004;15(4):227–32.
15. Achtari C, McKenzie BJ, Hiscock R, Rosamilia A, et al. Anatomical study of the obturator foramen and dorsal nerve of the Clitoris and their relationship to

minimally invasive slings. Int Urogynecol J Pelvic Floor Dysfunct. 2006;17(4):330–4.
16. Hinoul P, Vanormelingen L, Roovers JP, et al. Anatomical variability in the trajectory of the inside-out transobturator vaginal tape technique (TVT-O). Int Urogynecol J Pelvic Floor Dysfunct. 2007;18(10):1201–6.
17. Zahn CM, Siddique S, Hernandez S, et al. Anatomic comparison of two transobturator tape procedures. Obstet Gynecol. 2007;109(3):701–6.
18. Spinosa JP, Dubuis PY. Suburethral sling inserted by the transobturator route in the treatment of female stress urinary incontinence: preliminary results in 117 cases. Eur J Obstet Gynecol Reprod Biol. 2005; 123(2):212–7.
19. Delorme E, Droupy S, de Tayrac R, et al. Transobturator tape (Uratape): a new minimally-invasive procedure to treat female urinary incontinence. Eur Urol. 2004;45(2):203–7.
20. Deffieux X, Daher N, Mansoor A, et al. Transobturator TVT-O versus retropubic TVT: results of a multicenter randomized controlled trial at 24 months follow-up. Int Urogynecol J. 2007;21(11):1337–45.
21. deTayrac R, Deffieux X, Droupy S, et al. A prospective randomized trial comparing tension-free vaginal tape and transobturator suburethral tape for surgical treatment of stress urinary incontinence. Am J Obstet Gynecol. 2004;190:602–8.
22. Dietz JP, Foote AJ, Mak HLJ, et al. TVT and SPARC suburethral slings: a case control series. Int Urogynecol J. 2004;15:129–31.
23. Abdel-Fattah M, Ramsay I, Pringle S, et al. Evaluation of transobturator tension-free vaginal tapes in management of women with recurrent stress urinary incontinence. Urology. 2011;77(5):1070–5.
24. Castillo-Pine E, Sassoon A, Pons JE. Comparison of retropubic and transobturator tension-free vaginal implants for the treatment of stress urinary incontinence. Int J Gynaecol Obstet. 2010;110(1):23–6.
25. Richter HE, Albo ME, Zyczynski HM, et al. Urinary Incontinence Treatment Network. Retropubic versus transobturator midurethral slings for stress incontinence. N Engl J Med. 2010;362(22):2066–76.
26. Latthe PM, Singh P, Foon R, et al. Two routes of transobturator tape procedures in stress urinary incontinence: a Meta-analysis with direct and indirect comparison of randomized trials. BJU Int. 2010; 106(1):68–76.
27. Chen Z, Chen Y, Du GH, et al. Comparison of three kinds of mid-urethral slings for surgical treatment of female stress urinary incontinence. Urologia. 2010; 77(1):37–44.
28. Abdel-Fattah M, Ramsay I, Pringle S, et al. Randomized prospective single-blinded study comparing 'inside-out' versus 'outside-in' transobturator tapes in the management of urodynamic stress incontinence: 1-year outcomes from the E-TOT study. BJOG. 2010;117(7):870–8.
29. Nager CW, Sirls L, Litman HJ, et al. Urinary Incontinence Treatment Network. Baseline urodynamic predictors of treatment failure 1 year after mid urethral sling surgery. J Urol. 2011;186(2):597–603.
30. Miller JJ, Botros SM, Akl MN, et al. Is transobturator tape as effective as tension-free vaginal tape in patients with borderline maximum urethral closure pressure? Am J Obstet Gynecol. 2006;195(6): 1799–804.
31. Morey AF, Medendorp AR, Noller MW, et al. Transobturator versus trans-abdominal mid urethral slings: a multi-Institutional comparison of obstructive voiding complications. J Urol. 2006;175:1014–7.
32. Roumeguere T, Quackels T, Bollens R, et al. Transobturator vaginal tape (TOT) for female stress incontinence: one year follow-up in 120 patients. Eur Urol. 2005;48:805–9.
33. Amina MA, Randrianantenaina A, Michel F. Colic perforation as a complication of tension-free vaginal tape procedure. J Urol. 2003;170:2387.
34. Leboeuf L, Tellez CA, Ead D, et al. Complication of bowel perforation during insertion of tension-free vaginal tape. J Urol. 2003;170:1310–1.
35. Peyrat L, Boutin JM, Bruyere F, et al. Intestinal perforation as a complication of tension free vaginal tape procedure for urinary incontinence. Eur Urol. 2001;39:603.
36. Dyrkorn OA, Kulseng-Hanssen S, et al. TVT compared with TVT-O and TOT: results from the Norwegian National Incontinence Registry. Int Urogynecol J. 2010;21(11):1321–6.
37. Rajan S, Kohli N. Retropubic hematoma after transobturator sling procedure. Obstet Gynecol. 2005; 106(5):1199–202.
38. Siegel AL. Vaginal mesh extrusion associated with use of Mentor transobturator sling. Urology. 2005; 66(5):995–9.
39. Domingo S, Alama P, Ruiz N, et al. Diagnosis and management of vaginal erosion after transobturator suburethral tape procedure using a nonwoven thermally bonded polypropylene mesh. J Urol. 2005;173:1627–30.
40. Angioli R, Plotti F, Muzii L, et al. Tension-free vaginal tape versus transobturator suburethral tape: five-year follow-up results of a prospective, randomized trial. Eur Urol. 2010;58(5):671–7.
41. Novara G, Artibani W, Barber MD, et al. Updated systematic review and meta-analysis of the comparative data on colposuspension, pubovaginal slings, and midurethral tapes in the surgical treatment of female stress urinary incontinence. Eur Urol. 2010;58(2): 218–38.
42. Araco F, Gravante G, Sorge R, et al. Sedation with local versus general anesthesia for the tension-free vaginal tape Secur hammock procedure. Int J Gynaecol Obstet. 2011;113(2):108–11.
43. Delorme E. Surgery for female stress urinary incontinence with Transobturator tape. Ann Urol (Paris). 2005;39(1):10–5.
44. Abdel-Fattah M, Ramsay I, Pringle S. Lower urinary tract injuries after Transobturator tape insertion by different routes: a large retrospective study. BJOG. 2006;113(12):1377–81.

45. Ozel B, Minaglia S, Hurtado E, et al. Treatment of voiding dysfunction after transobturator tape procedure. Urology. 2004;64(5):1030.
46. Filocamo MT, Serati M, Frumenzio E, et al. The impact of mid-urethral slings for the treatment of urodynamic stress incontinence on female sexual function: a multicenter prospective study. J Sex Med. 2011;8(7):2002–8.
47. Rechberger T, Futyma K, Jankiewicz K, et al. Tape fixation: an important surgical step to improve success rate of anti-incontinence surgery. J Urol. 2011;186(1):180–4.
48. Abdel-fattah M, Ramsay I, Pringle S, et al. Evaluation of transobturator tapes (E-TOT) study: randomized prospective single-blinded study comparing inside-out vs. outside-in transobturator tapes in management of urodynamic stress incontinence: short term outcomes. Eur J Obstet Gynecol Reprod Biol. 2010; 149(1):106–11.
49. Teo R, Moran P, Mayne C, et al. Randomized trial of tension-free vaginal tape and tension-free vaginal tape-obturator for urodynamic stress incontinence in women. J Urol. 2011;185(4):1350–5.

Female SUI: Single-Incision Slings

5

Michael J. Kennelly and John P. Selph

Stress urinary incontinence (SUI) as defined by the standardization subcommittee of the International Continence Society is the complaint of involuntary leakage of urine on effort or exertion, or on sneezing or coughing [1]. SUI has been estimated to affect up to 50 % of women [2–5], with an estimated annual direct cost of 12 billion dollars for the treatment of female incontinence [6]. While various nonsurgical options exist to treat symptomatic patients, surgical options for women who fail conservative measures include retropubic colposuspension, needle suspension, periurethral injection therapy, fascial pubovaginal slings, and synthetic midurethral slings. As studies showing favorable outcomes and long-term results have emerged over the last 2 decades, the synthetic midurethral sling has become the most commonly performed and gold standard treatment of female SUI [7].

The pubovaginal sling, with autologous fascia placed at the bladder neck, was the initial sling procedure of choice, seeking to correct urethral hypermobility and modify pressure transmission caused by intra-abdominal straining. After studies in the early 1990s by Ulmsten and Petros described the integral theory, elucidating the importance of the midurethra in maintaining continence during stress, the first midurethral tension-free vaginal tape (TVT) was developed. The midurethral placement of the polypropylene synthetic sling reinforced the pubourethral ligament retropubically and provided sub-urethral support, and initial reports showed satisfactory continence results with decreased morbidity compared to traditional procedures [8, 9].

As evidence accumulated showing retropubic polypropylene tape (RPT) had cure rates similar to colposuspension, it became clear that RPT slings introduced a new set of potential complications. A review by Atherton et al. showed that RPT procedures are associated with a 0.2–1 % postoperative urinary retention rate, a 3–4 % risk of bladder, urethral, or intestinal perforation, and a 1–2.5 % risk of major vessel and nerve injury and hematoma in the retropubic space [10]. These complications, although infrequent, lead to further modifications and improvements in minimally invasive urinary incontinence surgery.

The next generation of sling procedures evolved from a retropubic to transobturator location, with the goal of maintaining success rates but avoiding complications (e.g., bladder, bowel, and vessel injury) associated with trocar passage through the retropubic space. Placement of transobturator tape (TOT) involved passing a trocar around the ischiopubic ramus and through the

M.J. Kennelly, M.D. (✉)
McKay Department of Urology, Women's Center for Pelvic Health, Charlotte Continence Center, Carolinas Medical Center, 2001 Vail Avenue, Suite 360, Charlotte, NC 28207, USA
e-mail: mkennelly@carolinas.org

J.P. Selph, M.D.
Department of Urology, UNC School of Medicine, Chapel Hill, NC, USA

G.H. Badlani (ed.), *Minimally Invasive Therapy for Urinary Incontinence and Pelvic Organ Prolapse*, Current Clinical Urology, DOI 10.1007/978-1-4939-0008-4_5,

obturator membrane, thus avoiding the retropubic vessels and viscera but still providing midurethral support. Passage of the trocar from an "inside-out" and "outside-in" approach was developed [10–12]. Multiple studies showed the new TOT technique to be not only comparable in efficacy to RPT slings [13–17], but also successful in reducing bowel and bladder complications. Despite these successes, reports of subjective groin pain, presumably from obturator nerve compression or muscle irritation, emerged [17].

While midurethral slings have been shown to have acceptable cure rates and low morbidity rates [9, 10, 17–23], the blind passage of a trocar through the transobturator or retropubic space affords the potential for bladder or bowel injury, groin or thigh muscle pain, injuries to nerves and blood vessels, and ureteral injury. Building on the success of RPT and TOT slings, the latest innovation in sling procedures, the single-incision sling (SIS), or mini-sling, seeks to reduce morbidity even further.

Single-Incision Slings

Single-incision slings (SIS) seek to build on the efficacy and safety of retropubic tape (RPT) and TOT procedures, yet reduce patient morbidity. SIS are designed to provide midurethral support through a single vaginal incision with a shorter sling that avoids the blind passage of a trocar through the transobturator or retropubic space, thereby reducing the potential complication rate and providing the patient with added benefits: limiting postoperative pain, no external incisions, local anesthesia only, and office-based procedures. Multiple companies have introduced SIS to the market. Each product is made of type 1 uncoated polypropylene mesh, but, importantly, they differ in their sling length, trajectory pathway, delivery device, fixation method, and fixation location, and thus they should not be considered interchangeable products (Table 5.1). Five products currently on the market are discussed below, including procedural steps, postoperative considerations, and results.

Appropriate patient selection is paramount to achieving satisfactory results with SIS. SIS are typically reserved for patients without prior anti-incontinence surgery, though experience with this method has led some surgeons to offer this technique to patients with previous anti-incontinence surgery. Renal insufficiency, coagulopathy, a compromised immune system, pregnancy or future planned pregnancy, and urinary tract obstruction or infection should be considered contraindications to SIS. As with all surgical procedures, informed consent should be obtained from patients before proceeding with intervention.

TVT-Secur System

Introduced in 2006, the first SIS was the Tension-Free Vaginal Tape-Secur™ System (TVT-S) (Ethicon Women's Health and Urology, Somerville, NJ, USA). The TVT-S is an 8 × 1.1 cm laser-cut macroporous polypropylene mesh with absorbable fixation tips that can be fixed to the urogenital diaphragm in a retropubic-like "U" position, or to the obturator internus muscle in a transobturator-like "hammock" or "H" position [24, 25] (Fig. 5.1). The "U" configuration replicates the RPT trajectory by anchoring the fixation tips against the periosteum of the pubis through the connective tissue of the urogenital diaphragm. The "hammock" configuration mimics the transobturator approach, securing the tips of the mesh to the obturator internus muscle along the posterior inferior ischiopubic ramus. Regardless of the technique chosen, early studies revealed the importance of anchoring the fixation tips in contact with the nearby bony structures, rather than the mobile muscular tissue, in order to provide long-term stability [25].

This product uniquely features 2-cm absorbable fixation tips that consist of a fleece layer composed of synthetic absorbable polyglactin 910 (Vicryl) and poly-p-dioxanone (PDS) yarn, which are sandwiched to the mesh using violet-dyed PDS in a thermal process. Once placed, these fixation tips provide immediate mechanical fixation similar to

Table 5.1 Single-incision slings

	TVT Secur™ System	MiniArc™	MiniArc Precise™	Solyx™ SIS System	Ajust™
Manufacturer	Ethicon	AMS	AMS	Boston Scientific	Bard
Needle	Two needles and driver	One needle with driver	One needle with driver	One needle with driver	One needle with driver
Needle diameter (mm)	8.1	2.3	2.3	3.81	5
Size (cm)	1.1×8	1.1×8.5	1.1×8.5	9	
Fixation	Absorbable tips coated with PDS™ and Vicryl™	Permanent self-fixating tips	Permanent self-fixating tips that are tapered and reinforced	Permanent polypropylene mesh carriers	Permanent self-fixating polypropylene anchors
Fixation location	Obturator internus muscle ("hammock") or urogenital diaphragm ("U")	Obturator internus muscle	Obturator internus muscle	Obturator internus muscle	Obturator membrane
Trajectory pathway	Transobturator or Retropubic	Transobturator	Transobturator	Transobturator	Transobturator
Tensioning method	By advancing only, prior to device release	Optional redocking feature	By advancing only, prior to device release	By advancing only, prior to device release	Bidirectional movement of adjustment mesh portion
Midline mark	No	Yes	Yes	No	Yes
Needle disengagement	Two-step process	One step	One step	One step	One step
Pull out force (lbs)	1.9	5.5	5.75	4.64	6.56

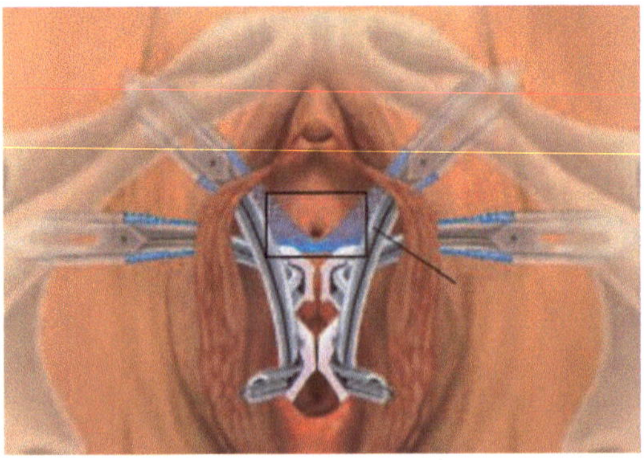

Fig. 5.1 TVT-Secur. The TVT-Secur's 8.0 × 1.1-cm polypropylene mesh with 2-cm absorbable fixation tips can be placed in either the "U" retropubic trajectory position or the "hammock" transobturator trajectory position (© Ethicon, Inc. Reproduced with permission)

the standard TVT system and are absorbed over a period of approximately 90 days [26]. During this time, the polypropylene mesh is encased by a thin fibrous layer of tissue that secures it to the surrounding tissue. Furthermore, as opposed to tanged mesh edges, the laser cut mesh edges impart the mesh with less stretch and a consistent width to facilitate proper placement.

Procedure

Placement of the TVT-Secur mesh can be performed under general, regional, or local anesthesia. The patient is positioned in the dorsal lithotomy position, taking care to pad all pressure points. After local infiltration, a 1.0–1.5 cm incision in the anterior vaginal wall is made along the midurethra, about 1 cm proximal to the urethral meatus. Because of the larger trocar size for the TVT-S compared to conventional slings, the incision is slightly larger to avoid gathering of vaginal tissue. Bluntly dissect with scissors in the paraurethral tissue on each side, taking care to maintain the original width of the incision as one dissects proximally so as to avoid dragging paravaginal tissue during insertion. The direction of the paraurethral dissection can be guided at a 45° angle from the sagittal midline if one desires a "U" placement or at the 3 and 9 o'clock positions if the "hammock" method is to be used.

"U" Position

Dissection is performed to the inferior edge of the pubic bone, ensuring that the scissors do not pierce the urogenital diaphragm and weaken the tissue to which the fixation tips will be anchored. A urethral catheter is placed with a rigid catheter guide to reduce risk of injury to the lower urinary tract. With a needle driver providing stabilization, the TVT-S inserter is then passed until the pubic bone is contacted. The surgeon's hand is then dropped until the inserter is parallel to the floor, and while aiming for the ipsilateral shoulder, the inserter is passed through the dense connective tissue of the urogenital diaphragm. Maintaining contact with the posterior pubic bone is critical to ensure appropriate anchoring. Once the mesh is firmly in the connective tissue, the procedure is repeated on the contralateral side. Adjustments to maintain tension-free placement of the mesh can be made by advancing or retracting the inserter for either the left or right side, ensuring that adequate contact with the pubic bone is maintained. A dynamic cough or crede stress test can be used to assist with tensioning. Unlike traditional midurethral slings, there should be no tissue left between the urethra and mesh, and because the sling is pushed rather than pulled through tissue, tension does not increase postoperatively with the TVT-Secur [25]. Careful separation of the inserters from the mesh is necessary to prevent unwanted withdrawal of the mesh. Once the release wires are pulled, the inserters cannot be reconnected to make adjustments. Cystoscopy is left at the surgeon's discretion, and once positioning is confirmed, the inserters are removed and the incision closed.

"Hammock" Position

Similar to TOT placement, dissection is performed laterally at the 3 and 9 o'clock positions to the lower edge of the ischiopubic ramus, avoiding penetration of the obturator internus muscle by the scissors. The TVT-S is placed flat to and in contact with the lower edge of the ischiopubic ramus while being pushed into the obturator internus muscle. Maintaining contact with the bony surface allows for adequate long-term fixation as well as limits risk of damage to other organs. The procedure is repeated on the contralateral side. As with the "U" positioning, tension-free placement is ensured with bilateral incremental advancement of the device, leaving no tissue between the mesh and urethra. Twisting of the mesh or rotating movements, multiple passes through or tearing of the obturator muscle, and placement away from the bony pelvis yield suboptimal results. Cystoscopy is left at the discretion of the surgeon.

Results

Studies regarding outcomes and complications from TVT-S are limited to short- and medium-term follow-up, with most studies having 1-year data. Initial studies suggested low complication rates but short-term cure rates of 69–88 %, which is lower than traditional cure rates for RPT and TOT slings [27–34]. These poor success rates were felt to be technical in nature as there was a significant learning curve associated with the procedure. Neuman noted a 20 % failure rate and 64 % complication rate in his first 50 patients compared to an 8 % failure rate and 26 % complication rate in the second fifty [25]. Modifications that generated better results included leaving no tissue between the urethra and sling, developing wider 12 mm tunnels due to the larger trocar, tunneling no further than the bone edge, and gently separating the locking mechanism to avoid unwanted tape removal when disconnecting the inserter. Another group noted improved results after the first 25 patients with modifications included tightening the sling such that no leakage of urine is noted during an intraoperative cough stress test and using a gentle rocking motion to release the inserter from the mesh [35].

Most initial reports have suggested a comparable success rate between the "U" and "hammock" type placement methods. Liapis et al. prospectively followed 82 patients who were alternately assigned to either the "U" or "hammock" technique. Objective cure rates based on cough test at 1 year were 62.8 and 71.8 % for the hammock and U technique, respectively, with an overall cure rate of 67.1 % for the TVT-Secur, which was notably less than success rates for traditional TVT procedures [36]. Kim et al. followed 115 women in a randomized comparative trial and reported no statistical difference in cure rate at 12 months based upon the Sandvik questionnaire (88.7 % cure for U-type and 87.1 % cure for hammock-type approach, $p=0.796$) [37]. Unlike Liapis's group's findings, cure rates in this trial were similar to 1-year cure rates in studies of traditional TVT procedures [38]. Another group found that the U-type technique (100 %, 22/22) had better cure rates at 6 months compared to the hammock technique (69 %, 11/16) [39]. Long-term results showing a significant difference between the two methods need to be further studied.

As more groups have published their experiences with TVT-Secur with longer follow-up, several systematic reviews of outcomes have been undertaken. Walsh reviewed the literature on outcomes at 1 year for the TVT-Secur and identified ten studies involving 1,178 patients [40]. Subjective and objective cure rate at 12 months was 76 %, with the U-type method showing a statistically significant higher objective cure rate at 12 months when compared to the "hammock" technique (OR 2.2, $p=0.0005$). Dmochowski et al. reported the outcomes at 12 months on 642 women undergoing the TVT-Secur procedure at 29 sites in eight countries—the objective cure rate at 1 year was 87.5 % [41]. A recent meta-analysis of nine randomized control trials (six TVT-Secur, two MiniArc, and one Ophira) involving SIS vs. standard midurethral slings found inferior objective and patient-reported cure rates in the SIS group [42]. Of the six trials involving TVT-Secur, subgroup analysis revealed a trend toward lower patient-reported and objective cure rates, though statistical significance was not reached. The authors concluded that the available literature on these SIS did not support their use in clinical practice. Two groups have published their experience with 3-year outcomes. Cornu's group showed a cure rate that fell to 40 % at a mean follow-up of 30 months for the TVT-Secur, compared to a 93.5 % success rate at

1 year [43]. In contrast to this dramatic fall in cure rate, Neuman noted a 90.9 % cure rate for the TVT-Secur at 36 months of follow-up in his series [44].

Recently, Hinoul and colleagues published a prospective, randomized, controlled trial of the TVT-Secur vs. TVT-Obturator (TVT-O) system [45]. From 2007 to 2009, 96 patients underwent TVT-Secur and 98 had a TVT-O, with 75 and 85 patients of each group having follow-up at 1 year, respectively. Using a standing cough stress test with 300 cc in the bladder or filled to at least 70 % of capacity based on voiding diary, SUI was present in 16.4 % vs. 2.4 % ($p<0.05$) of the TVT-Secur and TVT-O patients, respectively. Patients in the TVT-Secur experienced less postoperative pain and returned to work sooner, but the odds ratio for re-intervention for SUI 1 year after TVT-Secur vs. TVT-O was 2.3 (95 % CI 1.9–2.7).

Overall, efficacy rates of the TVT-S are mixed but tend to show lower efficacy rates than RPT and TOT slings in comparative trials. Clearly, surgical technique and surgeon skill play a key role in the providing patient success. Long-term data and advances in alternative SIS technologies have tempered the original enthusiasm for the TVT-S sling.

MiniArc

In August of 2007 the MiniArc™ (American Medical Systems, Minnetonka, MN, USA) became the second SIS released in the United States and Europe. It comprises an 8.5 × 1.1 cm type 1 polypropylene mesh with integrated self-fixation tips that anchor into the obturator internus muscle via a single 1.5 cm vaginal incision (Fig. 5.2). Unique design features include a narrower inserter, optional redocking feature, tanged mesh edges, a midline mesh mark, and the self-fixating tips.

An early criticism of the TVT-Secur was the difficulty in removing the inserter from the mesh, and the MiniArc was designed to allow a smoother engagement and disengagement of the needle and mesh, thereby reducing the risk of unwanted loosening of the mesh during inserter removal. This feature was achieved by not only utilizing a single 2.3 mm diameter needle that minimizes tissue trauma during placement, but also by creating permanent self-fixating tips that, based on cadaveric testing, require a pull-out force four times (5.5 lbs) higher than normal pelvic floor pressures (1.3 lbs) [46, 47]. The surgeon is also permitted to redock the needle and mesh, thus allowing for further tensioning after the sling is placed. In 2010, modifications to the MiniArc were made based on surgeon feedback, and AMS released the new and improved MiniArc Precise Sling. Changes included: (1) a snap fit needle-to-tip connection that prevents rotation of the mesh on the needle and secures the sling to the inserter; (2) a needle that retracts into the body of the inserter to help prevent displacement of the sling tip during inserter removal; and (3) tapered and reinforced mesh ends that minimize the potential for mesh twisting and ensure a flat placement on the urethra.

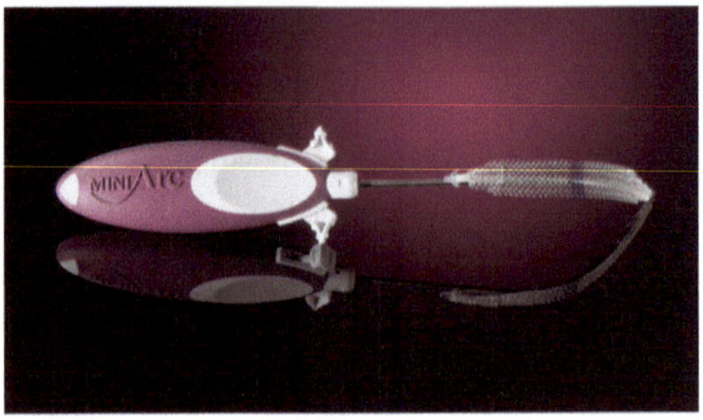

Fig. 5.2 MiniArc Precise. The MiniArc Precise's 1.1 × 8.5-cm macroporous polypropylene mesh fused to self-fixating tips is placed with a 2.3 mm needle (Courtesy of American Medical Systems, Inc., Minnetonka, MN)

Procedure

The sling is placed through a single 1.5 cm vaginal incision at the midurethra. Periurethral dissection is carried out with Metzenbaum scissors toward the interior portion of the inferior pubic ramus. The sling/needle assembly is advanced behind the ischiopubic ramus in a transobturator trajectory toward the obturator space bilaterally. The obturator internus fascia is pierced with the needle, and once the integrated self-fixating tip is fixed in the obturator internus muscle, the needle is removed. This step is repeated on the contralateral side. Should further tensioning be desired, redocking can be achieved by accessing the implanted tip on the initial side. The mesh should lie flat against the urethra with no mesh distortion or space left between the urethra and sling. Cough or Valsalva stress-testing or visual inspection of the tape assists with proper sling tensioning. Cystoscopy is left at the discretion of the surgeon, and the incision is irrigated and then closed.

Results

Initial studies showed promising results for the MiniArc, though other studies have shown mixed results at 1 year of follow-up. Moore and colleagues retrospectively reviewed 61 patients who had a MiniArc sling placed and found a 91.4 % cure rate with no intraoperative complications, pain, dyspareunia, or sling erosion [48]. In a multicenter prospective trial, Kennelly et al. assessed 157 of 188 women available for follow-up at 1 year and found 90.6 % of patients had a negative cough stress test [49]. There were no intraoperative complications, and 20 % of the cases were performed in the office setting. Pickens et al. noted a cure rate of 93.5 % (101/108) at 12 months in a prospective cohort of 108 patients who had follow-up, as well as significant improvement in quality of life based on the UDI-6 (65 of 100 vs. 13.32 of 100, $P<0.001$) and IIQ-7 (89.91 of 100 vs. 12.5 of 100, $P<0.001$) questionnaires [50]. In a retrospective cohort study at two centers comparing 75 patients undergoing the MiniArc and 56 patients undergoing the Monarc sling, 85 % of the MiniArc group vs. 89 % of the Monarc group had a negative cough stress test at 12 months [51]. Both groups saw significant improvement in subjective cure rates based on the IIQ-7 and UDI-6 questionnaires, and the authors concluded the MiniArc provides objective cure rates comparable to other slings, though longer follow-up is needed. In contrast to these findings, Hogewoning and colleagues noted a 56 % failure rate (not completely dry) and 68 % subjective cure rate (improvement in symptoms based on PGI-I questionnaire) at 1 year [52]. Others have noted lower efficacy rates of 77.8 % at 12 months and 75.7 % at 2 months [53, 54].

Overall, efficacy rates on the MiniArc are mixed but tend to show promising early results. Clearly, longer follow-up studies and ideally a long-term, prospective, randomized clinical trial are needed to help further elucidate the place of the MiniArc in the urologic armamentarium.

Solyx

The Solyx™ SIS system (Boston Scientific Corporation, Natick, MA, USA) was introduced in North America in 2009. The 9-cm polypropylene mesh is placed via a delivery device into the obturator internus muscle, where carrier barbs at each end of the mesh serve to anchor the sling in place while tissue ingrowth occurs over time (Fig. 5.3). The carriers snap on to the delivery device, and once passed into the obturator internus, minute adjustments to the sling can be made to gain

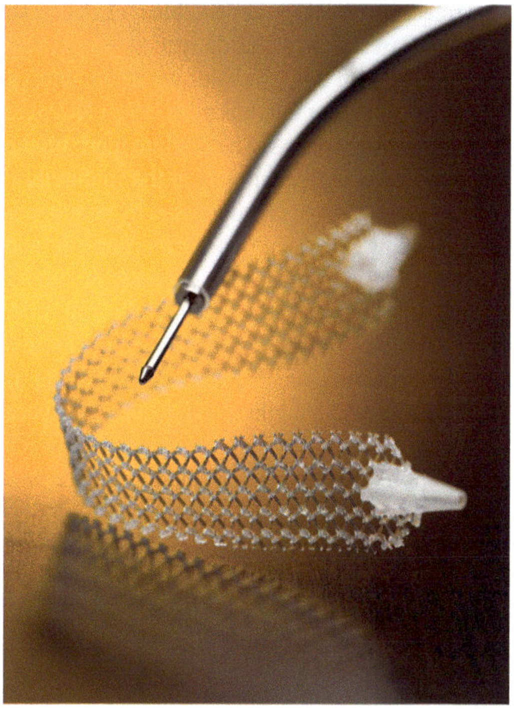

Fig. 5.3 Solyx Single Incision System. The 9.0 cm polypropylene sling fused to carrier barbs is placed in the obturator internus muscle with a snap-fit delivery device (Courtesy of Boston Scientific Corporation. Opinions expressed are those of the author alone and not of Boston Scientific)

appropriate tension. The lateral edges of the mesh are tanged in order to reduce loosening of the mesh as the delivery device is disconnected, and similar to the TVT-Secur, the delivery device cannot be reconnected to the carrier once they are detached. Additionally, the 4-cm central portion of the mesh is detanged and heat sealed to prevent irritation to the urethra and limit deformation.

Procedure

Anesthesia can be general, spinal, or local and is left to the surgeon's discretion. The patient is placed in the dorsal lithotomy position and prepped and draped in a sterile fashion. After local infiltration, a 1–1.5 cm vaginal incision is made at the level of the midurethra. Periurethral dissection with Metzenbaum scissors is directed at a 45° angle toward the inferior pubic ramus. Once an appropriate tunnel has been created, the mesh is attached flush to the delivery device tip, which is confirmed by hearing an audible "click." The device is inserted into the dissection tunnel and advanced toward the obturator foramen until it pierces the obturator internus muscle just lateral to the inferior pubic ramus. The midline mark on the mesh should be approximately at the midurethra. The carrier is released into the tissue by simultaneously holding the deployment mechanism and pulling the delivery device handle back. A similar procedure is repeated on the contralateral side. Appropriate tension is confirmed via cough stress test or visual assessment, ensuring the sling is placed against the urethra and leaving a space small enough to pass a small instrument in between or identifying "pillowing" of periurethral tissue through the mesh pores [55]. Slight adjustments to tension can be made prior to disconnecting the delivery device. Cystoscopy is left to the surgeon's discretion, the wound is irrigated, and the incision is closed in the usual fashion.

Results

There are limited data describing results regarding the Solyx SIS. Serels et al. published a retrospective review of 63 patients undergoing Solyx implantation at three US medical centers [55]. Patients had not undergone previous incontinence surgery, all had urethral hypermobility >30° with a Q-tip test, and stress incontinence was the predominant symptom (29 % had urge incontinence). Fifty-nine percentage of patients underwent concomitant procedures. At a mean follow-up of 6.5 months (range 5–8 months), 95 % of patients (60/63) were subjectively dry and had a negative cough stress test. Other than two patients experiencing transient urinary retention, no postoperative complications were noted. Like its predecessors, further study is needed to determine long-term efficacy.

Ajust

The AJUST™ Adjustable Single-Incision Sling system (CR Bard, Inc., Covington, GA, USA) entered the marketplace in 2008 in Europe and 2009 in North America. It too was designed to provide the benefits of TOT placement through a single vaginal incision. Design features include self-fixating polypropylene anchors, a midline mesh mark, a flexible stylet used to lock the sling after adjustment, and an introducer to insert the sling through the obturator membrane. The sling is unique in that it has a sub-urethral mesh section and an adjustment mesh portion that allows for post-insertion tightening or loosening without further insertion of the anchors (Fig. 5.4). This feature is achieved by having one fixed anchor and a second adjustable anchor through which the tubular adjustable mesh portion can be bidirectionally shifted. This setup gives the surgeon full view of the sling mesh during tensioning without any visual obstruction from the introducer. Once the appropriate tension is achieved, the flexible stylet is used to lock the sling in place.

Procedure

The patient is placed in the dorsal lithotomy position, and after local infiltration, a 1.5 cm incision is

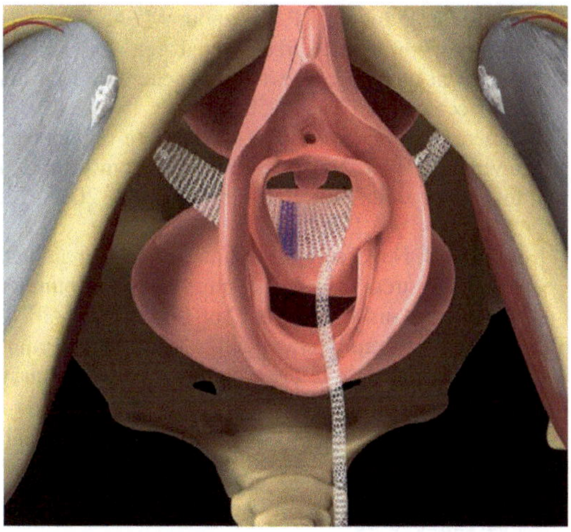

Fig. 5.4 AJUST adjustable single-incision sling. The AJUST is placed through the obturator membrane with self-fixating anchors. Post-insertion adjustments can be made by loosening or tightening the mesh relative to the fixed anchors (© 2013 C. R. Bard, Inc. Used with permission. Ajust is a registered trademark of C. R. Bard, Inc.)

made in the midurethra. Dissection is carried out horizontally toward the ischiopubic ramus. Starting with the fixed anchor side, the introducer is then passed toward the cephalad margin of the ischiopubic ramus. Once the fixed anchor passes the ischiopubic ramus, the surgeon halts the push maneuver and pivots the introducer handle past the midline and toward the obturator internus muscle. The fixed anchor is then pushed through the obturator internus muscle and membrane, ensuring the midline mark is at or slightly beyond midline on the side of insertion. The anchor is then released, the introducer is removed, and appropriate fixation is confirmed with a gentle tug on the mesh. The adjustable anchor is then loaded and placed on the contralateral side using the same technique. Once placed, the adjustment tab and tubular mesh are pulled until proper tensioning is achieved. If desired, gentle counter-traction on the sub-urethral sling will loosen the mesh. After proper tensioning, the flexible stylet is inserted in the adjustment tab opening and a sling lock is advanced up to the adjustable anchor to lock it in place. Excess adjustment mesh is then trimmed, the incision is irrigated, and the vaginal incision is closed. Cystoscopy is left to the discretion of the surgeon.

Results

Peer-reviewed literature describing results from the Ajust SIS is limited. One group recently published its 1-year outcomes of a multicenter, prospective cohort of 90 women undergoing Ajust-SIS placement [56]. Patients had SUI or mixed incontinence with predominant SUI symptoms, were not undergoing concomitant repairs, and did not have pelvic organ prolapse. At 12 months after surgery, 72/90 (80 %) patients reported being either "much improved" or "very much improved." One patient had sling placement converted to a standard midurethral sling for unclear reasons. Thirteen patients (14 %) were considered failures, that is, their symptoms were the same or worse or they had repeat incontinence surgery (five patients). Two patients had erosion of mesh into the vagina but were managed with local excision of eroded mesh. Of the 85 patients not requiring reoperation, 17 % (14/85) had a positive cough stress test at 1 year, while 82 % (70/85) had a negative stress test. Thirty-one patients underwent sling placement under local anesthesia: 97 % were completed, with 1 patient asking to be converted to general anesthesia due to pain. No patients had groin pain postoperatively. Meschia et al. published their data on 102 women undergoing Ajust sling placement, with an 85.7 and 91.4 % patient-reported and objective cure rates, respectively [57].

Conclusion

SUI is a common yet surgically correctable problem in many adult women. Traditional retropubic and transobturator slings have high success rates that have years of data to support their use. Nonetheless, blind passage of trocars during these procedures affords the opportunity for serious injury to visceral and vascular structures. SIS seek to provide the same benefit with lower morbidity. While the procedures are similar to traditional midurethral slings, SIS are not interchangeable and require attention to detail as each sling has unique characteristics and operative steps. Rather than replace RPT and TOT slings,

SIS seek to provide patients with an option for treatment that has decreased complications, high continence rates, and the potential for placement under local anesthesia in the office setting. To date, literature reviewing the efficacy of these slings is mixed, and further long-term and randomized controlled trials are needed to delineate the role of SIS in the treatment of SUI. An FDA panel convened in September of 2011 agreed with the need for further study. The group recommended that premarket evaluation of mini-slings should include clinical studies involving a control arm of women using a transobturator or retropubic sling. Furthermore, postmarket studies are necessary to study the efficacy and safety of currently available SIS. These studies should be randomized or have a rigorous cohort design, compare women with SIS to women with transobturator or retropubic slings, and have 3–5 years of follow-up [58].

References

1. Abrams P, Cardozo L, Fall M, et al. The standardization of terminology in lower urinary tract function: report from the standardization sub-committee of the International Continence Society. Urology. 2003; 61(1):37–49.
2. Hannestad YS, Rortveit G, Sandvik H, et al. A community-based epidemiological survey of female urinary incontinence: the Norwegian EPICONT Study. J Clin Epidemiol. 2000;53:1150–7.
3. Lara C, Nacey J. Ethnic differences between Maori, Pacific Island and European New Zealand women in prevalence and attitudes to urinary incontinence. N Z Med J. 1994;107:374–6.
4. Minassian V, Stewart WF, Wood GC. Urinary incontinence in women: variation in prevalence estimates and risk factors. Obstet Gynecol. 2008;111:324–31.
5. Peyrat L, Haillot O, Bruyere F, et al. Prevalence and risk factors of urinary incontinence in young and middle-aged women. BJU Int. 2002;89:61–6.
6. Chong EC, Khan AA, Anger JT. The financial burden of stress urinary incontinence among women in the united States. Curr Urol Rep. 2011;12(5):358–62.
7. Anger JT, Weinberg AE, et al. Trends in surgical management of stress urinary incontinence among female Medicare beneficiaries. Urology. 2009;74(2):283–7.
8. Petros PE, Ulmsten UI. An integral theory of female urinary incontinence. Experimental and clinical considerations. Acta Obstet Gynecol Scand Suppl. 1990;153:7–31.
9. Ulmsten U, Johnson P, Reqapour M. A three-year follow up of tension-free vaginal tape for surgical treatment of female stress incontinence. Br J Obstet Gynaecol. 1999;106:345–50.
10. Atherton M, Stanton S. The tension-free vaginal tape reviewed: an evidence-based review from inception to current status. Int J Obstet Gynaecol. 2005;112: 534–46.
11. de Leval J. Novel surgical technique for the treatment of female stress urinary incontinence: transobturator vaginal tape inside-out. Eur Urol. 2003;44:724–30.
12. Delorme E. Transobturator urethral suspension: mini-invasive procedure in the treatment of stress urinary incontinence in women. Prog Urol. 2001;6:1306–13.
13. Richter HE, Albo ME, Zyczynski HM, et al. Retropubic versus transobturator midurethral slings for stress incontinence. N Engl J Med. 2010; 362(22):2066–76.
14. Laurikainen E, Valpas A, Kivela A, et al. Retropubic compared with transobturator tape placement in treatment of urinary incontinence: a randomized controlled trial. Obstet Gynecol. 2007;109:4–11.
15. Barber M, Kleeman S, Karram M, et al. Transoburator tape compared with tension-free vaginal tape for the treatment of stress urinary incontinence. Obstet Gynecol. 2008;111:611–21.
16. Barry C, Lim Y, Muller R, et al. A multicentre randomized clinical controlled trial comparing the retropubic (RP) approach vs the transobturator approach (TO) for tension-free suburethral sling treatment of urodynamic stress incontinence: the TORP study. Int Urogynecol J Pelvic Floor Dysfunct. 2008;19:171–8.
17. Ogah J, Cody DJ, Rogerson L. Minimally invasive synthetic suburethral sling operations for stress urinary incontinence in women: a short version Cochrane review. Neurourol Urodyn. 2011;30(3):284–91.
18. Nilsson C, Palva K, Rezapour M, et al. Eleven years prospective follow-up of the tension-free vaginal tape procedure for treatment of stress urinary incontinence. Int Urogynecol J Pelvic Floor Dysfunct. 2008;19:1043–7.
19. Ward K, Hilton P, UK and Ireland TVT Trial Group. Prospective multicentre randomized trial of tension-free vaginal tape and colposuspensions as primary treatment for stress incontinence. BMJ. 2002;325:67.
20. Grise P, Droupy S, Saussine C, et al. Transobturator sling for female stress incontinence with polypropylene tape and outside in procedure: prospective study with 1 year follow up and review of transobturator tape sling. Urology. 2006;68:759–63.
21. De Leval J, Waltregny D. New surgical technique for treatment of stress urinary incontinence TVT-Obturator: new developments and results. Surg Technol Int. 2005;14:212–21.
22. Davila G, Johnson J, Serels D. Multicenter experience with the Monarc transobturator sling system to treat stress urinary incontinence. Int Urogynecol J Pelvic Floor Dysfunct. 2006;17:460–5.

23. Barry C, Lim Y, Muller R, et al. A multicentre randomized clinical controlled trial comparing the retropubic (RP) approach vs the transobturator approach (TO) for tension-free suburethral sling treatment of urodynamic stress incontinence: the TORP study. Int Urogynecol J Pelvic Floor Dysfunc. 2008;19:171–8.
24. Meschia M, Barbacini P, Ambrogi V, et al. TVT-Secur: a minimally invasive procedure for the treatment of primary stress urinary incontinence. One year data from a multicentre prospective trial. Int Urogynecol J Pelvic Floor Dysfunc. 2009;20:313–7.
25. Neuman M. Perioperative complications and early follow up with 100 TVT-Secur procedures. J Minim Invasive Gynecol. 2008;15:480–4.
26. Rezapour M, Novara G, Meier PA, et al. 3-month preclinical trial to assess the performance of a new TVT-like mesh (TVTx) in a sheep model. Int Urogynecol J. 2007;18:183–7.
27. Baracat F, Iglesias R, Pessoa R, et al. Unfavorable immediate outcome with the TVT Secure sling in twenty consecutive women with stress urinary incontinence. J Urol. 2008;179(4):535–6.
28. Karram M, Lucente V, Khandwala S, et al. An evaluation of the Gynecare TVT Secur System (tension-free support for incontinence) for the treatment of stress urinary incontinence [abstract]. Int Urogynecol J. 2007;18 Suppl 1:004.
29. Neuman M, Shaare-Zedek MC. Training TVT Secur: the first 150 teaching operations [abstract]. Int Urogyn J. 2007;18 Suppl 1:045.
30. Martan A, Masata J, Svabik K. Initial experience with TVT-Secur System procedure and the reason for persistent stress urinary incontinence [abstract]. Int Urogyn J. 2007;18 Suppl 1:044.
31. Marsh FA, Assassa P. An audit of the introduction of TVT Secur in clinical practice [abstract]. Int Urogyn J. 2007;18 Suppl 1:043.
32. Albrich S, Naumann G, Skala C, et al. TVT Secur ® First experiences after a follow-up of 17 months [abstract]. Neurourol Urodyn 2008;27
33. Saltz SM, Haff RE, Lucente VR. Short-term assessment of patients undergoing the new tension free vaginal tape Secur procedure for treatment of stress urinary incontinence [abstract]. Int Urogyn J. 2007;18 Suppl 1:046.
34. Debodinance P, Lagrange E, et al. TVT-Secur: more and more minimal invasive—preliminary prospective study on 40 cases [abstract]. Int Urogyn J. 2007;8 Suppl 1:239.
35. Molden S, Lucente V. New Minimally Invasive Slings: TVT Secur. Curr Urol Rep. 2008;9:358–61.
36. Liapas A, et al. Comparison of the TVT SECUR System "hammock" and "U" tape positions for management of stress urinary incontinence. Int J Gynaecol Obstet. 2010;111(3):233–6. Epub 2010 Sep 6.
37. Kim JJ, Lee YS, Lee KS. Randomized comparative study of the U- and H-type approaches of the TVT-Secur procedure for the treatment of female stress urinary incontinence: one-year follow-up. Korean J Urol. 2010;51(4):250–6.
38. Lee KS, Choo MS, Doo CK, Han DH, Lee YS, Kim JY, et al. The long term (5-years) objective TVT success rate does not depend on predictive factors at multivariate analysis: a multicentre retrospective study. Eur Urol. 2008;53:176–82.
39. Gagnon LO, le Tu M. Better short-term outcomes with the U-method compared with the Hammock technique for the implantation of the TVT-SECUR under local anesthesia. Urology. 2010;75(5):1060–4.
40. Walsh CA. TVT-Secur mini-sling for stress urinary incontinence: a review of outcomes at 12 months. BJU Int. 2011;108(5):652–7.
41. Dmochowski RR, Grier D, Franco N, et al. One year results from a World-Wide Registry of TVT-SECUR™ in women with stress urinary incontinence. J Urol. 2009;181:544.
42. Abdel-Fattah M, Ford JA, Lim CP, Madhuvrata P. Single-incision mini-slings versus standard midurethral slings in surgical management of female stress urinary incontinence: a meta-analysis of effectiveness and complications. Eur Urol. 2011;60(3):468–80.
43. Cornu JN, Sebe P, Peyrat L, et al. Midterm prospective evaluation of TVT-Secur reveals high failure rate. Eur Urol. 2010;58:157–61.
44. Neuman M, Sosnovski V, Kais M, et al. Transobturator vs single-incision suburethral mini-slings for treatment of female stress urinary incontinence: early postoperative pain and 3-year follow-up. J Minim Invasive Gynecol. 2011;18(6):769–73.
45. Hinoul P, Vervest HA, den Boon J, et al. A randomized, controlled trial comparing an innovative single incision sling with an established transobturator sling to treat female stress urinary incontinence. J Urol. 2011;185(4):1356–62.
46. Moore RD, Serels DR, Davila GW, et al. Minimally invasive treatment for female stress urinary incontinence (SUI): a review including TVT, TOT, and mini-sling. Surg Technol Int. 2009;18:157–73.
47. Howard D, Miller JM, Delancey JL, et al. Differential effects of cough, valsalva, and continence status on vesical neck movement. Obstet Gynecol. 2000;95:535–40.
48. Moore RD, Mitchell GK, Miklos JR. Single-center retrospective study of the technique, safety, and 12-month efficacy of the miniarc single-incision sling: a new minimally invasive procedure for treatment of female SUI. Surg Technol Int. 2009;18:175–81.
49. Kennelly MJ, Moore RD, Nguyen JN, et al. Prospective evaluation of a single incision sling for stress urinary incontinence. J Urol. 2010;184(2):604–9.
50. Pickens RB, Klein FA, Mobley III JD, White WM. Single incision mid-urethral sling for treatment of female stress urinary incontinence. Urology. 2010;77:321–4.
51. De Ridder D, Berkers J, Deprest J, Verguts J, Ost D, Hamid D, Van der Aa F. Single incision mini-sling versus a transobutaror sling: a comparative study on MiniArc and Monarc slings. Int Urogynecol J Pelvic Floor Dysfunct. 2010;21(7):773–8.

52. Hogewoning CR, Ruhe IM, Bekker MD. The MiniArc sling for female stress urinary incontinence: clinical results after 1-year follow-up. Int Urogynecol J. 2012;23(5):589–95.
53. Gauruder-Burmester A, Popken G. The MiniArc sling system in the treatment of female stress urinary incontinence. Int Braz J Urol. 2009;35:334–41.
54. Debodinance P, Delporte P. MiniArc: preliminary prospective study on 72 cases. J Gynecol Obstet Biol Reprod. 2009;38:144–8.
55. Serels S, Douso M, Short G. Preliminary findings with the Solyx single-incision sling system in female stress urinary incontinence. Int Urogynecol J. 2010; 21(5):557–61.
56. Abdel-Fattah M, Agur W, Abdel-All M, et al. Prospective multi-centre study of adjustable single-incision mini-sling (Ajust(®)) in the management of stress urinary incontinence in women: 1-year follow-up study. BJU Int. 2012;109(6):880–6.
57. Meschia M, Barbacini P, Baccichet R, et al. Short-term outcomes with the AjustTM system: a new single incision sling for the treatment of stress urinary incontinence. Int Urogynecol J. 2011;22(2): 177–82.
58. http://www.fda.gov/downloads/AdvisoryCommittees/CommitteesMeetingMaterials/MedicalDevices/MedicalDevicesAdvisoryCommittee/ObstetricsandGynecologyDevices/UCM271769.pdf

Fascial Slings: Is There Still a Place?

6

E. Ann Gormley

Indications

The gold standard sling, prior to the widespread adoption of the midurethral sling was the pubovaginal rectus fascial sling. The early operative descriptions of fascial slings by Aldridge and Millen in the 1940s describe the rectus fascia being left attached on one or both ends and a strip or two strips of fascia being passed under the urethra and either sutured to the other strip or being brought back through the space of Retzius on the other side and sutured to the underside of the rectus fascia [1, 2]. The fascial sling that is used today was introduced to the urologic community in 1978 by McGuire and Lytton [3]. They used a combined abdominal vaginal approach using rectus fascia. Fascial slings were initially advocated for complicated cases, patients who had failed multiple procedures such as Kelly plications, needle suspensions, or retropubic bladder neck suspensions and for patients with recognized intrinsic sphincter dysfunction (ISD). A number of publications in the last half of the 1990s, including the AUA guidelines for the surgical treatment of female stress urinary incontinence (SUI) in 1997 helped to fuel the use of the fascial sling as the main surgical procedure for virtually all stress incontinent patients [4]. With the advent of synthetic midurethral slings, many urologists, including some who exclusively practice female urology, have never performed a pubovaginal fascial sling.

Today in the era of synthetic slings, there remains a role for the pubovaginal fascial sling. Patients with pure ISD, however one defines that, should be offered a fascial sling or an injectable. Although there are studies that show success of midurethral slings in patients with ISD, one needs to be very cautious in the patient with a fixed urethra since according to Ulmsted's Integral theory a midurethral synthetic sling should not work without urethral mobility [5].

Synthetics should be avoided in any patients where sling tension might be beneficial, for example, the patient with myelodyplasia and a wide open bladder neck. If the goal of the sling is to close the bladder outlet, then this is better done at the bladder neck with fascia since putting tension on the midurethra with a synthetic may increase the risk of urethral erosion. In a female neurogenic patient undergoing an incontinent or continent catheterizable stoma, who requires a bladder neck closure, a fascial sling at the bladder neck can be utilized. This is advantageous compared to a formal bladder neck closure since the urethra can still be catheterized or scoped if there are problems with the stoma or catheterizable channel.

Synthetics are also avoided where there is a higher risk of infection because of contamination.

E.A. Gormley, M.D. (✉)
Department of Surgery, Dartmouth-Hitchcock Medical Center, 1 Medical Center Drive, Lebanon, NH 03756, USA
e-mail: ann.gormley@hitchcock.org

G.H. Badlani (ed.), *Minimally Invasive Therapy for Urinary Incontinence and Pelvic Organ Prolapse*, Current Clinical Urology, DOI 10.1007/978-1-4939-0008-4_6,

Examples of this would include the sling placed in a neurogenic patient who is also undergoing a bladder augmentation with bowel or the patient who is having a sling placed concomitantly with excision of a periurethral abscess or repair of a urethral diverticulum. Fascial slings are also the preferred sling material at the time of or following urethral reconstruction.

Patients with urethral mobility may also be offered a fascial sling. The ideal patient for a fascial sling who has urethral mobility is the patient who wishes to avoid a synthetic. This could be the patient who has failed a prior synthetic sling or had a synthetic complication or it may just be a patient who for some reason would prefer that her own tissue be used. As there is more scrutiny of the use of vaginal mesh for prolapse repairs an increasing number of patients are opting not to have any form of synthetic mesh implanted. The age of the patient must also be considered. Although synthetic midurethral slings offer the young woman a much quicker recovery we do not know the very long-term consequences of mesh in the vagina. This is of particular concern when a young woman is undergoing a second mesh sling or if the sling is being placed concomitantly with or following the placement of vaginal mesh for prolapse.

Preoperative counseling should consist of a discussion of the risks and benefits of autologous tissue vs. synthetic grafts, including potential for more abdominal wound discomfort or voiding problems with the use of their own fascia vs. complications of synthetics.

Results

Cure rates for fascial slings have generally been estimated to be in the range of 80–90 % [6]. In the AUA Guideline for the Surgical Management of Female Stress Urinary Incontinence in 2010, efficacy data were available for a variety of types of fascial slings but most of the available studies reviewed describe autologous fascia slings as described in this chapter [7]. In patients only undergoing a sling, the estimated cured/dry rates ranged between 90 % at 12–23 months and 82 % at 48 months or longer. The number of series reviewed where patients underwent a concurrent prolapse treatment were much smaller with far fewer patients but the cured/dry rates were similar and ranged from 85 to 92 %. In the Panel's meta-analysis of fascial slings alone, the estimated rates of postsurgical urge incontinence were 33 % in patients with preexisting urge incontinence and de novo urge incontinence was noted in 9 % of patients. The estimated rate of retention was 8 %. Complications were infrequent and included urinary tract infection (16 %), bladder injury (4 %), and wound complications (8 %). In those series where patients underwent a sling with a prolapse repair complication rates were similar.

The largest and most rigorous randomized trial involving fascial slings is the Urinary Incontinence Treatment Network's SISTeR Trial [8]. Using a very strict definition of continence, the SUI-specific treatment success for a sling which included a negative cough and Valsalva stress test, no self-reported stress symptoms and no retreatment for stress incontinence, was 66 % at 24 months. Overall treatment success at 24 months for a sling was 47 %. Both of these were superior to the success rate for a Burch colposuspension. Patient satisfaction with a sling at 24 months was 86 % which was significantly higher than the Burch which was 78 %. The most common complications in the sling group were urinary tract infections. Procedures to improve voiding occurred exclusively in the sling group and were required in 6 % of patients.

Although fascial slings are felt to be durable, there is a fall off in success rate over time. This was shown in an extension of the SISTeR trial (E-SISTeR) where patients who completed the SISTeR trial were followed for a total of 5 years [9]. The criteria for success in this trial was slightly different since patients did not do pad weight tests or undergo stress testing during the follow-up period. The success rate for fascial slings at 2 years was 52 % and 30.8 % at 5 years. The surgical retreatment rate for SUI was 2 %. At 5 years 83 % of all women in the fascial sling group were satisfied as compared to a satisfaction rate of 87 % at 2 years.

Technique

A combined abdominal and vaginal approach is used with the patient in the low lithotomy position. The lower abdomen, perineum, and vagina are prepped and draped to provide access to the lower abdomen and vagina. A Foley catheter is placed in the bladder to drain the bladder and to allow for palpation of the bladder neck. A 6–8 cm long transverse suprapubic incision is made 2–4 cm above the symphysis. The rectus fascia is exposed and incised transversely above the symphysis. The fascia is lifted off the rectus muscle bellies and a strip of fascia measuring 1.5–2 cm by 6–8 cm is harvested. Each end of the strip of fascia is whip stitched with a running 0 nonabsorbable suture and tied down leaving both ends as long as possible.

A weighted vaginal retractor, such as a Schurback, is inserted into the vagina. The anterior vaginal wall at the level of the bladder neck is infiltrated with a dilute vasopressin solution. A 4–5-cm vertical midline incision or an inverted U-shaped incision is made in the vaginal wall from the midurethra to the bladder neck. Using Metzenbaum or Church scissors, the vaginal wall is sharply dissected laterally off of the periurethral fascia which is identified as a glistening white color. Dissection in this plane is relatively bloodless and prevents inadvertent entry into the bladder or urethra. The vaginal wall is dissected laterally on both sides toward the ischium. Once the sling has been prepared, the pubocervical fascia is perforated sharply on either side of the urethra by keeping the scissors parallel to the perineum and aiming for the patient's ipsilateral shoulder thus gaining entry into the retropubic space. Finger dissection is used to create a tunnel for the sling into the retropubic space toward the rectus muscle bellies.

The retropubic space is entered via a suprapubic approach, by "popping" the index finger through the triangle bounded by the rectus muscle and the inguinal ligament. Retropubic tunnels are developed in continuity with the vaginal dissection by palpating the fingertip of the vaginal operator behind the rectus muscle. Via a vaginal approach the surgeon inserts an index finger into one side of the vaginal incision and up into the retropubic space. A curved clamp, such as a Crawford, is advanced through the retropubic tunnel from above down using the vaginal finger as a guide. The nose of the clamp is kept in constant contact with the posterior surface of the symphysis to avoid entering the bladder. Once the clamp is passed through the retropubic space and out the vaginal incision the clamp is opened and one end of the sling sutures is grasped and pulled retropubically into the abdominal wound. The same procedure is then repeated on the opposite side to draw up the other end of the sling suture into the abdominal wound. The Foley is removed and a cystoscopy is performed to rule out bladder, urethral, or ureteral injury. Bilateral ureteral jets should be seen to insure ureteral patency. If a bladder perforation has occurred, the sling is removed and a new retropubic tunnel is created. With the Crawford clamp in place, a cystoscopy is repeated. Visualization of a clamp in the bladder is very dramatic, whereas it is possible to miss seeing a piece of sling suture peeking through a small hole.

If no perforation is seen, the sling is gently pulled into the retropubic space bilaterally to seat the sling at the bladder neck. The sling is sutured to the periurethral fascia with one or two 3-0 absorbable sutures. The sling sutures are passed through two small stab wounds in the inferior leaf of the rectus fascia. The abdominal fascia is further dissected off of the rectus muscle so that it can be closed without tension and the vaginal wound is closed.

With a Foley catheter in the urethra, the sling tension is adjusted so that gentle traction on the Foley catheter does not result in inferior urethral mobility. The sling is generally tied very loosely so the surgeon can place 2–3 fingers between the fascia and the knot of the sling sutures. The suprapubic wound is closed and a vaginal pack placed. Abdominal pain and wound issues can be minimized by closing the fascia without tension and by meticulous hemostasis which may prevent seroma formation and subsequent wound break down.

An alternative method of obtaining fascia is to use a fascial stripper to harvest fascia lata.

Historically this was done through two or three transverse incisions on the lateral thigh and resulted in a very long strip of fascia. The main reason to consider using fascia lata today is in the patient with a large piece of mesh abdominally. In the patient with a hostile abdominal wall, abdominal dissection can be limited by passing the sling sutures using a Stamey or Peyrera type needle. A cystoscopy should be performed with the needle(s) in place.

Postoperative Problems

Urinary retention, which is usually the result of too much tension at the urethrovesical junction, is the greatest concern. Straining to void causes the sling to tighten. The patient must learn to void by relaxing and allowing the detrusor to contract. Clean intermittent catheterization is used until normal voiding occurs. If the patient is unable to resume normal voiding in 4–8 weeks, division of the sling vaginally will often result in resumption of normal emptying. Recurrent stress incontinence is very rare following sling incision.

In patients with mixed incontinence preoperatively, 20–35 % will have persistent urgency incontinence postoperatively. Fortunately most of these patients will respond to antimuscarinic treatment.

Persistent stress incontinence occurs if the sling is not tight enough to sufficiently compress the urethra particularly if there is excessive scarring from previous procedures. Rarely recurrent stress incontinence develops when the sling suture pulls out of the fascia or breaks in the early postoperative period. To prevent this, patients are advised to refrain from lifting for 4–6 weeks.

Urethral erosion with autologous fascial slings is exceedingly rare and in at least one of these cases the sling was inadvertently placed at the midurethra rather than at the bladder neck [10].

Wound problems, including wound seroma and infection, occur rarely but can be particularly problematic in the obese patient. Some patients may develop pain where the sling suture comes through the rectus. If this persists beyond 6 weeks, the sling suture can be removed under local through the prior abdominal incision.

Recurrent urinary tract infections do occur in the postoperative period and may be due to incomplete bladder emptying. Cystoscopy should be performed for persistent infections to insure that there is no sling or suture material in the bladder or urethra.

Conclusion

Ideally patients with SUI should be offered a choice of incontinence procedures and the choices should include a choice of sling material. To date the patient's own fascia is considered superior to cadaveric or xenograft tissue making it the best option for the patient who wishes to avoid a synthetic. There are also unique clinical situations where autologous tissue may offer an advantage to a synthetic sling including the need for tension on the sling and in cases where infection would be problematic.

References

1. Aldridge AH. Transplantation of fascia for relief of urinary stress incontinence. Am J Obstet Gynecol. 1942;44:398.
2. Millin T. Discussion on stress incontinence in micturition. Proc R Soc Med. 1947;40:361.
3. McGuire EJ, Lytton B. Pubovaginal sling procedures for stress incontinence. J Urol. 1978;119:82.
4. Leach GE, Dmochowski RR, Appell RA, et al. Female Stress Urinary Incontinence Clinical Guidelines Panel summary report on surgical management of female stress urinary incontinence. The American Urological Association. J Urol. 1997;158:875.
5. Petros PE, Ulmsten UI. An integral theory of female urinary incontinence. Experimental and clinical considerations. Acta Obstet Gynecol Scand Suppl. 1990;153:7–31.
6. Morgan TO, Westney OL, McGuire EJ. Pubovaginal sling: 4-year outcome analysis and quality of life assessment. J Urol. 2000;163:1845–8.
7. Dmochowski RR, Blaivas JM, Gormley EA, Juma S, Karram MM, Lightner DJ, Luber KM, Rovner ES, Staskin DR, Winters JC. Appell RA; Female Stress Urinary Incontinence Update Panel of the American Urological Association Education and Research, Inc. J Urol. 2010;183:1906–14.
8. Albo ME, Richter HE, Brubaker L, Norton P, Kraus SR, Zimmern PE, Chai TC, Zyczynski H, Diokno AC, Tennstedt S, Nager C, Lloyd LK, FitzGerald M, Lemack GE, Johnson HW, Leng W, Mallett V,

Stoddard AM, Menefee S, Varner RE, Kenton K, Moalli P, Sirls L, Dandreo KJ, Kusek JW, Nyberg LM, Steers W. Urinary Incontinence Treatment Network. Burch colposuspension versus fascial sling to reduce urinary stress incontinence. N Engl J Med. 2007;356:2143–55.
9. Brubaker L, Richter HE, Norton PA, Albo M, Zyczynski HM, Chai TC, Zimmern P, Kraus S, Sirls L, Kusek JW, Stoddard A, Tennstedt S, Gormley EA. Urinary incontinence treatment network. 5-Year continence rates, satisfaction and adverse events of Burch urethropexy and fascial sling surgery for urinary incontinence. J Urol. 2012;187(4):1324–30.
10. Handa VL, Stone A. Erosion of a fascial sling into the urethra. Urology. 1999;54:923.

Female Stress Urinary Incontinence Surgery Complications: Diagnosis, Evaluation, and Management

7

Eric S. Rovner and Alienor S. Gilchrist

Stress urinary incontinence (SUI) affects upwards of 40 % of American women [1]. Over the past several years, surgical treatment of SUI has evolved from mainly transvaginal needle suspensions, anterior vaginal wall plications, and retropubic suspensions to various types of slings, most commonly midurethral polypropylene slings. Sling surgeries for SUI can be classified by composition (autologous fascia, biologic or synthetic nonabsorbable materials), location of the sling (midurethral or beneath the bladder neck), and approach of placement (retropubic or transobturator). A full discussion of all the types of slings and sling complications is beyond the scope of this article but specific operations will be discussed where appropriate. The majority of the following discussion concerns midurethral slings via transobturator or retropubic approaches. Surgical treatment of SUI comprises some of the most commonly performed operations in the United States. Thus, it is important to understand how to avoid and, when necessary, diagnose and treat complications related to these surgeries.

Prevention of Complications

Although most complications are treatable and reversible, the optimal scenario is to prevent or minimize potential for adverse outcomes. This process begins in the preoperative period, initiated during the diagnostic evaluation and work-up. When determining the optimal surgical therapy for patients with urinary incontinence, many factors should be considered, including etiology and type of urinary incontinence and/or prolapse, bladder capacity, renal function, sexual function, medical comorbidities, or concurrent abdominal or pelvic pathology requiring surgical correction, prior abdominal and pelvic surgery, and finally, a patient's suitability for and willingness to accept the risks of surgery.

Standard preoperative evaluation of an individual with stress incontinence should include a focused history and physical, objective demonstration of SUI, an assessment of post-void residual urine volume and urinalysis and culture if warranted [2]. It is recommended that the incontinence be characterized and symptom impact and patient expectations be assessed. Additional studies may be indicated to evaluate the lower urinary tract, including pad tests and voiding diary, cystoscopy, and imaging. Furthermore, voiding function should be characterized, with noninvasive flow and post-void residual measurements, with invasive urodynamics reserved for patients with abnormal findings, mixed incontinence or

E.S. Rovner, M.D. (✉) • A.S. Gilchrist, M.D.
Department of Urology, Medical University of South Carolina, 96 Jonathan Lucas Street, CSB 644, Charleston, SC 29407, USA
e-mail: rovnere@musc.edu

G.H. Badlani (ed.), *Minimally Invasive Therapy for Urinary Incontinence and Pelvic Organ Prolapse*, Current Clinical Urology, DOI 10.1007/978-1-4939-0008-4_7,

history of neurologic abnormalities or dysfunctional voiding [2].

Reversible factors should be addressed. For those with postmenopausal, hypoestrogenic vaginal atrophy, topical estrogen replacement may reduce the incidence of postoperative vaginal wound dehiscence or extrusion of sling material. Urinary tract infection and genital tract infection (e.g., candidiasis) should likewise be treated prior to surgical intervention. Nutritional disorders should be assessed and corrected preoperatively prior to pursuing elective surgery, such as SUI surgery. Finally, any medical comorbidities that can be optimized (i.e., diabetic control, hypertension) should be pursued. For obese individuals, recent data suggests weight loss may be associated with improvement or resolution of SUI. In a recent large randomized trial, 52 % women with weight loss experienced 70 % improvement in frequency of stress incontinent episodes and 29 % of women had resolution of their SUI [3]. Weight loss may avoid surgery in this high risk group.

Choice of operative technique should be tailored to unique scenarios. For example, synthetic slings should be avoided in stress incontinent patients with the presence of intraoperative urethral injury, urethrovaginal fistula, or urethral diverticulum [2]. In the setting of concurrent prolapse, slings should be tensioned after prolapse repair is completed [2]. Cystoscopy should be performed intraoperatively in all patients undergoing sling surgery.

Complications occur for a variety of reasons. Petri et al. [4] looked at a series of 328 reinterventions following midurethral slings at four tertiary urogynecology centers in Europe. The indications for reoperation were varied and included obstruction, dysuria, and a host of others. The most common reason cited for failure of the previous operation was poor surgical technique, however, with the next most common reason being the wrong surgical indication. Both of these factors certainly can be addressed and minimized preoperatively. Operative experience with a given procedure has also been cited as an important factor contributing to the risk of operative complications. Kuuva and Nilsson [5] reviewed a nationwide database on midurethral slings and noted that operative complications varied inversely with surgical experience. As surgeons did more procedures, the incidence of complications declined dramatically. This supports the notion that surgeons who are relative novices at a given procedure are at risk for having more complications than their experienced colleagues.

Complications Related To SUI Surgery

Intraoperative Complications

Bleeding

Multiple blood vessels traverse the deep pelvis including large venous channels in the retropubic space. Named vessels in the obturator fossa along the pelvic sidewall including the iliac vessels and within the vascular pedicle of the bladder are at risk for injury especially during vaginal incontinence surgery due to lack of direct visualization of these structures during passage of trocars or needles. Major vascular injury can quickly lead to life-threatening hemorrhage if not recognized intraoperatively and may result in large retropubic hematomas postoperatively [6, 7]. In a series of over 5,000 midurethral slings, bleeding problems were seen in 2.7 % of cases [8]. Only 0.8 % of patients required intervention for bleeding; the vast majority of cases were managed conservatively without operative intervention. Less than 1 % of patients required transfusions. There were no deaths reported in this series as a result of bleeding. In a multicenter randomized controlled trial of 597 women undergoing retropubic versus transobturator sling for stress incontinence, the incidence of bleeding requiring blood transfusion was 6 % vs. 2.3 %, respectively [9].

The risk of bleeding during surgery can be minimized but not entirely eliminated by good operative technique. Bleeding during an open retropubic dissection, such as during Burch colposuspension, is usually easily visualized and controlled with a combination of cautery, suture ligature, and direct compression, if necessary.

In contrast to bleeding during retropubic surgery, bleeding during transvaginal surgery can be more problematic at times and more difficult to control. The initial dissection of the vaginal wall from the underlying fascia should be associated with minimal bleeding. Bleeding encountered during this early dissection may indicate an excessively deep and incorrect surgical plane within the wall of the bladder or urethra. In this circumstance, immediate recognition and reevaluation is necessary to avoid inadvertent entry into the urinary tract and to minimize bleeding. Following identification of this situation, dissection should proceed in the proper surgical plane; in reoperative surgery, however, this plane may be difficult to identify.

Another common site of bleeding during transvaginal anti-incontinence surgery occurs when traversing the endopelvic fascia from the vaginal side as during a retropubic urethrolysis. Entry into the retropubic space from the transvaginal side or placement of the suprapubic needles or trocars from the abdominal side may be associated with copious bleeding as the endopelvic fascia is perforated. If the bleeding is brisk, the vagina can be packed. It can be very helpful to manually elevate the anterior vaginal wall and compress it anteriorly directly against the posterior symphysis pubis for several minutes using the surgeon's hand, sponge stick, or a retractor. These maneuvers will effectively tamponade bleeding in the retropubic space. Packing and compression will result in adequate control in the majority of cases; if not, the surgeon should expeditiously complete the procedure, close the incisions, and pack the vagina [10]. Occasionally, in addition to vaginal packing, a Foley catheter placed per urethra with the balloon overinflated and then placed on traction will add additional security. Brisk bleeding that does not respond to manual compression for an extended period of time may suggest a major vessel injury and mandates further evaluation.

Urinary Tract Injury

During surgery, the urethra, bladder, or much more rarely the ureters may be injured. Although rare, major complications from slings remain under-reported in the literature [11]. The key to the management of each of these injuries is immediate recognition and repair. Long-term sequelae resulting from unrecognized urinary tract injury can be devastating to the patient, with potentially substantial medicolegal implications for the physician.

Urethra

From the transvaginal side, injury to the urethra may occur during initial dissection of the vaginal wall off the underlying fascia. Excessively deep dissection, especially in reoperative surgery, risks urethral injury. This is usually although not invariably heralded by an unexpected amount of bleeding. Placement of a urethral catheter prior to incision will help to identify the urethra intraoperatively, and in the case of urethral injury will allow immediate recognition as the catheter may become visible in the operative field. If a urethral injury is suspected, urethroscopy may be performed. The urethra should be repaired immediately and primarily in two layers using absorbable sutures in a watertight fashion. The urethra can be repaired over a 14F or larger catheter. It is not necessary to leave a drain other than the urethral catheter. Failure to recognize the injury or failure to repair it properly risks urethrovaginal fistula, erosion of sling material into the urethral lumen postoperatively (especially synthetic sling material), infection, and a multitude of other potential problems [12]. The urethra may also be perforated with trocar passage during midurethral sling procedures. This is reported in less than 1 % patients [12]. Countertraction during the initial dissection, maintaining good exposure, and a working knowledge of the anatomy are helpful in avoiding urethral injury.

In the event of a planned synthetic sling in the setting of a concomitant urethral injury, it is advisable to repair the urethra and abort the sling procedure until the urethra is completely healed [2]. An autologous sling may be considered a safer alternative than a synthetic sling at the time of a urethral injury as an anti-incontinence procedure, but insufficient data supports this notion [2].

The urethra is rarely injured during retropubic surgery as the middle and distal thirds are protected by the symphysis pubis.

Bladder

Intraoperative bladder injury may occur during transabdominal as well as transvaginal surgery. The potential for urinary tract injury varies considerably with the experience of the surgeon as well as operative approach [13]. Two recent large multicenter randomized controlled trials comparing retropubic versus transobturator midurethral slings demonstrated higher rates of bladder injury in the retropubic approach [9, 14]. In the Urinary Incontinence Treatment Network (UITN) trial of midurethral slings, Richter et al. reported a 5 % bladder perforation rate in the retropubic cohort but no perforations in the transobturator cohort [9]. Similarly, Barber et al. reported an 8 % rate of intraoperative bladder perforation in the retropubic midurethral sling approach, compared with 0 % in the transobturator approach [14]. The Cochrane review of midurethral slings analyzed 18 trials comparing retropubic versus transobturator approaches and found bladder perforation occurred significantly less frequently via the transobturator approach, 0.3 % vs. 5.5 % (RR 0.14, 95 % CI 0.07 to 0.26) [15].

Although the type of approach (transobturator vs. retropubic) seems to impact the risk of bladder injury [16], several recent papers have suggested that surgical inexperience is a risk factor for such injury as well [13, 17]. Upon reviewing 1,136 consecutive women who underwent a midurethral sling procedure (retropubic in 874 and transobturator in 262), Stav et al. reported 32 bladder perforations, with 94 % of these perforations occurring at the hands of inexperienced surgeons (defined as having performed fewer than 50 sling surgeries) [13]. Multivariate analysis revealed other significant independent risk factors for bladder perforation included the presence of rectocele (OR 6.2), local anesthesia (OR 5.9), body mass index less than 30 kg/m^2 (OR 5.6), previous Cesarean section (OR 3.7), and previous colposuspension (OR 3.2) [13]. McLennan et al. [17] reported that the risk of bladder perforation in a resident training program varied inversely with the number of cases done by the trainee. Redo surgery is almost certainly associated with a higher risk of urinary tract injury in patients undergoing midurethral sling surgery. Jeffry et al. [16] reported a bladder perforation rate during TVT of 71.4 % vs. 7.6 % in patients with prior surgery vs. those without. Likewise, in patients undergoing SPARC, Deval et al. [18] reported a 36.6 % vs. 7.5 % urinary tract injury rate in those with a history of prior surgery versus those without it.

Injury to the bladder during midurethral sling procedures is diagnosed intraoperatively by careful endoscopic examination of the bladder and bladder neck with a 70° lens following passage of the trocars. The bladder should be distended and then examined to ensure that a small injury does not go unrecognized in a fold of the bladder wall. To avoid injury during trocar needle passage, the urethra should be clearly palpated, the bladder drained prior to trocar passage, and the pelvic anatomy well delineated. If a bladder injury is noted intraoperatively, the trocar should be removed and reinserted. Bladder injury from a trocar usually does not require primary closure. Postoperative drainage of the bladder with a Foley catheter, however, is desirable to avoid urinoma, fistula formation, and pelvic abscess, though the optimal duration of catheter drainage in this setting is not well defined.

Ureter

In the era of midurethral slings, ureteric injury should be extraordinarily rare. Virtually all ureteric injuries can be identified by intraoperative cystoscopy. The administration of intravenous dyes such as indigo carmine permits obvious visualization of ureteral efflux confirming ureteral patency. Suspected ureteral injuries are confirmed by retrograde pyeloureterography. Ureteral obstruction from suture placement may be treated by removal of the offending suture and placement of a temporary indwelling ureteral stent. Ureteral transection requires ureteroneocystostomy.

Vagina

Perforation of the vaginal epithelium can occur during vaginal wall dissection or trocar passage for midurethral slings. Perforations from trocar passage, when unrecognized intraoperatively, will result in sling exposure in the vaginal cavity. This complication is often misclassified postoperatively as extrusion of the synthetic sling.

In the UITN trial of midurethral slings (TOMUS), Richter et al. reported a 4.3 % rate of vaginal epithelial perforations in the transobturator group compared with 2.0 % rate in the retropubic sling group [9]. Perforation from the trocar is identified intraoperatively by thorough visual inspection and palpation of the lateral fornices of the vagina following trocar passage. If perforation occurs, the trocar should be removed and repassed. The perforation may be oversewn with absorbable suture and does not preclude placement of a synthetic sling.

Bowel Injury

There exist multiple reports of bowel injury during urinary incontinence surgery [19–21]. Fortunately, this is a rare complication. Bowel injury may occur during entry into the retropubic space during an autologous pubovaginal sling or urethrolysis, or during passage of needle passers or trocars during midurethral slings. These can be devastating complications leading to sepsis, abscess, and even death [19]. Unfortunately, most of these injuries are not recognized until the postoperative period leading to considerable morbidity. Initial signs and symptoms heralding a bowel injury may be subtle including low-grade fever, abdominal pain, and ileus. If suspected, a diagnostic evaluation including plain and upright abdominal radiographs evaluating for the presence of intra-abdominal free air and cross-sectional imaging should be pursued expeditiously. Laparotomy, repair of the bowel injury, and possibly bowel resection are necessary for definitive treatment. In some cases, temporary proximal bowel diversion may be necessary.

Postoperative Complications

Voiding Dysfunction and Urinary Retention

Bladder outlet obstruction (BOO) following SUI may present as prolonged complete urinary retention, persistently elevated post-void residual urine volume, recurrent urinary tract infections, or as variably bothersome and poorly categorized lower urinary tract symptoms including combinations of obstructive symptoms and urinary urgency or urge incontinence. These last two groups are difficult to identify and are often not recognized as BOO by many authors. Unfortunately, development of postoperative voiding dysfunction can be unpredictable. Lemack et al. demonstrated that preoperative urodynamic parameters were unable to predict development of postoperative voiding dysfunction or risk for surgical revision in women undergoing pubovaginal sling [22].

The incidence of postoperative voiding difficulties across different sling approaches is variable and is difficult to compare. De novo urge incontinence rates at 12–23 months following autologous fascial sling is 6–13 % compared with 3–10 % with midurethral slings [2]. Historically, the incidence of postoperative retention lasting longer than 4 weeks or requiring intervention occurs in 2–8 % of patients undergoing autologous fascial slings, 5–15 % of patients undergoing synthetic slings at the bladder neck, and 2–4 % of those following midurethral slings [2]. The incidence of voiding dysfunction, including urinary retention and de novo urgency and urge incontinence, following midurethral slings ranges from approximately 3 to 21 % [9, 23–28]. Surgical intervention for voiding dysfunction and urinary retention has been reported in 0 to 4 % of patients undergoing midurethral slings [9, 24–27]. Short-term voiding difficulties and postoperative urgency following autologous pubovaginal sling appear more likely than following Burch [29]. The minimally invasive midurethral sling procedures are mechanistically tension-free and as such it is not surprising that they likely result in an overall lower incidence of postoperative voiding dysfunction than other types of open SUI procedures. When comparing the incidence of postoperative voiding dysfunction by midurethral sling approach, specifically transobturator vs. retropubic, the Cochrane review meta-analysis found no difference across 24 trials [15]. In 197 patients who underwent midurethral sling revision for voiding dysfunction, preexisting obstructive voiding symptoms, retropubic sling type, and concurrent surgery at the time of sling placement were found to be risk factors for sling revision [30].

In many individuals with lower urinary tract symptoms postoperatively who are not in frank urinary retention, the diagnosis of BOO is extremely difficult. Urodynamics, especially videourodynamics are often pursued diagnostically but may not be helpful in many cases as the classic "high pressure-low flow" pattern may not be present. Furthermore, there are no pressure-flow urodynamic criteria that accurately predict for successful voiding following urethrolysis. Various nomograms [31–33] have been developed for the diagnosis of female BOO but none are absolutely accepted as the gold standard. For patients not in frank urinary retention, the diagnosis of BOO is strongly suggested by postoperative onset of irritative voiding symptoms, recurrent urinary tract infections, and a poor urinary stream. Physical examination may be completely normal or suggest an oversuspended midvaginal segment or the lack of mobility of the urethra following insertion of a metal sound. A swan neck deformity may be seen during valsalva maneuver in some individuals. De novo prolapse should be excluded as a cause of postoperative BOO.

The timing of intervention associated with iatrogenic BOO is controversial. Indeed, most patients with transient postoperative urinary retention resume normal voiding following midurethral slings within 1–2 days of the procedure. Some patients may be delayed for 1–2 weeks, however, and those with a history of prior SUI surgery or those undergoing concomitant prolapse repair may be further delayed [34]. Some authors have recommended conservative therapy for postoperative voiding dysfunction for up to 3 months prior to attempting surgical revision [35]. However, a prolonged time to intervention for BOO may be associated with long-term, potentially irreversible bladder dysfunction, even following successful urethrolysis [36]. Compared with obstructive symptoms such as hesitancy, straining, and poor force of stream, overactive bladder symptoms caused by iatrogenically induced BOO following anti-incontinence surgery are less likely to improve despite a technically successful operation. In one series, voiding symptoms resolved in 82 % of obstructed patients following urethrolysis while OAB (storage) symptoms resolved in only 35 % [37]. In this series, increased time to intervention was not correlated with persistent detrusor dysfunction.

Once the diagnosis of BOO is considered or established, options include long-term intermittent urethral catheterization with or without antimuscarinic medication to reduce irritative symptoms, alpha-blocker pharmacotherapy (for which there is little or no evidence of efficacy in the setting of iatrogenic female BOO), and transvaginal incision of the sling. Anecdotal reports and small case series have suggested that urethral over dilation or re-exploration and "stretching" of the midurethral sling may have benefit for selected patients. Nevertheless, there is reasonable evidence that transvaginal incision of autologous pubovaginal slings as well midurethral slings is often highly successful in improving voiding dynamics [38–40]. This can be performed as short as one week from surgery, although there exists considerable variability among authors with respect to optimal timing of intervention. South et al. describe greater improvement in lower urinary tract symptoms when midline sling lysis is performed within one year after pubovaginal or midurethral sling [41]. The incision can be done under local anesthesia in some cases. Following isolation and division of the sling (Fig. 7.1), the edges of the cut sling often separate by 1–2 cm, indicating a satisfactory result. Iatrogenic obstruction due to autologous fascial slings is often treated in this manner as well [39].

For patients who fail transvaginal incision, a urethrolysis may be performed [42, 43]. Via a transvaginal or retropubic approach [42, 44, 45],

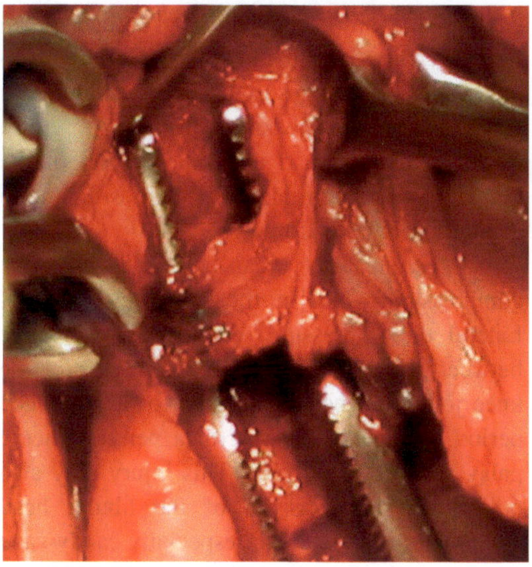

Fig. 7.1 Intraoperative isolation of obstructing midurethral sling

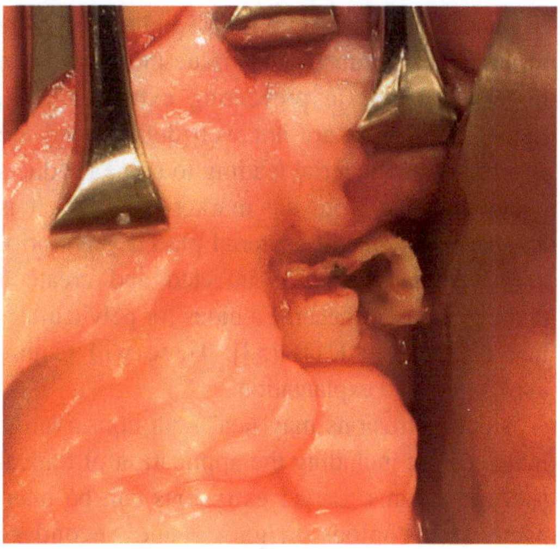

Fig. 7.2 Extruded multifilament sling

the retropubic space is entered and the urethra is sharply dissected off the posterior surface of the symphysis pubis and freed from the surrounding scar. The limbs of the sling or other retropubic attachments are isolated and divided in the retropubic space. Lateral attachments to the pelvic sidewall are incised as needed. A transvaginal, suprameatal approach to urethrolysis has also been described and may be particularly applicable when the anterior urethral surface is fixed to the symphysis, such as that following an MMK procedure. Recurrence of SUI symptoms following urethrolysis or sling incision may occur in 9–20 % of patients [39, 41]. Patients should be counseled regarding this possibility preoperatively as some may wish to continue on intermittent catheterization or other conservative therapy rather than risk recurrent SUI.

Vaginal Extrusion and Urinary Tract Erosion

Vaginal extrusion refers to finding exposed sling material in the vaginal canal postoperatively; erosion, however, suggests finding material within the lumen of the urinary tract at some time interval postoperatively that was clearly documented as not being within the urinary tract at the time of surgery. Reported rates of mesh extrusion and erosion range from 0 to 2 % [46].

Extrusion of material may be related to surgical technique, infection, or the physical properties of the implanted material. The extruded material may be located in the midline at the incision line or at the anterolateral vaginal wall. Midline extrusions imply wound dehiscence. Lateral extrusions may be caused by an unrecognized vaginal wall perforation or injury at time of sling placement.

Usually symptomatic, patient complaints suggesting an extrusion include a malodorous vaginal discharge, vaginal spotting, vaginal pain, and dyspareunia. Patients may present several days to months postoperatively. On physical examination the extruded material is often visible (Fig. 7.2), but physical findings may also be quite subtle [47]. Granulation tissue suggests the presence of an extrusion. Extruded synthetic mesh is often palpable within the vagina, although patient discomfort may preclude a complete examination.

Factors responsible for extrusion include the physical nature of the implanted material, quality of the vaginal tissues of the host, sling tension, wound healing, and infection [48]. It appears that multifilament materials are at greater risk for extrusion than monofilaments [49]. In addition, the pore size of the implanted sling material that is large enough to permit fibroblast and macrophage infiltration and subsequent tissue ingrowth is an important factor in preventing extrusion [50]. Some risk factors are not well defined and are specific to the material leading to some products being removed from the market [51, 52]. It is notable that synthetic material placed years prior may eventually become infected and create a draining sinus, or become a nidus for pelvic infection or recurrent UTIs [53]. These will require exploration and explantation.

Small extrusions may heal with conservative management including the application of topical estrogen creams. Larger extrusions can be managed with copious irrigation and secondary closure in the operating room. Some patients with large extrusions may benefit from excision and removal of the extruded segment of the sling.

Urinary tract erosion may occur with synthetic, biologic, or autologous materials [54]. This is a devastating complication that, unlike extrusion, is almost always managed operatively. Whether urinary tract erosion occurs as a result of a "missed" urinary viscus perforation at the time of surgery, or occurs as a result of migration of the material into the urinary tract sometime following surgery, is unclear. Patients may complain of irritative lower urinary tract symptoms, recurrent UTIs, hematuria, and dysuria, as well as pelvic pain. The definitive diagnosis is usually made endoscopically. For intravesical erosions, endoscopic scissor or laser transection of the intravesical portion of the eroded sling may permit the remaining sling material to retract outside the urinary tract [55]. If this fails or is technically not feasible, then open operative exploration, removal of the eroded material, closure of the urinary tract, and postoperative drainage will be necessary.

Nerve Injury

Several nerves traverse through the deep pelvis as well as superficially within the lower abdominal soft tissues. These nerves are at risk for injury during female incontinence surgery. Stretch or compression injury to the femoral nerve can occur as a result of positioning. Femoral nerve compression may occur at the level of the inguinal ligament caused by flexion of the hip joint, resulting in sensory changes to the anterior thigh or in more severe cases weakness of hip flexion [56]. Severe abduction and external rotation of the thigh should be minimized during positioning to avoid this complication.

The peroneal nerve can be injured by direct compression while in the lithotomy position. Lateral direct pressure on the peroneal nerve between the stirrup at the lateral aspect of the knee joint and the fibular head for a prolonged period of time may result in a peroneal nerve palsy and foot drop [56]. This injury may also occur with compression of the fibular head against the stirrup holder, especially candy-cane stirrups as the leg rotates externally after placement in the holders. The pudendal, ilioinguinal, and iliohypogastric nerves may be injured by suprapubic trocar placement or dissection resulting in pain in the suprapubic region [57, 58].

Bone Anchor-Related Complications

With the advent of minimally invasive midurethral slings, the use of bone anchors (BA) has declined; however, there are numerous reports of bone anchor-related complications, including osteitis pubis and osteomyelitis of the symphysis pubis [59–64]. Once diagnosed, osteomyelitis related to BAs requires operative exploration and removal of the bone anchor. BAs are often seated below the cortical bone, which mandates partial resection of the overlying bone, usually with fluoroscopic guidance, to locate and remove the BA.

Sexual Dysfunction

Historically, female sexual dysfunction following surgery for SUI has only infrequently been reported. Whether this is due to a generalized lack of understanding of the condition, lack of interest in reporting or investigating its occurrence, or whether it is due to an actual low incidence is unclear. Only recently has there been a trend to query female patients regarding sexual

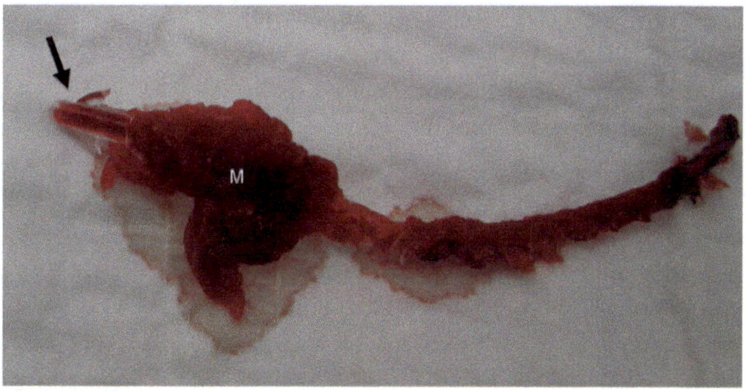

Fig. 7.3 Single incision sling removed from obturator muscle for obstruction and refractory groin pain (*arrow* indicates tissue anchor, *M* indicates obturator muscle)

dysfunction and to date only a few instruments exist [65].

Female sexual dysfunction is a complex and poorly understood phenomenon [66–68]. A full discussion is beyond the scope of this paper. Coital incontinence can be improved following successful sling surgery and sexual function score is likewise improved [69]; however, new onset sexual dysfunction following surgery unrelated to vaginal sling erosion has been reported in up to 20 % of individuals in some series [70, 71]. Shah et al. [72] reported no difference in female sexual function following distal urethral sling surgery. Brubaker et al. found that 2 years after pubovaginal sling surgery for SUI, patients reported improved sexual function with fewer incontinence episodes, less restriction of sexual activity as a result of fear of incontinence and no changes in rates of dyspareunia from baseline [69].

Dyspareunia is only one form of sexual dysfunction but it may occur following anti-incontinence surgery as vaginal anatomy is altered by these types of surgery. The vaginal axis can be shifted changing the angulation of the vaginal canal and narrowing of the vagina may occur as a result of aberrant scarring. Dissection along the anterior vaginal wall may result in nerve injury and neuroma formation. Band-like formation from the sling can also occur and may be palpable by the patient or partner. Ross et al. found that 52 of 85 women had a palpable sling on exam one year after TOT midurethral sling compared with only 15 out of 90 in the TVT group; however, only 11 and 9 subjects experienced tenderness with palpation, respectively [24]. De novo dyspareunia secondary to anterior vaginal wall banding in the paraurethral folds immediately adjacent to the midurethral sling was reported in 16 % of patients undergoing TOT but was absent in patients undergoing a retropubic midurethral sling approach [73].

Other poorly defined and poorly understood factors contributing to postoperative sexual dysfunction may exist. For example, in some series 4–5 % of patients following TVT or intravaginal slingplasty procedure experienced decreased libido [49, 70]. The reason for this decreased libido is unclear.

Postoperative dyspareunia should be assessed by a thorough physical examination. When vaginal scarring, banding, or narrowing, and especially sling extrusion have been excluded, other causes for new onset sexual dysfunction should be explored and treated [74].

Other Postoperative Complications

Refractory thigh or groin pain has been described following midurethral slings and may ultimately require surgical excision of the sling [75] (Fig. 7.3). Significantly higher rates of groin pain have been reported in the transobturator approach (12 %) compared with the retropubic approach (1.7 %) (RR 6, 95 % CI 3–11) in a recent Cochrane meta-analysis [15]. A recent study showing high initial incidence of postoperative thigh pain following transobturator tapes demonstrated almost complete resolution of pain after 6 months [76]. In a series of 32 patients undergoing sling removal for chronic pelvic and perineal pain, TVTs were removed via laparoscopic approach and TOTs with a combination of transvaginal and upper thigh incision, with 68 % of patients reporting improvement in pain and 22 % developing recurrent incontinence [77].

Rates of postoperative surgical site infection have generally remained low, between 1 and 15 % [9, 14] since monofilament mesh has largely supplanted multifilament mesh. However, thigh and pelvic abscesses have been reported with midurethral slings and require excision of the infected mesh in addition to debridement [14, 78].

Incisional hernia at the rectus fascia harvest site has been described in a patient undergoing autologous fascial sling [79]. Care must be taken during the harvest to avoid neurovascular injuries and prevent postoperative hernia formation during fascial closure.

Urinary fistula following anti-incontinence surgery is quite rare [80] yet an unrecognized and unrepaired intraoperative injury to the ureter, bladder, or urethra may result in ureterovaginal, vesicovaginal, or urethrovaginal fistula. Intraoperative recognition of the injury is critical to prevent fistula formation and thus the importance of a careful intraoperative endoscopic examination and confirmation of urinary tract patency cannot be overemphasized. Synthetic slings should be excised at the time of fistula repair and avoided when treating concomitant SUI, with options including autologous fascia slings and biological slings [2].

Conclusions

Surgery for SUI can be associated with numerous complications. Prevention of complications is paramount. SUI surgery repair is almost always elective and therefore careful attention to optimizing the patient preoperatively is paramount. Proper preoperative diagnosis and assessment will permit operative intervention only when indicated and appropriate. The spectrum of complications is changing as different approaches and newer synthetic materials are integrated into surgical repair. Rapid recognition, evaluation, and intervention are necessary to assure satisfactory resolution.

References

1. Norton P, Brubaker L. Urinary incontinence in women. Lancet. 2006;367(9504):57–67.
2. Dmochowski RR, Blaivas JM, Gormley EA, et al. Update of AUA guideline on the surgical management of female stress urinary incontinence. J Urol. 2010;183(5):1906–14.
3. Subak LL, Wing R, West DS, et al. Weight loss to treat urinary incontinence in overweight and obese women. N Engl J Med. 2009;360(5):481–90.
4. Petri E, Niemeyer R, Martan A, Tunn R, Naumann G, Koelbl H. Reasons for and treatment of surgical complications with alloplastic slings. Int Urogynecol J. 2006;17(1):3–13.
5. Kuuva N, Nilsson CG. A nationwide analysis of complications associated with the tension-free vaginal tape (TVT) procedure. Acta Obstet Gynecol Scand. 2002;81(1):72–7.
6. Rajan S, Kohli N. Retropubic hematoma after transobturator sling procedure. Obstet Gynecol. 2005;106(5 Pt 2):1199–202.
7. Walters MD, Tulikangas PK, LaSala C, Muir TW. Vascular injury during tension-free vaginal tape procedure for stress urinary incontinence. Obstet Gynecol. 2001;98(5 Pt 2):957–9.
8. Kolle D, Tamussino K, Hanzal E, et al. Bleeding complications with the tension-free vaginal tape operation. Am J Obstet Gynecol. 2005;193(6):2045–9.
9. Richter HE, Albo ME, Zyczynski HM, et al. Retropubic versus transobturator midurethral slings for stress incontinence. N Engl J Med. 2010;362(22):2066–76.
10. Ficazzola M, Nitti VW. Complications of incontinence procedures in women. In: Taneja S, Smith RB, Ehrlich RM, editors. Complications of urologic surgery. Philadelphia: Saunders; 2003. p. 482–98.
11. Deng DY, Rutman M, Raz S, Rodriguez LV. Presentation and management of major complications of midurethral slings: Are complications underreported? Neurourol Urodyn. 2007;26(1):46–52.
12. Morton HC, Hilton P. Urethral injury associated with minimally invasive mid-urethral sling procedures for the treatment of stress urinary incontinence: a case series and systematic literature search. BJOG. 2009;116(8):1120–6.
13. Stav K, Dwyer PL, Rosamilia A, Schierlitz L, Lim YN, Lee J. Risk factors for trocar injury to the bladder during mid urethral sling procedures. J Urol. 2009;182(1):174–9.
14. Barber MD, Kleeman S, Karram MM, et al. Transobturator tape compared with tension-free vaginal tape for the treatment of stress urinary incontinence: a randomized controlled trial. Obstet Gynecol. 2008;111(3):611–21.
15. Ogah J, Cody JD, Rogerson L. Minimally invasive synthetic suburethral sling operations for stress urinary incontinence in women. Cochrane Database Syst Rev. 2009;4, CD006375.

16. Jeffry L, Deval B, Birsan A, Soriano D, Darai E. Objective and subjective cure rates after tension-free vaginal tape for treatment of urinary incontinence. Urology. 2001;58(5):702–6.
17. McLennan MT, Melick CF. Bladder perforation during tension-free vaginal tape procedures: analysis of learning curve and risk factors. Obstet Gynecol. 2005;106(5 Pt 1):1000–4.
18. Deval B, Levardon M, Samain E, et al. A French multicenter clinical trial of SPARC for stress urinary incontinence. Eur Urol. 2003;44(2):254–8. discussion 258-259.
19. US Food and Drug Adminsitration: Manufacturer and User Facility Device Experience (MAUDE) Database. http://www.fda.gov/cdrh/maude.html. Accessed Jan 2011
20. Kobashi KC, Govier FE. Perioperative complications: the first 140 polypropylene pubovaginal slings. J Urol. 2003;170:1918–21.
21. Rooney KE, Cholhan HJ. Bowel perforation during retropubic sling procedure. Obstet Gynecol. 2010;115(2 Pt 2):429–31.
22. Lemack GE, Krauss S, Litman H, et al. Normal preoperative urodynamic testing does not predict voiding dysfunction after Burch colposuspension versus pubovaginal sling. J Urol. 2008;180(5):2076–80.
23. Rechberger T, Futyma K, Jankiewicz K, Adamiak A, Skorupski P. The clinical effectiveness of retropubic (IVS-02) and transobturator (IVS-04) midurethral slings: randomized trial. Eur Urol. 2009;56(1):24–30.
24. Ross S, Robert M, Swaby C, et al. Transobturator tape compared with tension-free vaginal tape for stress incontinence: a randomized controlled trial. Obstet Gynecol. 2009;114(6):1287–94.
25. Song PH, Kim YD, Kim HT, et al. The 7-year outcome of the tension-free vaginal tape procedure for treating female stress urinary incontinence. BJU Int. 2009;104(8):1113–7.
26. Ward KL, Hilton P, UK and Ireland TVT Trial Group. Tension-free vaginal tape versus colposuspension for primary urodynamic stress incontinence: 5-year follow up. BJOG. 2008;115(2):226–33.
27. Nazemi TM, Yamada B, Govier FE, Kuznetsov DD, Kodama K, Kobashi KC. Minimum 24-month followup of the sling for the treatment of stress urinary incontinence. J Urol. 2008;179(2):596–9.
28. Olsson I, Abrahamsson AK, Kroon UB. Long-term efficacy of the tension-free vaginal tape procedure for the treatment of urinary incontinence: a retrospective follow-up 11.5 years post-operatively. Int Urogynecol J. 2010;21(6):679–83.
29. Albo ME, Richter HE, Brubaker L, et al. Burch colposuspension versus fascial sling to reduce urinary stress incontinence. N Engl J Med. 2007;356(21): 2143–55.
30. Molden S, Patterson D, Tarr M, et al. Risk factors leading to midurethral sling revision: a multicenter case-control study. Int Urogynecol J. 2010;21(10):1253–9.
31. Chassagne S, Bernier PA, Haab F, Roehrborn CG, Reisch JS, Zimmern PE. Proposed cutoff values to define bladder outlet obstruction in women. Urology. 1998;51(3):408–11.
32. Blaivas JG, Groutz A. Bladder outlet obstruction nomogram for women with lower urinary tract symptomatology. Neurourol Urodyn. 2000;19(5):553–64.
33. Defreitas GA, Zimmern PE, Lemack GE, Shariat SF. Refining diagnosis of anatomic female bladder outlet obstruction: comparison of pressure-flow study parameters in clinically obstructed women with those of normal controls. Urology. 2004;64(4):675–9. discussion 679-681.
34. Mutone N, Brizendine E, Hale D. Factors that influence voiding function after the tension-free vaginal tape procedure for stress urinary incontinence. Am J Obstet Gynecol. 2003;188(6):1477–81. discussion 1481-1473.
35. Mishra VC, Mishra N, Karim OM, Motiwala HG. Voiding dysfunction after tension-free vaginal tape: a conservative approach is often successful. Int Urogynecol J. 2005;16(3):210–4. discussion 214.
36. Leng WW, Davies BJ, Tarin T, Sweeney DD, Chancellor MB. Delayed treatment of bladder outlet obstruction after sling surgery: association with irreversible bladder dysfunction. J Urol. 2004;172(4 Pt 1):1379–81.
37. Starkman JS, Duffy 3rd JW, Wolter CE, Kaufman MR, Scarpero HM, Dmochowski RR. The evolution of obstruction induced overactive bladder symptoms following urethrolysis for female bladder outlet obstruction. J Urol. 2008;179(3):1018–23.
38. Goldman H. Simple sling incision for the treatment of iatrogenic urethral obstruction. Urology. 2003; 62:714–8.
39. Nitti VW, Carlson KV, Blaivas JG, Dmochowski RR. Early results of pubovaginal sling lysis by midline sling incision. Urology. 2002;59(1):47–51. discussion 51-42.
40. Klutke C, Siegel S, Carlin B, Paszkiewicz E, Kirkemo A, Klutke J. Urinary retention after tension-free vaginal tape procedure: incidence and treatment. Urology. 2001;58(5):697–701.
41. South MM, Wu JM, Webster GD, Weidner AC, Roelands JJ, Amundsen CL. Early vs late midline sling lysis results in greater improvement in lower urinary tract symptoms. Am J Obstet Gynecol. 2009;200(5):564.e561–5.
42. Carr LK, Webster GD. Voiding dysfunction following incontinence surgery: diagnosis and treatment with retropubic or vaginal urethrolysis. J Urol. 1997; 157(3):821–3.
43. Romanzi LJ, Blaivas JG. Protracted urinary retention necessitating urethrolysis following tension-free vaginal tape surgery. J Urol. 2000;164(6):2022–3.
44. Anger JT, Amundsen CL, Webster GD. Obstruction after Burch colposuspension: a return to retropubic urethrolysis. Int Urogynecol J. 2006;17(5):455–9.
45. Petrou SP, Brown JA, Blaivas JG. Suprameatal transvaginal urethrolysis. J Urol. 1999;161(4):1268–71.
46. Daneshgari F, Kong W, Swartz M. Complications of mid urethral slings: important outcomes for future clinical trials. J Urol. 2008;180(5):1890–7.

47. Sweat SD, Itano NB, Clemens JQ, et al. Polypropylene mesh tape for stress urinary incontinence: complications of urethral erosion and outlet obstruction. J Urol. 2002;168(1):144–6.
48. Deval B, Haab F. Management of the complications of the synthetic slings. Curr Opin Urol. 2006;16(4): 240–3.
49. Glavind K, Sander P. Erosion, defective healing and extrusion after tension-free urethropexy for the treatment of stress urinary incontinence. Int Urogynecol J. 2004;15(3):179–82.
50. Amrute KV, Badlani GH. Female incontinence: a review of biomaterials and minimally invasive techniques. Curr Opin Urol. 2006;16(2):54–9.
51. Siegel A. Vaginal mesh extrusion associated with use of Mentor transobturator sling. Urology. 2005;66:995–9.
52. Yamada BS, Govier FE, Stefanovic KB, Kobashi KC. High rate of vaginal erosions associated with the mentor ObTape. J Urol. 2006;176(2):651–4. discussion 654.
53. Smith A, Rovner E. Long-term chronic complications from Stamey endoscopic bladder neck suspension: a case series. Int Urogynecol J. 2006;17(3):290–4.
54. Amundsen CL, Flynn BJ, Webster GD. Urethral erosion after synthetic and nonsynthetic pubovaginal slings: differences in management and continence outcome. J Urol. 2003;170(1):134–7. discussion 137.
55. Frenkl TL, Rackley RR, Vasavada SP, Goldman HB. Management of iatrogenic foreign bodies of the bladder and urethra following pelvic floor surgery. Neurourol Urodyn. 2008;27(6):491–5.
56. Schaffer B. Pearls and perils of patient positioning. AUA Update Series. 1995;14(178–183).
57. Fisher H, Lotze, PM. Nerve injury locations during retropubic sling procedures. Int Urogynecol J Pelvic Floor Dysfunction. 2011;22(4):439–441.
58. Boyles SH, Edwards R, Gregory W, Clark A. Complications associated with transobturator sling procedures. Int Urogynecol J. 2007;18(1):19–22.
59. FitzGerald MP, Gitelis S, Brubaker L. Pubic osteomyelitis and granuloma after bone anchor placement. Int Urogynecol J. 1999;10(5):346–8.
60. Franks ME, Lavelle JP, Yokoyama T, Chuang YC, Chancellor MB. Metastatic osteomyelitis after pubovaginal sling using bone anchors. Urology. 2000;56(2):330–1.
61. Rackley RR, Abdelmalak JB, Madjar S, Yanilmaz A, Appell RA, Tchetgen MB. Bone anchor infections in female pelvic reconstructive procedures: a literature review of series and case reports. J Urol. 2001;165(6 Pt 1):1975–8.
62. Enzler M, Agins HJ, Kogan M, et al. Osteomyelitis of the pubis following suspension of the neck of the bladder with use of bone anchors. A report of four cases. J Bone Joint Surg. 1999;81(12):1736–40.
63. Graham CW, Dmochowski RR, Faerber GJ, Clemens JQ, Westney OL. Pubic osteomyelitis following bladder neck surgery using bone anchors: a report of 9 cases. J Urol. 2002;168(5):2055–7; discussion 2057-2058.
64. Stember DS, Scarpero HM, Nitti VW. Vaginal granulation tissue secondary to bone anchors: experience in two patients. J Urol. 2003;169(6):2300–1.
65. Jones LR. The use of validated questionnaires to assess female sexual dysfunction. World J Urol. 2002;20(2):89–92.
66. Bancroft J. The medicalization of female sexual dysfunction: the need for caution. Arch Sex Behav. 2002;31(5):451–5.
67. Berman JR, Goldstein I. Female sexual dysfunction. Urol Clin North Am. 2001;28(2):405–16.
68. Moynihan R. The making of a disease: female sexual dysfunction. BMJ. 2003;326(7379):45–7.
69. Brubaker L, Chiang S, Zyczynski H, et al. The impact of stress incontinence surgery on female sexual function. Am J Obstet Gynecol. 2009;200(5):562.e561–7.
70. Lemack GE, Zimmern PE. Sexual function after vaginal surgery for stress incontinence: results of a mailed questionnaire. Urology. 2000;56(2):223–7.
71. Mazouni C, Karsenty G, Bretelle F, Bladou F, Gamerre M, Serment G. Urinary complications and sexual function after the tension-free vaginal tape procedure. Acta Obstet Gynecol Scand. 2004;83(10): 955–61.
72. Shah SM, Bukkapatnam R, Rodriguez LV. Impact of vaginal surgery for stress urinary incontinence on female sexual function: is the use of polypropylene mesh detrimental? Urology. 2005;65(2):270–4.
73. Cholhan HJ, Hutchings TB, Rooney KE. Dyspareunia associated with paraurethral banding in the transobturator sling. Am J Obstet Gynecol. 2010;202(5):481. e481–5.
74. Berman JR, Adhikari SP, Goldstein I. Anatomy and physiology of female sexual function and dysfunction: classification, evaluation and treatment options. Eur Urol. 2000;38(1):20–9.
75. Wolter CE, Starkman JS, Scarpero HM, Dmochowski RR. Removal of transobturator midurethral sling for refractory thigh pain. Urology. 2008;72(2):461. e461–3.
76. Teo R, Moran P, Mayne C, Tincello D. Randomized trial of tension-free vaginal tape and tension-free vaginal tape-obturator for urodynamic stress incontinence in women. J Urol. 2011;185(4):1350–5.
77. Rigaud J, Pothin P, Labat JJ, et al. Functional results after tape removal for chronic pelvic pain following tension-free vaginal tape or transobturator tape. J Urol. 2010;184(2):610–5.
78. Lee SYKJ, Park SJ, Kwon YW, Nguyen HB, Chang IH, Kim TH, Kim YS. Bilateral recurrent thigh abscesses for five years after a transobturator tape implantation for stress urinary incontinence. Korean J Urol. 2010;51(9):657–9.
79. Gomelsky A, Dmochowski RR. Incisional bladder hernia after rectus fascial sling. J Urol. 2003; 169(6):2299.
80. Estevez JP, Cosson M, Boukerrou M. An uncommon case of urethrovaginal fistula resulting from tension-free vaginal tape. Int Urogynecol J. 2010;21(7):889–91.

Part III

Male Incontinence

The Artificial Urinary Sphincter

8

Rose Khavari and Timothy Boone

History

Surgical techniques to restore or resemble urethral sphincter function date back to 1947 when Foley reported his experience with an external cuff placed around the urethra and manually operated by the patient using a pneumatic piston [1]. Thereafter, Berry in 1961 used an acrylic block underneath the bulbocavernosus muscle to cause permanent compression of the urethra [2] and similarly Kaufman used a silicone-gel prosthesis to compress the bulbar urethra in postprostatectomy patients [3]. Unfortunately, these devices were plagued with high rates of infection, urethral erosion, and poor continence rates. These complications led investigators to balance the pressure placed on the urethra, by trying to keep it less than the body's systolic blood pressure, while providing sufficient pressure to create continence. Eventually, in 1973, Scott implanted the first-generation artificial urinary sphincter known today as the AMS 800 Artificial Urinary Sphincter (American Medical Systems, Inc., Minnetonka, MN) [4] and since Scott's time this device has undergone minimal changes to its current AMS 800™ Urinary Control System configuration introduced in 1983. The AUS has proven to be an effective treatment for stress urinary incontinence and is regarded as the "gold standard" by many experts. The contemporary AUS device has many advantages over preceding devices: it functions in a non-obstructive pattern with voiding, the pressure in the system is regulated by the reservoir balloon and not the patient, and it can be used for incontinence in both male and female patients [5].

The AMS 800 AUS has three components: (1) The cuff placed around the bulbar urethra or the bladder neck, (2) the balloon reservoir with various pressures (51–60, 61–70, 71–80 cmH_2O), and (3) the scrotal or labial pump that contains the control mechanism and the deactivation button. Since all the three components can easily be connected and the system can be locked in a deactivated state, the AMS 800 AUS can be implanted in a single stage. After the recovery period, the AUS is activated by the pump allowing fluid in the system to fill the cuff and create a continent state. When the patient is ready to void, he or she can squeeze the scrotal or the labial pump and allow the fluid in the cuff to empty and return to the pressure regulating the balloon. After voiding the fluid automatically returns from the balloon to the cuff, repressurizing the system, thus closing the urethra.

Patient Selection, Evaluation, and Preoperative Workup

Although most artificial urinary sphincters are placed in postprostatectomy men with stress urinary incontinence, any male or female patient

R. Khavari, M.D. • T. Boone, M.D., Ph.D. (✉)
Department of Urology, Houston Methodist Hospital, 6560 Fannin, Suite 2100, Houston, TX 77030, USA
e-mail: tboone2@tmhs.org

G.H. Badlani (ed.), *Minimally Invasive Therapy for Urinary Incontinence and Pelvic Organ Prolapse*, Current Clinical Urology, DOI 10.1007/978-1-4939-0008-4_8,

with stress urinary incontinence can potentially be a candidate for AUS implantation. There is no strict lower limit or higher limit on the amount of incontinence. Females, children, patients with neurogenic bladder, or augmentation cystoplasty can be appropriately evaluated and potentially benefit from AUS. Along with counseling for AUS implantation, a history and physical exam, urodynamic testing, and cystourethroscopy is recommended.

During history taking, the urologist should determine the cause for the patient's incontinence (neurogenic, trauma, intrinsic sphincter deficiency, radiation, postprostatectomy, postcystectomy, etc.). Previous surgical procedures on the bladder and the urethra should be evaluated as well along with other comorbidities and conditions, including the patients overall health, anticoagulation use, skin conditions, meatal stenosis, urethral strictures, and mixed urinary incontinence (urge and stress). Furthermore, assuring that the patient is able to use his or her hands and has sufficient dexterity is an important part of the preoperative evaluation. The patient's willingness and cognition to operate the cuff every 4–6 h during the day should also be a part of preoperative discussion and counseling. One may also want to determine which hand is dominant for the patient in order to place the pump on that side of the scrotum or labia to facilitate operating the pump for the patient.

The physical examination should include a thorough genitourinary exam in males (skin infections, hernias, previous hernia surgeries, hydroceles, etc.) and a complete pelvic exam in females since concurrent pelvic organ prolase, or vaginal atrophy may be present. Presence of some of these findings may require repair at the same setting or require staging prior to AUS procedure.

Although the use of preoperative urodynamic testing in postprostatectomy patients undergoing AUS implantation is controversial, it can be used to confirm intrinsic sphincter deficiency, identify bladder capacity (we recommend a minimum of 250 mls), detrusor compliance, and voiding pressures and patterns [6]. Lai et al. in 2011 reported their experience with preoperative overactive bladder symptoms and mixed urinary incontinence in 129 postprostatectomy patients undergoing AUS implantation. They concluded that preoperative overactive bladder symptoms did not adversely impact the patient's outcome after AUS placement. Furthermore, most of the patients with mixed urinary incontinence will continue to have their overactive symptoms after surgery, making preoperative counseling imperative. Development of de novo overactive symptoms in our series was 23 % [7].

The authors recommend cystourethroscopy in all patients undergoing AUS. This will allow the physician to evaluate the urethra for any strictures, and the bladder for any foreign bodies, tumors, or stones. If any of these are discovered, they should be resolved prior to proceeding with AUS implantation.

Operative Techniques

Preoperatively, patients are counseled appropriately regarding the risks of infection, erosion, bleeding, and need for further procedures. A negative urine culture must be present. The perineum is examined in the preoperative setting to ensure that there are no signs of skin infection or breakdown. Perioperative deep vein thrombosis prophylaxis and perioperative antibiotics are administered based on AUA best practice guidelines [8]. Hair in the perineum is trimmed right before the surgery. If a bulbar urethral cuff is planned, the patient is positioned in lithotomy with appropriate padding. If a bladder neck cuff is anticipated, a frog leg position is suitable. The authors do a full 10 min skin preparation with iodophor-based solution. We also recommend copious irrigation with antibiotic solution throughout the procedure.

The cuff can be placed around the bulbar urethra which is the most common technique used in men, or around the bladder neck through a suprapubic approach in children, or using a vaginal approach in females.

For the bulbar urethral technique, the patient is placed in lithotomy position and we place a 12F Foley to have the bladder drained during the procedure. By palpating the catheter in the perineum, we identify the point of its turn through the pelvic floor and mark that as the middle of our incision. A vertical incision of about 5–6 cm is made and a Scott ring retractor (Lone Star Medical Products, Houston, TX) is used for exposure. Sharp dissection is used to expose the bulbocavernosus muscle which then is divided in the middle and retracted to the sides to expose the bulbous urethra. Using sharp dissection, the bulbar urethra is freed circumferentially. Care is taken to do the dissection distal to the turn of the urethra to avoid injuring the posterior urethra. When the dissection is done safely, a right angled clamp is passed and the circumference of the urethra is measured by a measuring tape. The integrity of the urethra is assured by using a small caliber soft angiocath and injecting the antibiotic solution at the meatus alongside the Foley while gently pulling on the Foley balloon to close the bladder neck. If the urethra distends and there is no leak, we proceed with the measurement and the implantation. At any point, if there is any injury to the urethra, the surgery needs to be stopped and the AUS implantation postponed to a later date. The high risk of erosion and infection in the presence of urethral perforation biases us to stop the elective procedure. Based on our experience, most bulbar urethras will require a 4.5 cm cuff (range 3.5–5 cm). From this point on, the sharp instruments on the field are used with care avoiding contact with the artificial urinary sphincter components.

Prior to implantation of the AUS, all components are irrigated with normal saline and air is aspirated from all components and tubing. This will ensure the hydraulic mechanism of the system runs smoothly and decreases the risk of air interfering with the pump locking mechanism. The cuff is pulled posterior to the urethra using a right angled clamp and wrapped around and secured in place by placing the plastic tab over the button, ensuring the button is seated securely. Then our attention is turned to create a pocket for the pressure balloon in the space of retzius. Since most of our patients are postprostatectomy individuals, the bladder is often adherent to the fascia. Therefore, we make a small suprapubic incision and carry it down to identify the fascia. The fascia is opened with sharp dissection under direct vision and a small pocket is created lateral to the midline incision underneath the rectus abdominus muscle. Usually a 61–70 cmH_2O pressure balloon reservoir is chosen which is filled with 22 cc of saline. Although various contrast media and dilutions were used in the past to fill the tubing and the device, we currently use normal saline in almost all cases. Then the rectus abdominus fascia is closed and a tunnel above the fascia, starting from the most caudal portion of the incision to the base of the scrotum, is created. A subdartos pocket in the most dependant part of the scrotum is made using a long clamp. A long nasal speculum is used to guide the pump into the scrotal pocket where it is held gently with a Babcock clamp placed across the tubing and skin above the pump. All the tubing is brought to the suprapubic incision, trimmed to fit without excess tubing, and connected under direct vision using quick-connect system after ensuring the pressure balloon is filled appropriately. After all connections are made, the tubing can be secured to the fascia with one or two interrupted sutures over the connectors to make the tubing less palpable by the patient. We have found that tubing fixation in this manner helps prevent pump migration. The artificial urinary sphincter is cycled under direct vision, and then locked in the deactivated position. The bulbocavernosus muscle is reapproximated and the perineal incision is closed using long-lasting absorbable sutures in multiple layers and approximating the bulbocavernosus muscle.

For bladder neck placement of the AUS cuff, the patient is placed in the frog leg position and a low midline or pfannenstiel incision is made. The bladder is mobilized and the endopelvic fascia is identified and opened under direct vision. The bladder neck is freed up posteriorly for about 2 cm separating it from the rectum in males and the anterior vagina in females. EEA Sizers™ in the vagina or the rectum can help to separate these organs during difficult dissections in previously operated or radiated fields. If identifying the bladder neck is difficult, one can make a small anterior cystotomy in a more cephalad part of the bladder to inspect and identify the bladder neck more precisely as long as this is well away from the cuff. Any small perforation to the bladder or the urethra can be closed primarily and the procedure could be continued to the conclusion as long as the cuff is not placed over the perforation. The authors prefer to postpone the cuff placement unless the cystotomy is anteriorly located and well away from the bladder neck. We also recommend waiting 6 weeks prior to activating the AUS system. On the contrary, if an injury to the rectum occurs, then placement of the AUS should be aborted. The cuff size used during this technique varies between 5 and 11 cm and the pressure balloon most commonly used is 71–80 cmH_2O which is placed in the retropubic space. The pump is placed in the labia or the scrotum as discussed previously. All tubing is brought anterior to the rectus fascia and connected securely where the device is cycled under direct vision.

The bladder neck cuff can also be placed through a vaginal incision in females. After placing the patient in lithotomy and placing a Foley catheter, an inverted U incision is made with the apex at the bladder neck. The vaginal flap is completely freed up and the endopelvic fascia is identified bilaterally and perforated. The bladder neck and the proximal urethra is freed up and a measuring tape is used to measure the circumference of the bladder neck. A cuff is placed and we recommend cystoscopy to ensure that the cuff is placed distal to the ureteral orifices. The bladder is tested for any inadvertent cystotomies which are repaired if identified. The rest of the procedure is similar to the one described above.

Postoperative Care

We recommend continuing the intravenous antibiotic for 24 h per AUA best practice guidelines and early ambulation. Strict glucose control in the perioperative period is imperative in diabetic patients. The catheter is removed 24 h postoperatively and we ensure the patients can empty their bladder without any difficulty prior to being discharged. We activate the AUS in 4–6 weeks in the clinic and provide appropriate patient education. Patients are instructed to recognize signs and symptoms of infections in the skin or the urine and immediately notify their physician. In addition they are counseled to notify other health care providers of their implant and they are educated that the AUS needs to be deactivated when a catheter must be inserted in their urethra.

Complications

Urethral Atrophy

The most common cause for revision surgery following AUS placement is urethral atrophy reported at 9.6 % [9]. This is defined as failure of the urethra below the cuff to completely coapt which can be visualized during cystoscopy, along with low Valsalva leak point pressures during urodynamics, loss of visibility of contrast in the cuff on X-ray (in circumstances where contrast is used), and ultimately confirmed by urethral thinning during surgical exploration. Various techniques are used to address this complication which are discussed in a later part of this chapter in more detail.

Infection

Despite all precautions taken, some patients will develop infections which can be abrupt or chronic and may require intravenous antibiotics or explantation of the device. In 1995 Martins and Boyd reported their experience with postoperative infection-erosion patients by isolating a pleomorphic group of organisms, specifically enteric, Gram-positive, and anaerobic organisms by culture [10]. Although, most experts believe *Staphylococcus epidermidis* is the most common organism, Magera et al. showed that *Staphylococcus aureus* was the most common organism in their series [11]. Unlike other infections, infections involving AUS can occur without any fever, leukocytosis, fluctuance, or purulence. Patients with an AUS infection usually present with inflammation, erythema, edema, and pain in the perineum or the pump. Having a high index of suspicion will prompt the diagnosis and immediate treatment can be helpful in improving patient outcomes.

Usually new onset pain is a sign of AUS infection. In select patients social continence can be restored with reinsertion of the AUS following removal for infection or erosion [12]. Lai et al. reported their experience with 21 secondary reimplant cases following explantation due to erosion or infection. The authors reported a fourfold increased risk of future cuff erosion when compared to virgin cases. However, overall good functional outcome with an acceptable continence rate was achieved in their reoperative series [13].

Device Failure

Most experts would agree that the life of the AUS is usually between 10 and 15 years. However, various mechanical or functional defects can lead to AUS dysfunction. Leak in the device is one of the most common mechanical failures wherein patients complain of recurrent incontinence, a completely flat pump or the feeling of air in the system. In our experience the pressure control pump is the most common site to fail probably due to bending the pump to open the cuff over many years. The silicone-coated cuff, tubing, and the reservoir are less likely to be the source of fluid leak. The leak can be identified in the operating room by using an ohmmeter to identify the leaking component and revise the individual component as needed when the device is only several years old.

Debris, air, or kinks in the tubing can also lead to malfunction. Patients may report that they need to use the pump more often to completely empty their bladder over many years with the AUS. Concurrent changes in bladder function with age must be taken into account as well. These issues can be minimized by meticulous primary surgical techniques and careful evaluation later on, however, revisions may be needed.

Special Circumstances

Artificial Urinary Sphincter in Children

The functional results of implanting the artificial urinary sphincter in children are variable. Cattie et al. in 2008 reported their experience in 44 children (age range 8.6–29.5 years) who had undergone an AUS implantation for severe urinary incontinence secondary to neuropathic bladder dysfunction. They reported frequent complications of urinary retention (24), urethral erosion (2), scrotal erosion (5), and mechanical dysfunction (7). This led to 9 removals, 5 deactivations, 6 revisions, and 5 total replacements [14]. In another study from Ruiz et al., presenting their 14-year experience of AUS implantation in children and adolescents, they reported a 86.3 % survival rate of the implant and a 26.3 % revision rate with overall continence of 87 % [15]. They noted more complications with extrophy patients who had multiple previous procedures on their bladder and bladder neck.

Artificial Urinary Sphincter in Neurogenic Bladder, Spinal Cord Injury, and Neobladder

In most pediatric and adolescent patients who have undergone AUS implantation, a neurogenic cause has been the primary reason for their stress urinary incontinence. The adult literature also supports implantation of AUS in selected patients who have appropriate bladder compliance and capacity with good outcomes and acceptable complications. Kastler in 2011 reported their experience in a multicenter-retrospective study on 51 adult patients where 31 % (16/51) had spina bifida and 69 % (35/51) had spinal cord injury with a 74 % continence rate after 10 years of follow-up [16]. Patients with severe stress urinary incontinence who have undergone cystoprostatectomy with a continent ileal neobladder can regain continence by implanting an artificial urinary sphincter. O'Connor et al. reported their experience with five patients who showed a decrease in pad use from 6.2 to 0.6 per day making them completely continent or socially continent [17]. Westney et al. also reported their experience in nine post-cystectomy patients with a continent ileal neobladder where the average pad use decreased from 6 to 1 per day ($p < 0.005$) with two explantations, suggesting the AUS can improve quality of life with comparable complication rates to other series in selected patients [18].

Controversies

Recurrent Urinary Incontinence (Urethral Atrophy)

Recurrent incontinence can be due to multiple factors including device malfunction, erosion, detrusor over activity, and urethral atrophy. Recurrent incontinence secondary to urethral atrophy can be managed by downsizing or repositioning the cuff, placement of an additional tandem cuff, or placement of a male sling [19–21]. Each approach, while effective in selected patients, can also have complications such as postoperative infection, erosion, or need for further procedures.

Some degree of urethral atrophy is expected with AUS placement. Normally the pressure-regulating balloon chosen is the 61–70 cmH_2O for bulbar urethral cuffs, reserving the 71–80 cmH_2O pressure balloons for bladder neck cuffs. In urethral atrophy patients, over time more fluid is needed in the cuff to maintain the desired inflation and coaptation. In general, the volume of urethral tissue under the cuff contributes to effective luminal coaptation. Eventually, the pressure in the balloon would not be able to provide sufficient pressure to provide coaptation for continence and therefore recurrent incontinence occurs. The patient may notice that gradually more pumps are needed to deflate the cuff. The cuff placed at the bulbar urethra and the bladder neck is usually filled with 0.75 cc and 2 cc, respectively. In the setting of urethral atrophy there is usually more fluid in the cuff and the patient may need to pump more to deflate the cuff.

Down-Sizing, Transcorporal Placement, or Repositioning the Urethral Cuff

In 1995, Stone et al. reported a small series of patients with urethral atrophy treated by proximally repositioned cuffs with an 83 % success rate [22]. The authors believed that this approach may have less risk of erosion.

More recently in 2003, Stone et al. followed a slightly larger group of patients for 7 years after downsizing their bulbar urethral cuffs from a 4.5 to 4 cm using the existing space and pseudocapsule. Their patient satisfaction and continence scores improved suggesting this approach is an effective and safe method to manage urinary incontinence secondary to cuff-induced urethral atrophy [19]. Minimal dissection is needed during this approach and the other components of the device are not manipulated, thus decreasing the risk of infection and the time to reactivate the AUS.

Some experts argue that during AUS revisions the urethra is vulnerable to injury and most commonly the cuff is placed in a more distal location inadvertently requiring a much smaller size. Therefore, transcorporal placement of the cuff has become popular among some implanters with the belief that this will allow for more bulk around the urethra and more appropriate cuff sizing with less risk of erosion. In 2002, Webster et al. reported their experience in 31 patients, with a mean follow-up of 17 months, in patients who underwent AUS revision using a transcorporal cuff showing that 84 % of the patients had occasional stress urinary incontinence [23]. This technique can only be an option in the patient with preexisting erectile dysfunction since entry of the corpora will damage tumescence.

Insertion of a Tandem Cuff

Originally, Brito et al. in 1993 described placement of tandem bulbar urethral cuffs in patients with severe urinary incontinence who still suffered from persistent leakage following AUS placement. They increased their continence rate from 85 to 95 % [9]. In another series with longer follow-up of 74.1 and 58.0 months for single and double cuff patients, respectively, O'Connor et al. reported no significant improvement with a double cuff placement. However, the patients with double cuff insertion had a higher complication rate and required further interventions [9].

Placing a tandem cuff as a salvage procedure for recurrent stress urinary incontinence with longer follow-up (mean of 3.3 years) was reported by Elliott et al. in 2003. The authors reported improved continence and patient satisfaction in their series. Their reoperation rate due to leakage and erosion was 1 and 2 % in 18 patients, respectively [24].

Furthermore, in a selective group of patients with a high risk of infection and erosion, salvage transcorporal tandem cuff placement has been proposed. In 2007 Elliott et al. reported a small number of patients who had undergone tandem transcorporal cuff placement suggesting yet another effective alternative for approaching this complicated group of patients [20].

Male Sling after Urethral Atrophy Following Artificial Urinary Sphincter

More recently several investigators have proposed the use of a non-bone-anchored transobturator suburethral sling such as the AdVance Sling (American Medical Systems, Minnetonka, MN) to manage recurrent urinary incontinence secondary to urethral cuff-induced atrophy. This approach may decrease entry to the capsule formed by the urethral cuff, therefore less risk of infection. In addition the downtime of AUS activation after a second AUS cuff placement or a revision is eliminated with this technique. Non-bone-anchored transobturator male slings work by elevating the urethra rather than compression. Christine et al. have suggested that in selected patients in whom the external sphincter is still partially functional by external compression during cystoscopy may experience improvement in their recurrent incontinence with salvage AdVance Sling. Furthermore, in their small retrospective report, the authors showed that in over 50 % of their patients continence was obtained without reactivation of the AUS [21].

Artificial Urinary Sphincter Following a Failed Male Sling

The literature does not have sufficient data regarding implantation of AUS following a failed non-bone-anchored transobturator male sling. Most likely this can be explained by the fact that these slings are recent to the field and a long-term follow-up is still pending. However, Fisher et al. reported their experience with 11 patients having failed a bone-anchored male sling who subsequently underwent an artificial urinary sphincter placement. In their small series, with a mean follow-up of 14.2 months, they reported feasibility of this procedure with high patient satisfaction and no intraoperative complications or urethral injuries. However, one AUS had to be explanted due to infection [25].

Nocturnal Deactivation

There is some controversy among experts regarding nocturnal deactivation of the AUS which may provide a "rest period" and decrease the incidence of urethral atrophy. In 2001, Boone et al. reported a retrospective comparison, with a long term follow-up, comparing patients at Mayo Clinic who deactivate their AUS at night compared to Baylor patients who keep their AUS activated at all times except during voids. It appears that the risk of urethral atrophy and recurrent incontinence was less in nocturnal deactivation group (10 % vs. 21 %). Therefore, the authors suggest nocturnal deactivation for motivated patients who are dry at night and would like to decrease the risk of urethral atrophy [26].

External Bulking Agents

In cases of severe urethral cuff atrophy, when the maximal circumference of the urethra is less than 4 cm, some experts have tried using external bulking agents. Lue et al. in 2005 reported their experience with wrapping an external urethral bulking material (Surgisis ES, Cook Urological, Spencer, IN) in patients with a small urethra in order to enhance the diameter of the urethra prior to placing a 4 cm cuff. In their series of five patients they reported this technique to be feasible and well-tolerated with satisfactory results [27].

Radiation and AUS

External Radiation Therapy

Only a few studies pertaining to radiation in patients with postprostatectomy incontinence requiring an AUS focus on preoperative evaluation, complications, success, and other specific considerations. Radiation is known to affect the urethra, bladder, and the surrounding tissues making the area more susceptible to infection and erosion secondary to tissue hypo-vascularity [28]. In addition, the bladder exposed to radiation may become smaller in capacity and experience more overactivity. Hemorrhagic cystitis, another potential complication following radiation therapy, can be a challenge for radiated patients who are being evaluated for AUS placement. In 1995, Boyd et al. reported their outcomes of AUS placement in patients undergoing major pelvic surgery with or without radiotherapy. Thirty four out of their eighty one patients had received radiation either in an adjuvant setting or as a primary treatment. They recommended waiting 12 weeks prior to activating the AUS and had acceptable overall results [28]. In another small series a social continence rate of 87 % with an overall complication rate of 25 %, and erosion/infection rate of 12.5 % was reported [29]. In one review, with a mean follow-up of 31 and 36 months in two groups of postprostatectomy patients who did not and did receive radiation, respectively, Boone et al. reviewed their results of continence, urodynamic testing, complication rate, overall satisfaction, and quality of life. Their radiation group included patients who had external beam radiation as their primary treatment with or without salvage prostatectomy, or radiation given in an adjuvant setting. They reported similar continence rates, urgency with or without urge incontinence, and satisfaction rates in both patient groups. They also report that their rate of infection, erosion (14 %), and reoperations were similar in these two groups [30]. Based on their findings, the authors recommend that no special precautions or consideration is necessary in patients who have received radiation compared to the patients who have not. These reasonable results with AUS placement in patients with prior radiation history may argue that the bulbar urethra is outside of the radiated field. In addition, current external beam radiation is much more precise and with a smaller treatment target, the affected field is much more limited.

In our experience, and by consulting the literature, AUS implantation following radiation therapy alone is rare. Most data available and experiences mentioned above apply to patients with adjuvant or salvage radiation therapy. Our unpublished experience shows radiotherapy after implantation to be well tolerated in the setting of biochemical recurrent disease.

Another topic of concern and discussion is the functional bladder change that occurs in patients who have undergone radiation. Prior radiation may promote bladder fibrosis and instability. In the study reported by Hadley et al., radiated patients had more bladder instability, smaller bladder capacity (less than 300 ml), low compliance (less than 20 ml/cm water), and early bladder sensation (at a volume less than 85 ml) but the difference was statistically significant only for bladder instability ($p < 0.05$) [29].

Minimally Invasive Therapy for Localized Prostate Cancer Treatment

Traditionally, the treatment choices for prostate cancer had been prostatectomy or radiation therapy. Recent sophisticated technology has introduced alternative methods in managing localized prostate cancer. These include proton beam therapy, cryoablation of the prostate, brachytherapy, and high-intensity focused ultrasound (HIFU). Although some promising results have been suggested by these techniques with a short-term follow-up, their complication rates, including urinary incontinence of 4–40 % is variable and concerning [31].

Data regarding artificial urinary sphincter implantation following these techniques is very limited in the literature. Benoit et al. reported placement of AUS in 4 men out of 2,124 men in Medicare population that had undergone brachytherapy [32]. Instrumentation across the AUS for recurrent prostate obstruction or chronic sloughing of necrotic tissue can be very difficult.

Recurrent Bladder Neck Contracture and AUS

Obstruction of the outlet in postprostatectomy or cystectomy patients due to bladder neck contracture can be managed by transurethral electrocautery resection, laser ablation, or direct visual internal urethrotomy. If the patient responds to this management and establishes an open bladder neck, a subsequent artificial urinary sphincter can be inserted. However, in many cases the bladder neck contracture is recurrent and does not respond to endoscopic management and the insertion of a urethral wall stent becomes an option. Use of a urethral stent is reserved for very selected cases. Elliott et al. also reported their experience with successful placement of AUS following Urolume™ placement with minimal morbidity and 89 % patient satisfaction after 17.5 months of follow-up [33]. Magera et al. report a median of three failed endoscopic management of recurrent bladder neck contracture in their series. They were able to stabilize the bladder neck in 13 out of 25 patients with one stent and in 6 out of 25 patients with 2–4 stents. Urinary continence was then achieved by placement of artificial urinary sphincter with satisfactory results [34]. Lai et al. also showed that a staged UroLume™ stent with delayed artificial urinary sphincter implantation provided good continence control in 8 out of 11 patients with recurrent bladder neck contractures [35]. In conclusion the authors believe that in highly selected patients the bladder neck contracture can be stabilized with UroLume™ stent followed by implantation of artificial urinary sphincter. Early studies using Mitomycin C as an adjuvant to internal urethrotomy may provide another tool in managing the recurrent bladder neck contracture prior to AUS placement [36].

Conclusion

Since the first implantation of the artificial urinary sphincter in 1973, thousands of men, women, and children have regained urinary continence, thanks to Dr. Brantley Scott. With long-term data now available, the AUS has become widely used with satisfactory outcomes. Multiple large series have confirmed the AUS to be a durable treatment for sphincter deficiency patients even in patients with neurogenic bladder, radiation treatment, bladder neck contracture, failed slings or injectables, mixed urinary incontinence, or low detrusor pressures [35, 37]. More experience is needed to evaluate the AUS in men with incontinence following minimally invasive treatment of prostate cancer with more contemporary technologies such as brachytherapy, proton therapy, or HIFU.

References

1. Foley FE. An artificial sphincter; a new device and operation for control of enuresis and urinary incontinence. J Urol. 1947;58:250.
2. Berry JL. Evaluation of a new procedure for correction of postprostatectomy urinary incontinence. Bull N Y Acad Med. 1964;40:790.
3. Kaufman JJ. Treatment of post-prostatectomy urinary incontinence using a silicone gel prosthesis. Br J Urol. 1973;45:646.
4. Scott FB, Bradley WE, Timm GW. Treatment of urinary incontinence by implantable prosthetic sphincter. Urology. 1973;1:252.
5. Light JK. Complications of surgery for male urinary incontinence. In: Smith RB, Ehrlich RM, editors. Complications of urologic surgery, prevention and management. Philadelphia: WB Saunders; 1990.
6. Lai HH, Hsu EI, Boone TB. Urodynamic testing in evaluation of postradical prostatectomy incontinence before artificial urinary sphincter implantation. Urology. 2009;73:1264.
7. Lai HH, Boone TB. Implantation of artificial urinary sphincter in patients with post-prostatectomy incontinence, and preoperative overactive bladder and mixed symptoms. J Urol. 2011;185:2254.
8. Wolf Jr JS, Bennett CJ, Dmochowski RR, et al. Best practice policy statement on urologic surgery antimicrobial prophylaxis. J Urol. 2008;179:1379.
9. Brito CG, Mulcahy JJ, Mitchell ME, et al. Use of a double cuff AMS800 urinary sphincter for severe stress incontinence. J Urol. 1993;149:283.
10. Martins FE, Boyd SD. Post-operative risk factors associated with artificial urinary sphincter infection-erosion. Br J Urol. 1995;75:354.
11. Magera Jr JS, Elliott DS. Artificial urinary sphincter infection: causative organisms in a contemporary series. J Urol. 2008;180:2475.
12. Kowalczyk JJ, Nelson R, Mulcahy JJ. Successful reinsertion of the artificial urinary sphincter after removal for erosion or infection. Urology. 1996;48:906.
13. Lai HH, Boone TB. Complex artificial urinary sphincter revision and reimplantation cases-how do they fare compared to virgin cases? J Urol. 2012; 187:951.
14. Catti M, Lortat-Jacob S, Morineau M, et al. Artificial urinary sphincter in children–voiding or emptying? An evaluation of functional results in 44 patients. J Urol. 2008;180:690.
15. Ruiz E, Puigdevall J, Moldes J, et al. 14 years of experience with the artificial urinary sphincter in children and adolescents without spina bifida. J Urol. 2006; 176:1821.
16. Chartier Kastler E, Genevois S, Game X, et al. Treatment of neurogenic male urinary incontinence related to intrinsic sphincter insufficiency with an artificial urinary sphincter: a French retrospective multicentre study. BJU Int. 2011;107:426.

17. O'Connor RC, Kuznetsov DD, Patel RV, et al. Artificial urinary sphincter placement in men after cystectomy with orthotopic ileal neobladder: continence, complications, and quality of life. Urology. 2002;59:542.
18. Westney OL, Hinh P, Lee D. Outcomes of artificial urinary sphincter prosthesis implantation for treatment of stress urinary incontinence in patients with ileal neobladder. In: AUA, 2011. Abstract 1170.
19. Saffarian A, Walsh K, Walsh IK, et al. Urethral atrophy after artificial urinary sphincter placement: is cuff downsizing effective? J Urol. 2003;169:567.
20. Magera Jr JS, Elliott DS. Tandem transcorporal artificial urinary sphincter cuff salvage technique: surgical description and results. J Urol. 2007;177:1015.
21. Christine B, Knoll LD. Treatment of recurrent urinary incontinence after artificial urinary sphincter placement using the AdVance male sling. Urology. 2010; 76:1321.
22. Couillard DR, Vapnek JM, Stone AR. Proximal artificial sphincter cuff repositioning for urethral atrophy incontinence. Urology. 1995;45:653.
23. Guralnick ML, Miller E, Toh KL, et al. Transcorporal artificial urinary sphincter cuff placement in cases requiring revision for erosion and urethral atrophy. J Urol. 2002;167:2075.
24. DiMarco DS, Elliott DS. Tandem cuff artificial urinary sphincter as a salvage procedure following failed primary sphincter placement for the treatment of post-prostatectomy incontinence. J Urol. 2003; 170:1252.
25. Fisher MB, Aggarwal N, Vuruskan H, et al. Efficacy of artificial urinary sphincter implantation after failed bone-anchored male sling for postprostatectomy incontinence. Urology. 2007;70:942.
26. Elliott DS, Barrett DM, Gohma M, et al. Does nocturnal deactivation of the artificial urinary sphincter lessen the risk of urethral atrophy? Urology. 2001; 57:1051.
27. Rahman NU, Minor TX, Deng D, et al. Combined external urethral bulking and artificial urinary sphincter for urethral atrophy and stress urinary incontinence. BJU Int. 2005;95:824.
28. Martins FE, Boyd SD. Artificial urinary sphincter in patients following major pelvic surgery and/or radiotherapy: are they less favorable candidates? J Urol. 1995;153:1188.
29. Wang Y, Hadley HR. Experiences with the artificial urinary sphincter in the irradiated patient. J Urol. 1992;147:612.
30. Gomha MA, Boone TB. Artificial urinary sphincter for post-prostatectomy incontinence in men who had prior radiotherapy: a risk and outcome analysis. J Urol. 2002;167:591.
31. Alan J, Wein LRK, Novick Andrew C, Partin Alan W, Peters Craig A, editors. Campbell-Walsh urology. 10th ed. Philadelphia: Elsevier Expert Consult; 2012.
32. Benoit RM, Naslund MJ, Cohen JK. Complications after prostate brachytherapy in the Medicare population. Urology. 2000;55:91.
33. Elliott DS, Boone TB. Combined stent and artificial urinary sphincter for management of severe recurrent bladder neck contracture and stress incontinence after prostatectomy: a long-term evaluation. J Urol. 2001; 165:413.
34. Magera Jr JS, Inman BA, Elliott DS. Outcome analysis of urethral wall stent insertion with artificial urinary sphincter placement for severe recurrent bladder neck contracture following radical prostatectomy. J Urol. 2009;181:1236.
35. Lai HH, Hsu EI, Teh BS, et al. 13 years of experience with artificial urinary sphincter implantation at Baylor College of Medicine. J Urol. 2007;177:1021.
36. Mazdak H, Meshki I, Ghassami F. Effect of mitomycin C on anterior urethral stricture recurrence after internal urethrotomy. Eur Urol. 2007;51:1089.
37. Peterson AC, Webster GD. Artificial urinary sphincter: lessons learned. Urol Clin North Am. 2011;38:83.

Complications of Male Incontinence Procedures: Diagnosis, Evaluation, and Management

9

Andrew C. Peterson

Urinary incontinence (UI), the complaint of any involuntary leakage of urine [1], may be the result of congenital anomalies, injury, genitourinary surgery, and other conditions. The most common etiology of UI in men is radical prostatectomy (RP), with the primary mechanism being failure to store urine secondary to inadequate function of the outlet-sphincter. Despite improvements in surgical technique that have reduced the rate of post-prostatectomy UI, the burden of disease in the United States remains high and is expected to rise because of increasing numbers of RP performed annually [2].

UI significantly compromises heath-related quality of life in men [3] and can be improved by surgical treatment using bulbar urethral slings, and the artificial urinary sphincter (AUS). Although bulking agents have been used in the past as a first-line treatment for male UI, the severity of incontinence and postsurgical scarring in the vesicourethral region after prostatectomy have made surgical correction the first-line treatment for the majority of cases.

The AUS is one of the best available treatments for UI in males. It has proven long-term durability and effectiveness across the spectrum of moderate and severe degrees of urinary loss. Despite this, several other treatments such as the urethral slings, including the transobturator bulbar sling and the perineal bone-anchored sling have emerged as viable treatment options for the male with UI. Herein, we discuss the possible complications that these treatments may pose and their evaluation and management in men with UI after surgical treatment.

Evaluation and Diagnosis of Problems After Initial Surgical Treatments for Male UI

Because of the wide range of possible complications from these types of surgical interventions for UI (the various types of the male sling and the AUS) patients may present after surgery with a wide range of problems including difficulty with urination, pain, hematuria, infection, erosion, and damage to other structures such as the rectum, ureters, and bladder. Therefore, the evaluation of all men with problems after initial surgery for UI requires a detailed history, physical examination, and urinalysis. Many cases will also require cystoscopy and pressure flow urodynamics.

For those presenting with continued loss of urine after surgical intervention, it is imperative to clearly differentiate between stress and urge incontinence. For this, the 72-h voiding diary and the 24-h pad test are inexpensive, simple tools that are invaluable in the assessment prior to proceeding with any invasive testing [4]. The voiding diary

A.C. Peterson, M.D., F.A.C.S. (✉)
Division of Urology, Duke University Medical Center, DUMC 3146, Rm 1113, Green Zone, Davison Bldg, Durham, NC 27710, USA
e-mail: drew.peterson@duke.edu

G.H. Badlani (ed.), *Minimally Invasive Therapy for Urinary Incontinence and Pelvic Organ Prolapse*, Current Clinical Urology, DOI 10.1007/978-1-4939-0008-4_9,

reliably and objectively assesses the complaint and may uncover significant urgency and urge incontinence that may not be related to the incontinence surgery [5]. Self-reported daily pad usage varies considerably with only moderate concordance with urinary incontinence volume [6]. Thus the 24-h pad weight test, which objectively measures the volume of the incontinence, may be helpful in comparing the patient's preoperative urine loss volume to the postoperative urine loss thereby aiding in the direction of appropriate therapy.

Laboratory

Urine analysis and culture when the UA is suggestial of infection are required prior to the initial surgical correction of male UI as well as prior to any revision surgeries. They are also extremely important when evaluating any patient with any problem after surgery. The presence of blood, white blood cells, and any evidence of infection may indicate erosion of mesh or material such as the urethral cuff into the urethra.

Cystoscopy

Because unrecognized urethral pathology can significantly complicate all of the surgical options for UI, endoscopic evaluation is recommended prior to any intervention for problems after initial surgical management of urinary incontinence [7–9]. Furthermore, in patients with recurrent incontinence after AUS implantation, cystoscopy may aid in differentiating mechanical failure from other causes such as urethral atrophy. Finally, when an AUS or sling [10] has been removed due to infection or erosion, repeat evaluation of the urethra prior to reimplantation is essential to rule out urethral stricture, diverticulum, fistula, and other urethral complications that may hinder replacement of a new cuff at a later time.

Urodynamics

Although a careful history and voiding diary may be sufficient to confirm the adequacy of bladder function in patients with problems after initial management of UI, formal pressure flow urodynamics may permit an accurate assessment of the bladder function and incontinence type and severity. Detrusor overactivity, while not a contraindication to surgery for UI if discovered initially, requires realistic counseling regarding the likelihood of persistence or exacerbation after treatment of incontinence. Likewise, reduced bladder compliance presents a more serious concern, because prolonged storage at high pressures may lead to deteriorating renal function and continued leakage. Therefore, urodynamics may be indicated in patients with continued or recurrent incontinence after appropriate initial surgical management.

Artificial Urinary Sphincter

The AUS is still one of the most well-established devices for the treatment of male UI. The AUS (AMS 800) is a complex mechanical device consisting of a fluid-filled cuff placed around the bladder neck or bulbar urethra, a control pump placed in the scrotum or labia in the female, and a pressure-regulating balloon (PRB) placed in a preperitoneal location. The tubing is connected by quick connect devices supplied from the company. Fluid transfer from the cuff to the PRB is accomplished by active "pumping" while refilling occurs passively by a pressure gradient from the reservoir that traverses a resistor implanted in the pump. Therefore, one can see that there are many aspects to the device that may lead to malfunction, failure, erosion, and infection.

Long-term durability of the AUS is well established, although this device still has a revision rate of 16 and 28 % at 2 and 5 years, respectively [11]. In addition, these mechanical devices will all ultimately fail and need revision approximately 7–10 years after placement with 72 % of the original sphincters functioning in place at a mean follow-up of 69 months [12].

Artificial Urinary Sphincter Cuff

The AUS cuff is most commonly placed around the bulbar urethra via a perineal incision, although a transscrotal approach has been popularized by

Wilson and associates [13] (see below). The aim is to place the cuff as proximal on the bulbar urethra as possible. This is the area with the largest diameter of corpus spongiosum and provides protection of the cuff from activation while sitting because it is protected by the split corporal bodies. When circumferentially mobilizing the urethra at the cuff location, blunt spreading dissection is discouraged in this area because it risks injury to the urethra, especially in reoperative cases. Rarely, when an injury is made to the urethra during this dissection, it can be closed with interrupted fine absorbable suture and a new site more distally can be chosen without needing to abort the case. However, in complicated or severe cases of injury (lacerations greater than 1 cm) we find it is the better part of valor to abort the case relegating the patient to catheter drainage for 2–3 weeks with a re-attempt at placement after complete healing.

The circumference of the urethra is measured around the corpus spongiosum to guide selection of cuff size, some authors advocate selecting a cuff size 0.5–1 cm smaller than the measured circumference of the urethra in order to compensate for compression of the spongiosum. If a cuff is selected and placed around the urethra but is obviously incorrect (too large or too small), the best option is to discard that cuff and replace with the appropriate size.

Pressure-Regulating Balloon

The placement of the pressure-regulating balloon (PRB) may be achieved through a scrotal, perineal, or abdominal incision, depending on prior surgical incisions, body habitus, and surgeon preference. The PRB is filled with 20–23 mL of sterile normal saline or contrast material, unless a bladder neck cuff is used, which requires additional fluid volume. In order to provide an isotonic solution, contrast solutions should always be diluted with sterile water. Failure to fill the device with isotonic solution may result in fluid leach from the system and therefore malfunction.

It is important to note that precise placement of the PRB behind the abdominal wall in the preperitoneal space is paramount to its correct functioning. In morbidly obese patients when the PRB is placed in the subcutaneous fat, we have found that it does not transmit adequate rises in intra-abdominal pressures to the cuff therefore contributing to significant urinary leakage with stress. In these cases, the PRB should be moved to a preperitoneal space with a revision operation. We prefer to use a second incision in the right lower quadrant to place the balloon in all cases as we found that placement through the inguinal canal may predispose it to herniation and malfunction requiring a revision surgery in the future.

Control Pump

The pump assembly is placed into the anterior scrotum from the inguinal, scrotal, or perineal incision. Care must be taken to avoid leaving excessive tubing in the scrotum as this may result in malpositioning of the pump making it difficult to manipulate.

Connections are typically made in the abdominal incision. This allows exploration at a later date if needed for revision by placing all the connections in one easily accessible spot. The quick connectors supplied by the manufacturer provide secure, connections for newly implanted devices. In these cases when the entire device is not being replaced, it is recommended to use the hand-tied connectors that are provided by the company in the accessory kit utilizing, securing the connections with 3-0 Prolene suture.

Tandem Cuff AUS

Despite improvements in AMS 800 design and implantation techniques, as many as 11 % of patients may have significant incontinence after single-cuff AUS placement [14]. In cases of persistent UI from incomplete urethral occlusion despite the use of the smallest cuff (3.5 cm), the addition of a second cuff around the bulbar urethra can yield satisfactory continence [15–17]. However, the indiscriminate use of the tandem cuff approach as first-line surgical treatment is to be discouraged because of higher rates of erosion associated with the distal cuff [18].

Placement of the second cuff is performed via the perineal incision. After circumferential dissection around the bulbar urethra, at least 1.5–2 cm distal to the primary cuff, a new cuff is placed. Connection to the existing device requires division of the existing cuff tubing and use of a Y-connector, securing it with either the quick connector clamps provided by the company or a hand-tied connection with 3-0 Prolene suture as indicated. When adding a new cuff to an existing system, as described above an additional 3 mL of fluid should be added to the system to fill the second cuff without depleting the fluid in the PRB. Doing so may significantly change the pressure that is generated by the PRB and placed on the urethral cuff.

Transcorporal AUS Cuff

The transcorporal placement of the AUS provides another option when dealing with difficult initial or revision surgery [19]. Rather than dissecting between the corpus spongiosum and the ventral cavernosa, parallel longitudinal incisions in the tunica albuginea of the corpora cavernosa allow the plane of dissection to pass through the septum of the corpora from one side to the other. This technique leaves the ventral tunica albuginea attached to the dorsum of the spongiosum. The lateral edges of the tunica albuginea are then closed dorsal to the cuff to help with postoperative bleeding. Advantages of the transcorporal approach include reduced risk of urethral injury during reoperation after prior erosion or urethra injury; better cuff fit because of the increased bulk of the urethra; and potential reduction in erosion risk. The technique is particularly useful when proximal cuff atrophy occurs in cases where the smallest cuff has been already used. Transcorporal placement 2–3 cm distally, leaving an intervening segment of normal urethra, may yield AUS continence results similar to those in non-revision placement surgeries. Webster and associates reported a cure and improvement rate of 84 % without intraoperative urethral injuries or postoperative urethral erosions at a mean follow-up of 17 months [19].

Transscrotal AUS

Wilson described this technique in which all components of the AUS are placed through a transverse scrotal incision. Originally developed for reoperative surgery due to urethral atrophy, it allowed placement of a more distal cuff in tandem or with the transcorporal technique. Although the initial report was favorable in terms of continence outcomes, several later reports suggest that the transscrotal technique yields inferior continence results [20, 21]. One possible explanation is that it does not allow equivalent placement of the cuff around the proximal, larger diameter bulbar urethra when compared to the perineal approach. Because of this, we prefer to use the perineal approach in all cases to decrease the possible risk of intermittent unintended activations of the device due to the distally located cuff.

Complications of the AUS

Urinary Retention

We do not routinely leave catheters in after placement of an AUS, leaving the device deactivated and the patient simply incontinent. If the patient develops urinary retention in the immediate postoperative period, this should be managed by transurethral bladder drainage with a small (10 or 12 Fr) catheter for 24–48 h. Cuff deactivation must be confirmed before catheterization. If the patient fails a voiding trial at 48–72 h, suprapubic drainage is recommended to reduce the risk of urethral erosion. It is important to limit the time an indwelling urethral catheter is left in place because even very small ones may result in erosion of the cuff secondary to abrasion from the sawing motion of the catheter along with compression. Therefore, one must be extremely cautious in patients with an AUS and catheter in place and not be falsely assured that erosion will not happen simply because the catheter is small. When placing a suprapubic tube, ultrasound or fluoroscopic guidance is recommended to prevent puncture or potential contamination of the PRB and tubing that may lie in the area.

Very rarely, retention that lasts several weeks implies under sizing of the cuff; in such cases reoperation and cuff replacement may be required. Correlation with preoperative urodynamic findings is advised to establish preoperative function of the bladder, another reason that preoperative urodynamics evaluation in all patients undergoing surgical treatment for UI is important. Late-onset urinary retention that occurs more than 2–4 weeks after surgery mandates endoscopic and urodynamic evaluation to rule out proximal urethral obstruction, erosion, or detrusor failure.

AUS Infection

Device infection remains a serious and possibly devastating complication of any implant surgery. The rate of infection with initial AUS surgery is 1–3 % [14, 22–24] but may be as high as 10 % in reoperative cases and when placed into those who have had pelvic radiation and multiple reoperations [25]. Skin pathogens are the most commonly cultured organism, usually *Staphylococcus epidermidis* and *S. aureus* [26]. The introduction of InhibiZone©, a coating consisting of rifampin and minocycline hydrochloride, has led to a reduction in the infection rates in implant surgery [27]. Late infections (>4 months) may represent indolent organisms introduced at the time of operation or by hematogenous spread.

The first initial presentation of an early postoperative AUS infection is usually scrotal pain at the pump, although erythema, edema, and frank purulence will commonly accompany this symptom (Fig. 9.1). Often, these infections may be smoldering and take time to declare themselves. These cases often are seen as chronic pain after AUS implantation often without overt evidence of infection such as induration, swelling, and fever. In these cases we will place the patient on

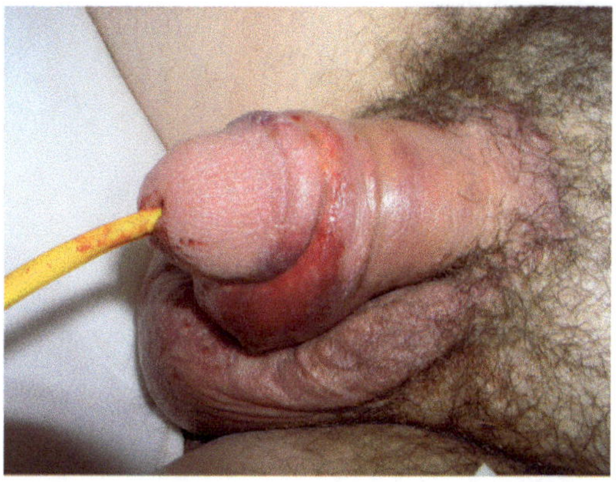

Fig. 9.1 Erythema, edema, and frank purulence will commonly accompany scrotal pain on early postoperative AUS infection

antibiotics that cover gram-positive organisms (oral cephalexin) in addition to an antibiotic that has good penetration of the biofilm layer (rifampin) [28]. Because implant infections are most often not amenable to antibiotic therapy, AUS infection will almost always require explantation. Traditional management includes device removal followed by a waiting period of several months with delayed reimplantation.

Immediate salvage of the infected non-eroded AUS may be accomplished with complete device removal, antiseptic irrigation, and immediate reimplantation [18, 29, 30]. This procedure includes an irrigation regimen used in penile prosthesis salvage protocols [30, 31]. Mulcahy and associates used this approach to salvage 7 of 8 patients with infected non-eroded AUS in a total of 9 operations [30]. In all cases the entire AUS was removed and the wounds were copiously irrigated according to a seven-solution protocol just prior to but during the same operation in that a new system is implanted. This procedure consists of irrigating sequentially with bacitracin and gentamicin in 0.9 % normal saline, half strength hydrogen peroxide, half strength povidine-iodine, pressure irrigation with 1 g vancomycin and 80 mg gentamicin in 5 L of normal saline, half strength povidine-iodine, half strength hydrogen peroxide, bacitracin and gentamicin in 0.9 % normal saline. They also recommend a stepwise approach to the procedure first removing

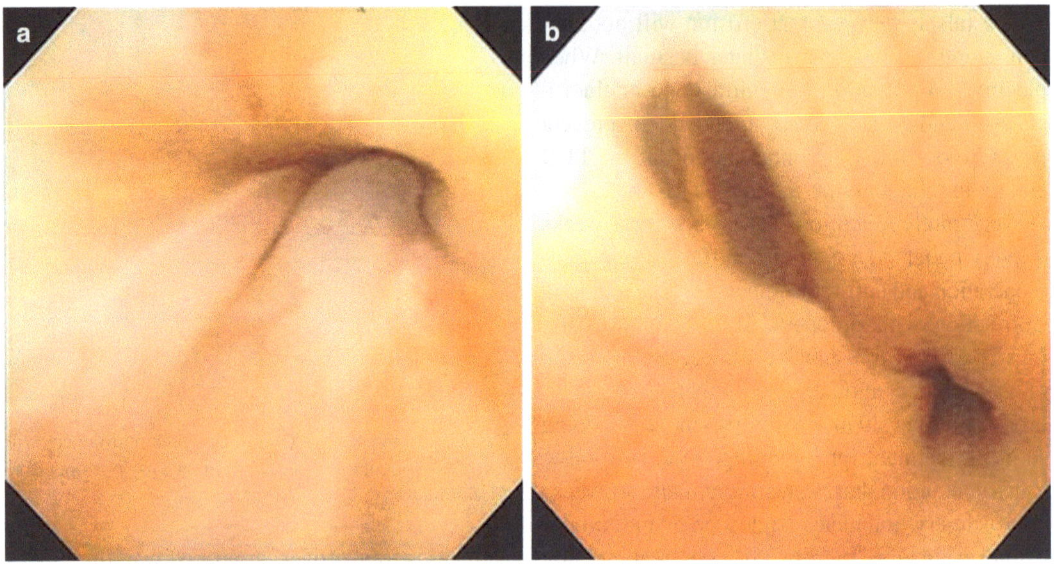

Fig. 9.2 (**a**) Eroded closed AUS. (**b**) Eroded open AUS

all prosthetic parts and foreign material, irrigating with the seven antiseptic solutions as listed above, changing gowns, gloves, surgical drapes and instruments, inserting the new prosthesis, then closing the wounds with no drains or catheters and treating with oral antibiotics for 1 month. Contraindications to prosthesis salvage include sepsis, ketoacidosis, necrotizing infection, immunosuppression, and the finding of gross purulent material at the time of explantation.

Urethral Erosion

Urethral erosion is reported in up to 5 % of AUS implantations [14, 22–24, 32]. In an analysis of their 13-year experience in patients with urethral erosions, Webster and associates determined that patients with hypertension, coronary artery disease, prior radiation therapy, and prior AUS revisions were more than twice as likely to suffer secondary urethral erosions [33]. Furlow introduced the concept of postoperative deactivation during the healing process to decrease pressure-induced ischemia and necrosis [34]. While Motley and Barrett did see a decrease in secondary urethral erosion from 18 to 1.3 % with this technique [35] we have not found this procedure particularly useful in our practice.

Cystoscopy is the diagnostic procedure of choice in evaluating men with suspected AUS erosion. It is indicated in any cases of recurrent urinary tract infections, hematuria, new onset urinary retention, pain with voiding, pain at the AUS pump, and sometimes in cases of prolonged catheterization. Erosion may be subtle with little external manifestations when the AUS has not yet become infected so sometimes one must have a very high index of suspicion whenever there is the possibility of AUS problems. Careful and systematic cystourethroscopy must be performed as some erosions can be very subtle. We perform urethroscopy up to the closed AUS cuff and cycle the cuff under direct vision with full flow of the irrigation in order to aid in the complete evaluation of the site (Fig. 9.2).

Immediate removal of all the components of the AUS is imperative in cases of erosion, because they are assumed to be infected. There is currently a debate on how to appropriately manage the urethra in cases of eroded sphincter cuff. Some authors advocate a formal primary anastomotic urethroplasty if the tissues are amenable. There is some evidence that simple catheter placement, time, and/or suprapubic cystostomy allows healing without subsequent significant stricture formation [18, 36]. Because these erosions are often large and complex (Fig. 9.3),

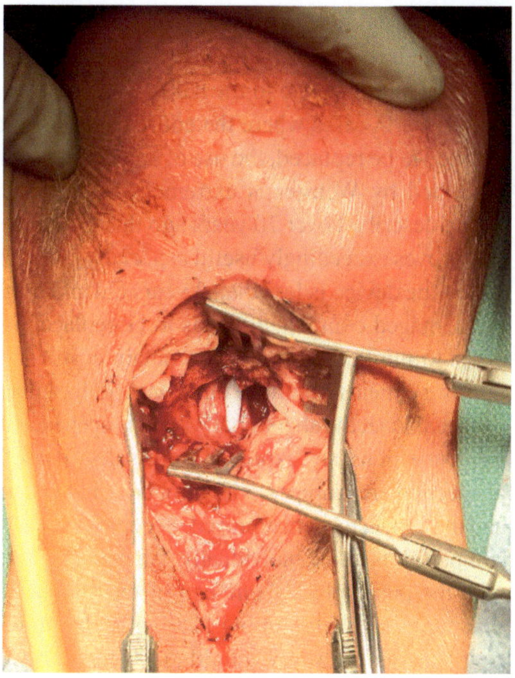

Fig. 9.3 For large and complex erosions, a Foley catheter is left in for 3 weeks with removal after a pericatheter urethrogram shows no extravasation of contrast

we prefer to primarily close the capsule with interrupted fine absorbable suture, leaving a Foley catheter in for 3 weeks with removal after a pericatheter urethrogram shows no extravasation of contrast. Perineal wounds are considered infected and loosely approximated or allowed to close by secondary intention. Reimplantation is considered only after urethral healing is confirmed by urethrography and a delay of 3–6 months is observed.

In preparation for reimplantation, urethral patency is confirmed by cystoscopy or retrograde urethrogram (Fig. 9.4) [31, 35, 37]. A new cuff should be placed in a new location either proximal or distal to the previous site because scarring as well as a compromised vascular supply makes replacement of the cuff at the erosion site difficult and risky [35]. Frank et al. [37] reported a successful outcome in 87 % of reimplantation after erosion or infection, with recurrent urethral erosion in 8.7 %. More recently, in a series of 46 patients with prior AUS erosion who underwent reimplantation, 35 % suffered another erosion

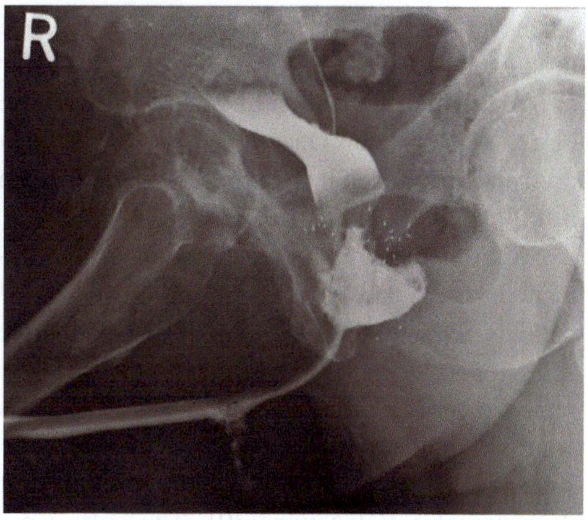

Fig. 9.4 Retrograde urethrogram confirms urethral patency in preparation for reimplantation

within an average of 6.7 months [33]. Use of the transcorporal approach in such cases may reduce the risk of urethral injury during the secondary surgery as well as potentially provide greater protection against subsequent erosion [19, 38].

Urethral Atrophy

Urethral atrophy results from the chronic compression of the spongy tissue under the occlusive cuff. This is the most common reason for revision of the AUS [39]. The evaluation for this must include a combination of the voiding diary, pad test, radiographic evaluation of the cuff in the closed and cycled state and cystourethroscopy to rule out erosion and cuff malfunction. Treatment options include cuff downsizing, movement of the cuff to a more proximal or distal location where the urethra may be thicker, or placement of a second cuff in tandem. In our practice, the simple replacement of the PRB with a higher-pressure reservoir to overcome urethral atrophy is no longer recommended due to risk of erosion [39].

Our approach is to downsize the cuff in the same location when possible. If the existing cuff is already 3.5 cm, we place the cuff more proximally, when feasible, or distally using the transcorporal technique if necessary. Because there are a finite number of locations for the artificial sphincter cuff we attempt to use the same location whenever possible for downsizing. We advance to the smallest size cuff available (3.5 cm) prior to moving to new location or considering the use of a tandem system. Once a single site has been used and abandoned it is no longer safe to replace a cuff at a later time in that same spot.

Saffarian et al. reported a significant improvement in daily pad usage from 3.9 to 0.5 in 17 patients with urethral atrophy [40]. In a large series of secondary AUS surgery, the cuff was replaced in 142 cases of which 33 % of cuffs were placed distal to the original location, 11 % were placed proximal and 52 % were placed at the original cuff location [39]. The cuffs were downsized in 56 % of cases, unchanged in 30 % and upsized in 13 %, reflecting the new locations. In cases of urethral atrophy, several prominent centers have successfully added a second cuff in tandem to salvage continence [15, 16].

Mechanical Failure

The rate of mechanical failure has diminished substantially after introduction of the narrow-backed cuff. Because of the inherent design of the device, when they fail they do so in the open position resulting in recurrent incontinence and rarely urinary retention. Elliott and Barrett [12] reviewed the long-term durability of the AMS 800 in 323 patients that were implanted at the Mayo clinic between 1983 and 1994. The change in design resulted in a decrease in nonmechanical failure from 17 to 9 %. This was thought to be primarily due to a reduction in urethral atrophy. A decrease in mechanical failure from 21 to 7.6 % was primarily thought to be due to a reduction in cuff leak along with improvements in the synthetic material, which lessened the risk of fracture or kinking of the device. In the absence of infection or erosion, replacement of an isolated malfunctioning component of the AUS (pump, cuff, balloon) may be feasible if the revision occurs within 3 years of implantation. However, a slow leak from the PRB may be difficult to diagnose intraoperatively, and if in doubt total device replacement is always recommended. When older than 3 years the entire device should be replaced completely.

Troubleshooting the device in the operating room can be challenging because leaks may often be small and invisible to the naked eye! We have found that in cases where the entire device is not planned to be replaced, the use of an ohmmeter as described by Webster is extremely useful [41]. While described over 20 years ago this technique still proves exceedingly useful especially in cases where the device is less than 3 years old and only the damaged component needs to be replaced in order to minimize morbidity, contain costs, and improve patients' return of functionality. To utilize this technique, the abdominal wound is opened and all connections are exposed. Both sides of each connection are clamped with a rubber shod clamp and the connectors are removed. Sequentially, each component is tested individually. We prefer to start with the pump placing one end of the ohmmeter sensor inside of the tubing leading to the pump so it's in contact with the fluid inside the system. If there is a break in the system, touching the second, grounding probe to the patient's body will elicit a circuit. Any reading on the ohmmeter indicates a leak is present in the system. Each component is sequentially tested in the same manner. One must understand that if a device has leaked all of its fluid that the component may need to be filled with saline in order to produce a circuit.

Special Circumstances

The management of urethral and vesicourethral anastomotic stricture encountered after AUS implantation proposes a unique challenge. Stricture at the site of the AUS cuff may result from compression or ischemia and may indicate impending urethral erosion. These may be managed with periodic filiform and follower dilation [42]. However, strictures proximal to an AUS may need to be addressed with balloon dilation [43] or holmium laser incision through a flexible ureteroscope [44].

In the event significant endoscopic manipulation is required, such as transurethral resection proximal to the cuff site; our practice is to surgically uncouple the cuff for the duration of the endoscopic procedure. In this procedure an incision is

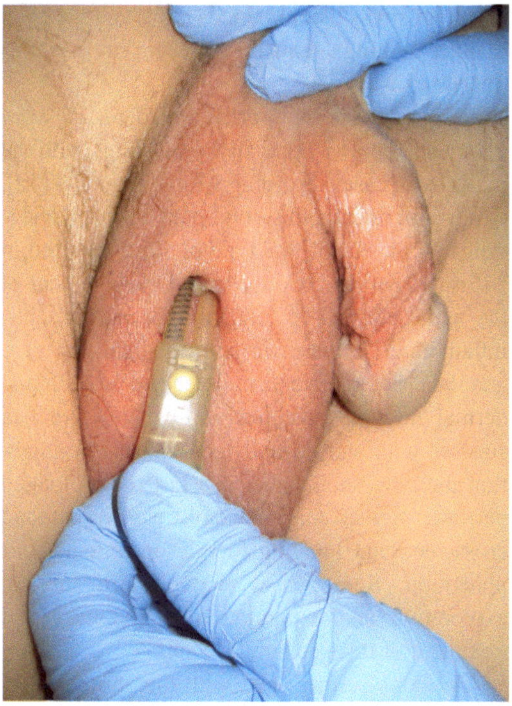

Fig. 9.5 Rarely, a component of the device, such as a pump, may erode through the skin, exposing itself

made over the perineal wound and the urethral cuff is identified and dissected free. After copious irrigation, it is uncoupled allowing unhindered endoscopic access to the urethral pathology proximal to the AUS cuff. During the transurethral portion of the procedure, the perineal wound is packed with an antibiotic-soaked gauze sponge. At the termination procedure, the cuff is reattached ensuring that it is securely fashioned and left deactivated as required. Because of the need to manipulate the device, we prefer to give preoperative antibiotics consisting of vancomycin and gentamycin in these cases.

Component Extrusion

Rarely, a component of the device may erode through the skin, exposing itself. These events are usually associated with a preexisting infection, leading to skin edema and inflammation. Rarely, eroded components may appear relatively benign (Fig. 9.5). In all cases, we recommend immediate removal of all components of the device. Because of the tubing that connects the system as one, it is assumed that once one part of the device is exposed and infected, the entire system is at risk.

Male Slings for Incontinence

Male sling procedures represent a significant addition to the surgical armamentarium for UI by providing an alternative to the AUS [45]. These two procedures; the bone-anchored sling and transobturator sling may be considered in cases with mild incontinence [36].

Bone Anchor Bulbourethral Sling

The bone-anchored sling is performed through a single perineal incision that results in short operative times and low erosion rates [46, 47]. Titanium screws provide fixation of the sling to the inferior pubic ramus. A 4 by 7-cm piece of mesh or organic material is secured to the bone-anchored sutures and then tied down. Sling tension is increased until a retrograde leak pressure of 60 cmH_2O is achieved by checking backflow pressures. While the results of this technique have been generally positive, long-term follow-up has revealed that this procedure is not without problems.

Transobturator Bulbourethral Sling

The transobturator sling has been shown to be effective in short-term follow-up of multiple well-preformed series [48]. In selected populations approximately 75 % of patients are cured or significantly improved, with results durable up to a year. Bulbar urethral slings can be used as an alternative in those that refuse the AUS from fear of infection, erosion, or mechanical failure as well as those with limited physical or cognitive capacity [49]. The trade-off between risk and efficacy must be considered, with most authors recommending the AUS for more severe UI but for mild UI the bulbar sling procedure is a viable alternative.

In contrast to the bone-anchored approach, the transobturator sling is designed to reposition and lengthen the membranous urethra [48]. After exposing the corpus spongiosum in a manner identical to the AUS described above, the space between the corpus spongiosum and corpora cavernosa is developed on each side. Using the provided trocars, the sling is brought through the obturator foramen as close as possible to the superior aspect of the triangle formed by the corpus spongiosum and the pubic ramus. With tensioning, the proximal bulbar urethra should move approximately 3–4 cm cephalad [48]. The tail ends of the sling are trimmed and buried under the skin.

Sling Complications

With the two types of slings now available (the transobturator bulbar urethral sling and the bone-anchored sling) the complication profile for these slings has become slightly more clear. The infection/erosion rate for both types of slings ranges from 2 to 15 % and the need for revision have been previously reported to range 2–4.2 %. While effective as discussed above, both slings have slightly different problems associated with them.

Complications of the Bone-Anchored Sling

The most common complications of the bone-anchored male slings include perineal pain, urinary retention, infection, anchoring complications from bone anchors, and mesh erosion. Styn et al. reported their experience with 119 men who underwent 140 bone-anchored sling for the treatment of male stress incontinence [50]. In this series, the overall complication rate was 58.8 and 26.9 % required reoperation. While the authors did not report any significant intraoperative complications, they do note that recurrent stress incontinence may be as high as 25.2 %, and up to 17.6 % will develop new urge incontinence. Wound infections (16 %) were the most commonly reported immediate postoperative complications. Many patients in this study required reoperation for various reasons including dislodgment of bone screws (5.9 %), revision for recurrent stress incontinence (5 %), and the need to place bulking agents for recurrent stress incontinence (5.9 %).

Perineal pain is reported in up to 74 % of patients [51] after bone-anchored slings with the majority of cases resolving within 3 months [52]. Chronic perineal and scrotal pain has been a significant concern of this type of sling reported in 2–5 % of patients. Conservative management of the pain consists of aggressive use of anti-inflammatories, narcotic pain medications, rest, and time. Some patients may require use of transdermal lidocaine patches and others have had success with steroid and local anesthetic injection therapy. Should the pain last for prolonged periods, greater than 90 days we recommend cross-sectional imaging to rule out infection or phlegmon. Some cases may require surgical exploration and explantation of the mesh for treatment of this problem.

The bone screws used with this system offer their own specific set of problems. As discussed prior, up to 5.9 % of patients will need reoperation because of problems associated with the screws. Dislodgment, bone infection, and pain have all been reported with this type of anchoring system. While these tend to be reported sporadically, this has been a significant issue. Most often these may result in recurrent incontinence [53] and osteitis pubis. Patients should be counseled that when considering the bone-anchored sling that bone infection (osteitis pubis) may require removal of the entire sling along with the involved bone. Cultures of the infected bone should be sent as some patients will require long-term intravenous antibiotics after removal of the hardware.

Wound infections have been reported to occur in 7.9–16 % of cases. These may range from superficial inflammatory conditions to severe deep wound infections needing sling explantation with extensive debridement and wound care. If not treated rapidly, these may lead to erosion into the urethra with significant urethral damage.

Acute urinary retention after surgery occurs in up to 15 % of patients undergoing these slings. In most series these cases resolve with the improvement of postoperative edema on an average of 10–14 days. Isolated cases have required release of the sling.

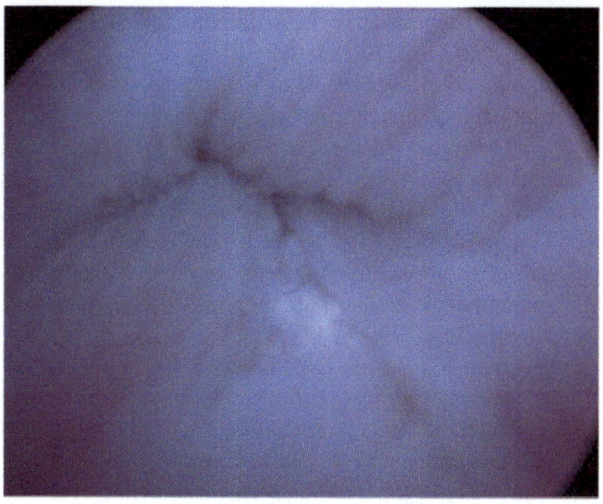

Fig. 9.6 Eroded mesh sling

Transobturator Male Sling

Gaining approval in 2006 and just recently achieving wide scale acceptance, the complications resulting from this device had not previously been well described. In 2009, Bauer and her group reviewed their experience with over 230 patients who underwent placement of the transobturator male sling [54]. After a median follow-up of 17 months, the complication rate was 23.9 %. Interestingly, there were no intraoperative complications such as rectal perforation, bleeding, or urethral and bladder injuries. Postoperative urinary retention was described in 49 patients (21.3 %). Wound infection (0.4 %), urinary tract infections (0.4 %), and persistent perineal pain (0.4 %) were also described. Two patients (0.9 %) had to undergo sling explantation for various reasons including incorrect placement (the authors attributed this to either an erosion into the urethra or an intraoperative urethral injury at the time of placement) and symphisitis thought to be from preexisting Guillain–Barre syndrome.

Others have reported sporadic cases of erosion of the sling into the urethra (Fig. 9.6) [10]. In some cases sling removal with a combined reconstructive procedure such as urethroplasty may be required. While erosion is a theoretically possible event, many of these cases may actually be unrecognized injury at the time of placement of the sling. Therefore, careful systematic cystoscopy with urethroscopy at the time of sling placement is imperative to rule out intraoperative injuries and prevent these cases of erosion.

Of the 49 patients (21.3 %) who presented with acute urinary retention, all except one resolved within 12 weeks (mean 27 days). The one patient who did not begin voiding spontaneously underwent transection of the sling after 4 months which resulted in the ability to void. Because of the high rates of short-term urinary retention that we have observed immediately after surgery, we currently send all patients home with a catheter in place from the anesthesia recovery unit teaching them how to remove it themselves. After initiating this procedure, we have not had any patients returning with urinary retention greater than 24 h after surgery.

The authors did note that they could find no risk factors for postoperative retention when looking at preoperative evaluation. They also note in the discussion that of the 230 patients, only three required reoperation (1.3 %) requiring sling explantation or transection. These results were also verified by Cornu et al. who looked at the results of 102 patients finding similar rates of complications [55]. Overall, these rates are significantly less than those seen with the artificial sphincter or the other urethral compressive slings such as the bone-anchored slings. The patient who presented with a wound infection and febrile urinary tract infection were treated successfully with antibiotics with no further problems or symptoms.

References

1. Abrams P, Cardozo L, Fall M, et al. The standardisation of terminology of lower urinary tract function: report from the Standardisation Sub-committee of the International Continence Society. Neurourol Urodyn. 2002;21(2):167–78.
2. Stanford J, Steophenson R, Coyle L, et al. Prostate Cancer Trends 1973–1995, SEER Program, National Cancer Institute. NIH Pub 99-4543; 1999.
3. Coyne KS, Zhou Z, Thompson C, Versi E. The impact on health-related quality of life of stress, urge and mixed urinary incontinence. BJU Int. 2003;92(7):731–5.
4. Flynn BJ, Webster GD. Evaluation and surgical management of intrinsic sphincter deficiency after radical prostatectomy. Rev Urol. 2004;6(4):180–6.
5. Groutz A, Blaivas JG, Chaikin DC, et al. Noninvasive outcome measures of urinary incontinence and lower

urinary tract symptoms: a multicenter study of micturition diary and pad tests. J Urol. 2000;164(3 Pt 1): 698–701.
6. Dylewski DA, Jamison MG, Borawski KM, Sherman ND, Amundsen CL, Webster GD. A statistical comparison of pad numbers versus pad weights in the quantification of urinary incontinence. Neurourol Urodyn. 2007;26(1):3–7.
7. Erickson BA, Meeks JJ, Roehl KA, Gonzalez CM, Catalona WJ. Bladder neck contracture after retropubic radical prostatectomy: incidence and risk factors from a large single-surgeon experience. BJU Int. 2009;104(11):1615–1619.
8. Krambeck AE, DiMarco DS, Rangel LJ, et al. Radical prostatectomy for prostatic adenocarcinoma: a matched comparison of open retropubic and robot-assisted techniques. BJU Int. 2009;103(4):448–53.
9. Wasson JH, Reda DJ, Bruskewitz RC, Elinson J, Keller AM, Henderson WG. A comparison of transurethral surgery with watchful waiting for moderate symptoms of benign prostatic hyperplasia. The Veterans Affairs Cooperative Study Group on Transurethral Resection of the Prostate. N Engl J Med. 1995; 332(2):75–9.
10. Harris SE, Guralnick ML, O'Connor RC. Urethral erosion of transobturator male sling. Urology. 2009;73(2):443.e19–20.
11. Dalkin BL, Wessells H, Cui H. A national survey of urinary and health related quality of life outcomes in men with an artificial urinary sphincter for post-radical prostatectomy incontinence. J Urol. 2003; 169(1):237–9.
12. Elliott DS, Barrett DM. Mayo Clinic long-term analysis of the functional durability of the AMS 800 artificial urinary sphincter: a review of 323 cases. J Urol. 1998;159(4):1206–8.
13. Wilson SK, Delk JR, Henry GD, Siegel AL. New surgical technique for sphincter urinary control system using upper transverse scrotal incision. J Urol. 2003;169(1):261–4.
14. Montague DK, Angermeier KW. Postprostatectomy urinary incontinence: the case for artificial urinary sphincter implantation. Urology. 2000;55(1):2–4.
15. Brito CG, Mulcahy JJ, Mitchell ME, Adams MC. Use of a double cuff AMS800 urinary sphincter for severe stress incontinence. J Urol. 1993;149(2):283–5.
16. DiMarco DS, Elliott DS. Tandem cuff artificial urinary sphincter as a salvage procedure following failed primary sphincter placement for the treatment of post-prostatectomy incontinence. J Urol. 2003;170(4 Pt 1): 1252–4.
17. O'Connor RC, Gerber GS, Avila D, Chen AA, Bales GT. Comparison of outcomes after single or DOUBLE-CUFF artificial urinary sphincter insertion. Urology. 2003;62(4):723–6.
18. Kowalczyk JJ, Spicer DL, Mulcahy JJ. Erosion rate of the double cuff AMS800 artificial urinary sphincter: long-term followup. J Urol. 1996;156(4):1300–1.
19. Guralnick ML, Miller E, Toh KL, Webster GD. Transcorporal artificial urinary sphincter cuff placement in cases requiring revision for erosion and urethral atrophy. J Urol. 2002;167(5):2075–8.
20. Stone AR, Nguyen M, Tse V. Re: new surgical technique for sphincter urinary control system using upper transverse scrotal incision. J Urol. 2003;170(2 Pt 1): 550–1.
21. Henry GD, Graham SM, Cleves MA, Simmons CJ, Flynn B. Perineal approach for artificial urinary sphincter implantation appears to control male stress incontinence better than the transscrotal approach. J Urol. 2008;179(4):1475–9.
22. Gundian JC, Barrett DM, Parulkar BG. Mayo Clinic experience with use of the AMS800 artificial urinary sphincter for urinary incontinence following radical prostatectomy. J Urol. 1989;142(6):1459–61.
23. Marks JL, Light JK. Management of urinary incontinence after prostatectomy with the artificial urinary sphincter. J Urol. 1989;142(2 Pt 1):302–4.
24. Litwiller SE, Kim KB, Fone PD, White RW, Stone AR. Post-prostatectomy incontinence and the artificial urinary sphincter: a long-term study of patient satisfaction and criteria for success. J Urol. 1996; 156(6):1975–80.
25. Montague DK. The artificial urinary sphincter (AS 800): experience in 166 consecutive patients. J Urol. 1992;147(2):380–2.
26. Licht MR, Montague DK, Angermeier KW, Lakin MM. Cultures from genitourinary prostheses at reoperation: questioning the role of Staphylococcus epidermidis in periprosthetic infection. J Urol. 1995;154(2 Pt 1):387–90.
27. Carson III CC, Mulcahy JJ, Harsch MR. Long-term infection outcomes after original antibiotic impregnated inflatable penile prosthesis implants: up to 7.7 years of followup. J Urol. 2011;185(2):614–8.
28. Choong S, Whitfield H. Biofilms and their role in infections in urology. BJU Int. 2000;86(8):935–41.
29. Bell BB, Mulcahy JJ. Management of cuff erosion of the double cuff artificial urinary sphincter. J Urol. 2000;163(1):85–6.
30. Bryan DE, Mulcahy JJ, Simmons GR. Salvage procedure for infected noneroded artificial urinary sphincters. J Urol. 2002;168(6):2464–6.
31. Kowalczyk JJ, Nelson R, Mulcahy JJ. Successful reinsertion of the artificial urinary sphincter after removal for erosion or infection. Urology. 1996; 48(6):906–8.
32. Singh G, Thomas DG. Artificial urinary sphincter for post-prostatectomy incontinence. Br J Urol. 1996; 77(2):248–51.
33. Raj GV, Peterson AC, Webster GD. Outcomes following erosions of the artificial urinary sphincter. J Urol. 2006;175(6):2186–90.
34. Furlow WL, Barrett DM. Recurrent or persistent urinary incontinence in patients with the artificial urinary sphincter: diagnostic considerations and management. J Urol. 1985;133(5):792–5.
35. Motley RC, Barrett DM. Artificial urinary sphincter cuff erosion. Experience with reimplantation in 38 patients. Urology. 1990;35(3):215–8.

36. Flynn BJ, Webster GD. Evaluation and surgical management of intrinsic sphincter deficiency after radical prostatectomy. Rev Urol. 2004;6(4):180–6.
37. Frank I, Elliott DS, Barrett DM. Success of de novo reimplantation of the artificial genitourinary sphincter. J Urol. 2000;163(6):1702–3.
38. Aaronson DS, Elliott SP, McAninch JW. Transcorporal artificial urinary sphincter placement for incontinence in high-risk patients after treatment of prostate cancer. Urology. 2008;72(4):825–7.
39. Raj GV, Peterson AC, Toh KL, Webster GD. Outcomes following revisions and secondary implantation of the artificial urinary sphincter. J Urol. 2005; 173(4):1242–5.
40. Saffarian A, Walsh K, Walsh IK, Stone AR. Urethral atrophy after artificial urinary sphincter placement: is cuff downsizing effective? J Urol. 2003;169(2):567–9.
41. Webster GD, Sihelnik SA. Troubleshooting the malfunctioning Scott artificial urinary sphincter. J Urol. 1984;131(2):269–72.
42. Debell M, Wessells H. Recurrent bulbar urethral stricture in the region of an artificial urinary sphincter. J Urol. 2001;166(3):1006–7.
43. Westney OL, Del Terzo MA, McGuire EJ. Balloon dilation of posterior urethral stricture secondary to radiation and cryotherapy in a patient with a functional artificial urethral sphincter. J Endourol. 1999; 13(8):585–6.
44. Anger JT, Raj GV, Delvecchio FC, Webster GD. Anastomotic contracture and incontinence after radical prostatectomy: a graded approach to management. J Urol. 2005;173(4):1143–6.
45. Comiter CV. Surgery Insight: surgical management of postprostatectomy incontinence—the artificial urinary sphincter and male sling. Nat Clin Pract Urol. 2007;4(11):615–24.
46. Comiter CV. The male sling for stress urinary incontinence: a prospective study. J Urol. 2002;167(2 Pt 1): 597–601.
47. Madjar S, Jacoby K, Giberti C, et al. Bone anchored sling for the treatment of post-prostatectomy incontinence. J Urol. 2001;165(1):72–6.
48. Rehder P, Gozzi C. Transobturator sling suspension for male urinary incontinence including post-radical prostatectomy. Eur Urol. 2007;52(3):860–6.
49. Kumar A, Litt ER, Ballert KN, Nitti VW. Artificial urinary sphincter versus male sling for post-prostatectomy incontinence—what do patients choose? J Urol. 2009;181(3):1231–5.
50. Styn NR, McGuire EJ, Latini JM. Bone-anchored sling for male stress urinary incontinence: assessment of complications. Urology. 2011;77(2):469–73.
51. Giberti C, Gallo F, Schenone M, Cortese P, Ninotta G. The bone anchor suburethral synthetic sling for iatrogenic male incontinence: critical evaluation at a mean 3-year followup. J Urol. 2009;181(5):2204–8.
52. Comiter CV. The male perineal sling: intermediate-term results. Neurourol Urodyn. 2005;24(7): 648–53.
53. Mahdy A, Elmissiry M, Ghoniem G. Recurrent stress urinary incontinence after dislodged screws in patient with bone-anchored suburethral sling. Urology. 2008;72(5):1185.e11–3.
54. Bauer RM, Mayer ME, May F, et al. Complications of the advance transobturator male sling in the treatment of male stress urinary incontinence. Urology. 2010;75(6):1494–8.
55. Cornu JN, Sebe P, Ciofu C, et al. The advance transobturator male sling for postprostatectomy incontinence: clinical results of a prospective evaluation after a minimum follow-up of 6 months. Eur Urol. 2009; 56(6):923–7.

Stem Cells for the Treatment of Stress Urinary Incontinence

10

Ervin Kocjancic, Karan Motiani, and Jaspreet Joneja

Stress urinary incontinence (SUI) is the most common form of urinary incontinence, which affects approximately 200 million people worldwide [1]. SUI is defined as the involuntary loss of urine associated with physical activities that increase intra-abdominal and bladder pressure. Intrinsic urethral rhabdosphincter deficiency and urethral hypermobility are the most commonly cited etiologies of SUI, which are targets for treatment [1, 2]. Current treatment modalities include pharmacotherapy, injectable bulking agents, pelvic floor muscle therapy, weight loss, and slings [3]. The current standards of care have varying rates of success, failure, and significant side effect profiles that differ from patient to patient. As a result, there has been a push for new therapies to treat SUI. One of the most promising areas of current research into SUI therapy is the use of stem cell-based therapy for urethral rhabdosphincter regeneration as current research shows that age-related apoptosis of the sphincter is a predominant etiology of SUI.

Briefly, stem cells are undifferentiated cells that have the ability to self-renew or differentiate based upon the organism's needs. Self-renewal occurs to ensure that the stem cell population is maintained while differentiation occurs in order to produce more specialized cells that can be used for necessary biological functions. Furthermore, there are two broad types of stem cells: embryonic and adult. Embryonic stem cells (ESCs) are obtained from the inner cell mass of embryonic blastocysts and have the greatest ability to differentiate into many tissue types. The use of these cells is challenging due to ethical and regulatory issues. Adult stem cells are obtainable from various tissues such as bone marrow stroma, muscle, adipose, and blood but are limited in their abilities to differentiate into various tissue types [4]. The benefit with these cells is derived from the ease with which they are obtained as well as the lack of regulatory issues. Once obtained, the cells are cultivated in a laboratory-based environment where they can be grown, replicated, and selected for the desired cell type. Once the selected cell type is extracted, it must be reimplanted in the desired location where regenerative repair will occur [4].

With regard to SUI therapy, the goal of treatment is to cause regenerative repair of the deficient urethral rhabdosphincter by using stem cells to replace, repair, and enhance the biological function of the damaged tissue [4]. Adult stem

E. Kocjancic, M.D. (✉)
Department of Urology, Pelvic Health and Reconstructive Urology, College of Medicine, University of Illinois at Chicago, 722 W. Maxwell St. Suite 224, Chicago, IL 60607, USA
e-mail: ervkoc@gmail.com

K. Motiani, M.D.
Department of Surgery, University of Cincinnati, College of Medicine, Cincinnati, OH, USA

J. Joneja, M.D.
Department of Urology, University of Illinois at Chicago, Chicago, IL, USA

G.H. Badlani (ed.), *Minimally Invasive Therapy for Urinary Incontinence and Pelvic Organ Prolapse*, Current Clinical Urology, DOI 10.1007/978-1-4939-0008-4_10,

cells are of the greatest interest in current research studies due to aforementioned reasons. Additionally, adult stem cells can differentiate into myogenic cells that are transplantable back into the host that they were harvested from. Bone marrow stromal cells have been cited as a common source of multipotent mesenchymal adult stem cells. These cells are able to differentiate into adipogenic, osteogenic, chondrogenic, and, most importantly, myogenic cells [4]. The limitations of using this source are the pain and complications associated with procurement. Furthermore, the yield of myogenic cells from bone marrow has been shown to be lower than other sources [5]. Adipose-derived stem cells have gained much attention as these cells are relatively easy to harvest from fat tissues and can differentiate into adipogenic, chodrogenic, osteogenic, myogenic, and neurogenic cells. When transplanted, these cells can act as bulking agents as well as induce myogenic regeneration [5]. The final source of adult stem cells that is commonly used in SUI therapy is muscle-derived. These cells are taken from muscle biopsies that can be performed with local anesthesia. The cell types that can be obtained from this source include myoblasts, satellite cells, muscle progenitor cells, and muscle-derived stem cells [4]. Periurethral transplantation of these cells allows for formation of new myofibers and innervations due to the release of neurotrophins [4]. The limitations of using these types of cells include poor survival of injected cells, which is currently being investigated in the literature [1].

Why Stem Cells

In the last decade the use of human stem cells has been presented as a potential breakthrough in the treatment of several different types of lower urinary tract diseases. The regenerative medicine held great expectations in the treatment of functional disorders of lower urinary tract system such as urinary incontinence, neurogenic bladder, and urethral trauma. While these approaches hold much promise, the practical results and treatments available to patients have been slow to materialize. We did not see the rapid translation of research done in the labs into the clinical treatments.

The initial concept of cell-based therapy for SUI was based on the hypothesis that injection of skeletal myoblasts into a dysfunctional urethra could "recharge" the sphincter muscle [6]. The further evolution was the injection of stem cells derived from skeletal muscle cells. In 2002 Yiou et al. published their results on skeletal-derived stem cells injection in a murine model of urethral sphincter lesion [7]. These initial results were followed by other preclinical and clinical studies (Table 10.1). The next step was represented by the utilization of nonskeletal stem cells such as those derived from adipose tissue or stem cells derived from bone marrow [8].

Sources of Stem Cells

There are two groups of stem cells that have been investigated for a clinical use. They are the pluripotent ESCs and the multipotent adult stem cells. Due to ethical concerns and the possible teratogenicity, the use of ESC has been limited in most of Western Europe and North America.

The adult, somatic, stem cells can be obtained from any vascularized tissue as it is currently thought that they constitute the pericytes of the vessels within the tissue [9]. The common donor sites for adult stem cells are the bone marrow, the skeletal muscle, and the adipose tissue. Each of the above sources has advantages and limitations as summarized in the schematic below.

Bone Marrow

Bone marrow has three types of Stem cells [10]: hemopoietic, endothelial, and mesenchymal (potentially useful for SUI regenerative therapy). The advantages are that they are easy to isolate, easy to cultivate, multipotent, and leak of MHC class I cell surface marker (invisible to the host immune system and as such can potentially be used as "Universal" cells from one donor to a different recipient). Disadvantages are that a bone

Table 10.1 Clinical trials for stem cell use in stress urinary incontinence

Study	Patients	Stem cell type	Administration method	Follow-up
Se`be P, Doucet C et al.	12 females	Autologous mesenchyme-derived stem cells (MDSC)	Intrasphincteric injection	1 year: 3 patients dry, 7 patients improved on 24 h pad test but not on voiding diary, 2 patients slightly worse
Lee CN, Jang JB et al.	39 females	Allogenic human umbilical cord blood stem cells	Urethral submucosal injection	1 year: the effectiveness was similar to conventional bulking agents
Herschorn S, Carr L et al.	29 females	Autologous MDSCs	Intrasphincteric injections; two doses given	1 year: showing 50 % success rate with no leakage
Mitterberger A, Pinggera GM et al.	20 females	Skeletal muscle-derived autologous fibroblasts and myoblasts	Transurethral U/S-guided injections of fibroblasts into urethral submucosa and myoblasts into sphincter	1 year: 18/20 patients were cured while the remaining 2 were improved. 2 years: 16/20 were still cured, 2 others were improved, 2 lost to follow up
Carr LK, Steele D et al.	8 females	Autologous MDSC	Transurethral injection	1 year: 1/8 cured, 5/8 improved, no serious adverse reactions reported
Strasser H, Marksteiner R et al.	42 females	Autologous myoblasts and fibroblasts from skeletal muscle	TUUS-guided injection into rhabdosphincter	1 year: 38/42 completely continent
Blaganje M, Lukanović A et al.	38 females	Autologous myoblast from skeletal muscle	Ultrasound-guided injection into the external urethral sphincter followed by electrical stimulation (ES)	6 week: 78.4 % had negative urinary stress test, 13.5 % considered themselves cured

marrow biopsy is required to harvest the cells, and they represent only a small % of cells in the bone marrow.

Muscle-Derived Stem Cells

Muscle-derived stem cells have the advantages of being easy to harvest (simple muscular biopsy and they have good integration with host muscle tissue. Disadvantage include that it is difficult to obtain a sufficient number of stem cells and keep the cells alive after the transplant. The process requires a specific plating technique and cell expansion technique. It is also a time-consuming process (up to 6 weeks are required from the harvesting to the reimplantation of the stem cells). Also, they express the surface antigens (only autologous transplant is possible).

Adipose-Derived Stem Cells

Advantages are that they are easy to harvest (simple liposuction) and large numbers of multipotent cells are present in the adipose tissue. Disadvantages are that they are difficult to manage, have less favorable homing and implantation, and they express the surface antigens (only autologous transplant is possible).

Are Stem Cells Safe?

Many of the earliest stem cell studies were conducted on cells isolated from tumors rather than from embryos. Of particular interest was research on embryonic carcinoma cells (EC), a type of stem cell derived from teratocarcinoma. The EC research laid the foundation for the later discovery of and subsequent work on ESC. Both ESCs isolated from the mouse (mESCs) and then later from humans (hESCs) shared not only pluripotency with their EC cousins, but also robust tumorigenicity as each readily form teratoma. Surprisingly, decades after the discovery of mESCs, the question of what drives ESCs to form tumors remains largely an open one. This gap in the field is particularly serious as stem cell tumorigenicity represents the key obstacle to the safe use of stem cell-based regenerative medicine therapies [11].

The molecular basis of the tumorigenicity of pluripotent cells lies in their cancer-resembling properties, namely their ability to self-renew and proliferate, lack of contact inhibition, and telomerase activity which are promoted by several molecular processes and have been described in detail by Blum and Benvenisty [12, 13]. On closer examination of the karyotype of ESCs, polyploidy has been observed in mESCs despite an intact spindle assembly checkpoint (SAC) [14]; Mantel and co-workers demonstrated that mESCs and hESCs have an intact SAC, but that mitotic failure-induced polyploidy does not lead to apoptosis of these cells. Mitotic errors often occur in rapidly proliferating cells and the SAC, typically leading to apoptosis of these cells and the necessity for genome maintenance. Uncoupling of this mechanism will lead to karyotypic abnormalities in ESC culture. In addition, when inducing double-strand breaks in the DNA of mouse ESCs and mouse embryoid bodies (EBs) by the DNA-damaging agent etoposide, ESCs were resistant to apoptosis whereas the EBs underwent caspase-3-dependent apoptosis. This suggests that polyploidy tolerance in ESCs will give way to apoptosis upon lineage-specific differentiation. This hypothesis has been confirmed for mouse as well as human mononuclear polyploid/aneuploid cells, indicating that checkpoint–apoptosis uncoupling is an intrinsic behavior of mESCs and hESCs [15].

The examination of gene expression in several human tumors has shown that the pluripotency markers used in reprogramming somatic cells to induced pluripotent stem cells (iPSCs) are directly oncogenic (e.g., c-*Myc* and *Klf4*) or are involved in tumorigenesis (e.g., *Sox2*, *Nanog*, and *Oct3/4*). Targets of *Nanog*, *Sox2*, and *Oct4* that encode for transcription regulators are overexpressed and prove especially active in high-grade breast tumors [11, 16]. Upregulation of *Nanog* and *Oct4* is also associated with poor outcomes in patients with oral cancer [17, 18]. The pluripotent genes *Oct3/4*, *Sox2*, *Nanog*, c-*Myc*, and *Klf4* were also present in prostate tumor cell lines, as well as in primary prostate tumor tissue. Furthermore, injection of these tumor cells containing the pluripotent genes created strong tumorigenicity in immunodeficient mice [19].

The biological link between pluripotency and tumorigenicity can perhaps best be described by c-*Myc*. Although not required for the induction of pluripotency in iPSCs, c-*Myc* augments the reprogramming ability of *Oct4*, *Sox2*, and *Klf4*, inhibits differentiation, and promotes proliferation. Myc proteins have been shown to influence several thousand genes. The majority of these are upregulated and involved in cell growth; the few genes that are downregulated are involved in cell cycle arrest, cell adhesion, and cell–cell communication. The influence of *Myc* on these nuclear processes is oncogenic [20, 21].

However, not all members of the *Myc* family possess the same properties. L-*Myc*, for instance, has a decreased transformation activity and only few human cancers are associated with an aberrant expression of L-*Myc*. A recent study reported the creation of iPSCs with L-*Myc* instead of c-*Myc* and chimeric mice derived from these L-*Myc* iPSCs showed reduced tumorigenicity [19].

Recently, 21 genes were found to be highly expressed in hESCs as well as in teratomas [13]. These genes were then credited as known oncogenes, if they were involved in cell cycle progression, inhibition of apoptosis, signal transduction, transcription, or translation. Of these 21 genes, *Survivin* (*BIRC5*) was found to be the strongest candidate gene. *Survivin* is an anti-apoptotic gene that is also involved in mitotic regulation and is expressed in the majority of cancers [22]. It was highly expressed in hESCs and teratomas and downregulated in mature EBs [23].

From these insights into the gene expression of hESCs and iPSCs, it can be concluded that tumor formation is not dependent on the presence of EC-like cells, but is more an intrinsic property of pluripotent cells. Furthermore, this tumorigenicity of pluripotent cells is reduced upon differentiation. The dilemma now facing investigators is that in reducing the tumorigenicity of stem cells, the very essence of stem cells that makes them useful also has to be reduced, namely self-renewal and pluripotency. The "best" ESCs are often considered to be those that grow fairly rapidly, form tightly packed colonies, have a low rate of spontaneous differentiation, and are readily passageable. The simplest way to slow or even eliminate the tumorigenicity of normal stem cells prior to transplantation may be to take advantage of their natural "brakes" or pluripotency by partially differentiating them into progenitors [24].

Introduction of a Stem Cell-Specific Suicide Gene

The stable genetic introduction of a suicide gene such as thymidine kinase (tk) into stem cells has been reported to be effective in combination with Ganciclovir (*Gan*) treatment [25].

Directed Killing of Residual Stem Cells Based on a Nongenetic Method

The most promising approach to this end is to use killer antibodies directed against antigens present on the surface of hESC such as SSEA-4 or a member of the TRA family [26].

Use Stem Cells Themselves for Transplant, but First Eliminate Tumor Forming Potential Without Genetic Modification

In theory, the simplest approach to regenerative medicine and the one expected to lead to robust regenerative tissue growth would seem to be to use stem cells themselves, but ones that had been treated in such a way that they were no longer tumorigenic [27].

Clinical Experience

Once the tissue is harvested, the stem cells are isolated and proliferated in the lab and the cells have to be reinjected in the patients' body.

In the literature several different options have been presented:

- Transurethral injection
- Peri urethral injection
- Ultrasound-guided transurethral injection into the striated sphincter,
- Ultrasound-guided injection followed by electrical stimulation.

The different options are summarized in Table 10.1.

In the past, one major problem and limitation in these therapies, regardless of the source of stem cells, is represented by the poor survival of the injected cells [28]. These problems have partially been solved with new seeding technique such as pre-plating and the use of specific growth factors [29].

The working principles on how stem cells can restore the damaged urethral sphincter function are still not completely clear. For instance, research in animal suggests urethral recovery after injection of bone marrow-derived mesenchymal stem cell secretions as after injection of paracrine factors of the stem cells themselves. Therefore, weather the improvement results from the injection of the stem cells or from their secretion of specific proteins is unclear [30]. This might actually represent a possibility for future treatment of SUI. Some authors are speculating that in the future some patients may have SUI prevented with immediate postpartum injection of "off the shelf" proteins into the urethra, while others who have already developed SUI may undergo injection of genes to reawaken the homing potential of the damaged tissue, or undergo a small biopsy and return few weeks later to for injection of stem cells into the urethra.

The use of growth factor that regulates the proliferation and differentiation of skeletal myoblasts to promote healing seems fascinating in the process of enhancing healing process. However, their short biologic half-lives, the rapid clearance of these molecules from the circulation, and the difficulty to maintain a sufficient concentration in the specific anatomic side is currently preventing from its routine clinical use [29].

Conclusion

Currently, midurethral tapes represent the gold standard in the treatment of SUI. The tapes, regardless of the route through which they are deployed, restore the supporting function of ligaments and fascia structure that stabilize urethra during sudden increase in the intra-abdominal pressure. Despite excellent success rates the tapes are not risk-free. One of the concerns with these procedures is related to the fact that the vast majority of the slings are made of polypropylene and are currently under FDA scrutiny. The stem cells injected in the urethra have the potential to restore the functional, contractile response of the striated sphincter. The potential advantage is enormous as this therapy could treat SUI with a minimal risk. The initial results are promising; however, there are many questions that remain unanswered. Larger and longer clinical trials are necessary to move from a promising cure to the new gold standard and a permanent cure of SUI.

References

1. Nikolavsky D, Chancellor MB. Stem cell therapy for stress urinary incontinence. Neurourol Urodyn. 2010;29:S36–41.
2. Lin C, Lue TF. Stem cell therapy for stress urinary incontinence: a critical review. Stem Cells Dev. 2012;21(6):834–43.
3. Cameron A, Haraway AM. The treatment of female stress urinary incontinence: an evidenced-based review. Res Rep Urol. 2011;3(1):109–20. http://dx.doi.org/10.2147/RRUS10541.
4. Smaldone MC, Chancellor MB. Muscle derived stem cell therapy for stress urinary incontinence. World J Urol. 2008;26(4):327–32.
5. Ho CP, Bhatia NN. Development of stem cell therapy for stress urinary incontinence. Curr Opin Obstet Gynecol. 2012;24(5):311–7.
6. Chancellor MB, Yokoyama S, Tirney S, Matteas CE, Ozawa H, Yoshimura N, de Groat WC. Preliminary results of myoblasts injection into the urethra and bladder wall: a possible method for treatment of stress urinary incontinence and impaired detrusor contractility. Neurourol Urodyn. 2000;19:279–87.
7. Yiou R, Dreyfus P, Chopin DK, Abbou CC, Lefaucher JP. Muscle precursor cell autografting in a murine model of urethral sphincter injury. BJU Int. 2002;89:298–302.
8. Yamamoto T, Gotoh M, Hattori R, Toriyama K, Kamei Y, Iwaguro H, Matsukawa Y, Funahashi Y. Periurethral injection of autologous adipose-derived stem cells for treatment of stress urinary incontinence in patients undergoing radical prostatectomy: report of two initial cases. Int J urol. 2010;17:75–82.
9. Meirelles L, Fontes AM, Covas DT, et al. Mechanisms involved in the therapeutic properties of mesenchymal stem cells. Cytokine Growth Factor Rev. 2009;20:419–27.
10. Stem cell treatment- Stem cell research- stem cell therapy. Stemcelltreatments.org. http://www.stemcelltreatment.org/.
11. Knoepfler PS. 2009 Deconstructing stem cell tumorigenicity: a roadmap to safe regenerative medicine. Stem Cells. 2009;27(5):1050–6.
12. Blum B, Benvenisty N. The tumorigenicity of human embryonic stem cells. Adv Cancer Res. 2008;100:133–58.
13. Blum B, Benvenisty N. The tumorigenicity of diploid and aneuploid human pluripotent stem cells. Cell Cycle. 2009;8:3822–30.
14. Malashicheva AB, Kisliakova TV, Savatier P, Pospelov VA. Embryonal stem cells do not undergo cell cycle arrest upon exposure to damaging factors. Tsitologiia. 2002;44:643–8.
15. Mantel C, et al. Checkpoint-apoptosis uncoupling in human and mouse embryonic stem cells: a source of karyotypic instability. Blood. 2007;109:4518–27.
16. Palma I, Peña R-Y, Contrerasb A, Ceballos-Reyesc G, Coyoteb N, Erañab L, Kofman-Alfaroa S, Queipoa G. Participation of OCT3/4 and b-catenin during dysgenetic gonadal malignant transformation. Cancer Lett. 2008;263:204–11.
17. Ben-Porath I, Thomson MW, Carey VJ, Ge R, Bell GW, Regev A, Weinberg RA. An embryonic stem cell-like gene expression signature in poorly differentiated aggressive human tumors. Nat Genet. 2008;40:499–507.
18. Chiou S-H, et al. Positive correlations of Oct-4 and Nanog in oral cancer stem-like cells and high-grade oral squamous cell carcinoma. Clin Cancer Res. 2008;14:4085–95.
19. Bae KM, et al. Expression of pluripotent stem cell reprogramming factors by prostate tumor initiating cells. J Urol. 2010;183:2045–53.
20. Takahashi K, Tanabe K, Ohnuki M, Narita M, Ichisaka T, Tomoda K, Yamanaka S. Induction of pluripotent stem cells from adult human fibroblasts by defined factors. Cell. 2007;131:861–72.
21. Eilers M, Eisenman RN. Myc's broad reach. Genes Dev. 2008;22:2755–66.

22. Ambrosini G, Adida C, Altieri DC. A novel antiapoptosis gene, survivin, expressed in cancer and lymphoma. Nat Med. 1997;3:917–21.
23. Blum B, Bar-Nur O, Golan-Lev T, Benvenisty N. The anti-apoptotic gene survivin contributes to teratoma formation by human embryonic stem cells. Nat Biotechnol. 2009;27:281–7.
24. Brederlau A, Correia AS, Anisimov SV, et al. Transplantation of human embryonic stem cell-derived cells to a rat model of Parkinson's disease: effect of in vitro differentiation on graft survival and teratoma formation. Stem Cells. 2006;24: 1433–40.
25. Schuldiner M, Itskovitz-Eldor J, Benvenisty N. Selective ablation of human embryonic stem cells expressing a 'suicide' gene. Stem Cells. 2003;21: 257–65.
26. Choo AB, Tan HL, Ang SN, et al. Selection against undifferentiated human embryonic stem cells by a cytotoxic antibody recognizing podocalyxin-like protein-1. Stem Cells. 2008;26:1454–63.
27. Alvarnas JC, Forman SJ. Graft purging in autologous bone marrow transplantation: a promise not quite fulfilled. Oncology. 2004;18:867–76.
28. Qu Z, Bakir L, van Deutekom JC, Robins PD. Development of approaches to improve cell survival in myoblast transfer therapy. J Cell Biol. 1998;142: 1257–67.
29. Florini JR, Ewton DZ, Magri KA. Hormons, growth factors and myogenic differentiation. Annu Rev Physyol. 1991;53:201–16.
30. Goldman HB, Sievert KD, Damser M. Will we ever use stem cells for the Treatment of SUI: ICI-RS 2011. Neurourol Urodyn. 2012;31:386–9.

11 Treatment of Overactive Bladder Refractory to Medications

Rajveer S. Purohit and Jerry G. Blaivas

Approach to Management

Conservative therapy for overactive bladder (OAB) has been shown to be a viable stand alone or adjunctive option to antimuscarinic agents (AMAs). Typically nonsurgical options such as behavioral therapy, pelvic floor muscle therapy (PFMT), and biofeedback have been recommended prior to more invasive options such as electrical stimulation, intravesical Botox, or augmentation enterocystoplasty, ileovesicostomy, and urinary diversion. We believe this standard step-wise algorithmic approach to treatment is reasonable, but in some instances may subject patients to unnecessary expense and delay in treatment. Rather, we prefer to individualize our approach to maximize the likelihood of success in each patient while appropriately weighing relative risks with potential benefits. So, for example, a patient with severe neurogenic OAB refractory to AMA may opt for augmentation cystoplasty rather than intradetrusor injection of Botox or neuromodulation.

Treatment of associated conditions such as prostatic obstruction in men or vault prolapse in women should be considered prior to starting a nonsurgical regimen for OAB. When referred a patient with OAB refractory to AMAs, clinicians should begin a thorough history with a detailed account of the nature of the patient's urinary symptoms with each symptom characterized and quantified as accurately as possible by the patient. A physical exam may help elucidate refractory causes of OAB; for example, many patients may report unsuccessful treatment of OAB symptoms with AMAs by their primary doctor, but may be unaware that they have pelvic prolapse causing urethral obstruction that causes the OAB symptoms. Questionnaires, bladder diaries, and pad tests (for incontinent patients) are also useful.

In patients with OAB refractory to AMAs we believe that cystoscopy and videourodynamics (VUD) should be considered to look for (1) remediable causes of OAB (urethral obstruction, urethral diverticulum, bladder cancer, etc.) and (2) to classify the Type of OAB. A VUD-based classification system can help determine which patients would maximally benefit from BT and PFMT [1]. In this system, *Type 1* OAB refers to sensory urgency in which patients essentially have a normal VUD without evidence of involuntary

R.S. Purohit, M.D., M.P.H. (✉)
Department of Urology, Weill Cornell Medical College of Cornell University, 445 E. 77th Street, New York, NY 10075, USA
e-mail: rajpu@yahoo.com

J.G. Blaivas, M.D.
Department of Urology, Weill Cornell Medical College of Cornell University, 445 E. 77th Street, New York, NY 10075, USA

Department of Urology, SUNY Downstate College of Medicine, Brooklyn, NY, USA

Institute for Bladder and Prostate Research, New York, NY, USA

G.H. Badlani (ed.), *Minimally Invasive Therapy for Urinary Incontinence and Pelvic Organ Prolapse*, Current Clinical Urology, DOI 10.1007/978-1-4939-0008-4_11,

detrusor contractions but complain of urinary urgency. *Type 2* refers to patients whose urgency can be correlated to a VUD finding of involuntary detrusor contractions but who are able to prevent incontinence by contracting their urinary sphincter. *Type 3* refers to those patients who are able to contract their sphincter in response to an involuntary bladder contraction but are ultimately unable to abort the contraction and prevent incontinence. *Type 4* refers to those patients who are either unaware or completely unable to prevent any incontinence from developing during a bladder contraction. For patients with Type 1 OAB, behavioral modification will both identify behavioral patterns and external stimuli that trigger the sensory urgency and teach patients to modify it. Type 2 and Type 3 OAB patients can be instructed with the aid of BT and PFMT to identify the onset of a detrusor contraction and contract their striated sphincter in response. For Type 2 patients, who are ideal candidates for BT, this will often cause the contraction to subside preventing incontinence and decreasing urinary frequency; in Type 3 patients, the sphincteric contraction may provide enough of a time window to urinate in the bathroom. BT and PFMT are rarely successful in Type 4 patients.

Surgical treatment of OAB is considered under two circumstances: when there is an underlying remediable condition, and when the OAB symptoms have proven refractory to nonsurgical treatments. For refractory OAB unassociated with a remedial condition, Botox injections, neuromodulation, enterocystoplasty, and urinary diversion may be considered.

Behavioral Therapy

Behavioral therapy (BT) is a process of teaching patients to measure and empirically alter observable behaviors that cause or exacerbate their OAB symptoms. There is consensus among experts that it is effective [2] and may be even more effective than AMAs [3]. The use of behavioral therapy in conjunction with AMAs may be more efficacious than either therapy alone [4, 5]. BT is most often used when the etiology of OAB is unknown, but it may also be effective when OAB is secondary to an underlying condition such as prostatic obstruction or even neurogenic conditions such as multiple sclerosis or Parkinson's disease [6]. But successful outcomes require a motivated patient committed to the regimen prescribed by the behavioral therapist which can sometimes require substantial changes in behavior.

BT should begin with a careful history, which is crucial in understanding potential behavioral influences on OAB. The patient should be queried in regard to his daytime and nocturnal urinary patterns and his or her ability to postpone micturition once an urge develops. Causes for voiding (e.g., severe urgency or convenience voiding) and contributing factors such as caffeine usage should also be determined.

The primary tools used to measure outcomes and evaluate the nature and severity of OAB symptoms is the 24-h bladder diary whose reproducibility has been previously confirmed (Fig. 11.1) [7, 8]. The diary measures the volume and time of each void and annotates associated symptoms. The bladder diary that we prefer, also records the reason for and the severity of urgency for each void—the urge perception score (Table 11.1) [9]. It can distinguish polyuria with normal volume voids from patients who effectively have a small bladder capacity. For patients who complain of OAB symptoms and are found to have polyuria, fluid restriction may be sufficient to alleviate symptoms, but changing ingrained behaviors can be difficult and diaries can assess the degree of compliance with fluid restriction. Critical for behavioral modification, repeat diaries provide data on the effects that changes to variables, such as caffeine, may have on urination.

Behavioral modification can be used for patients with both sensory urgency without detrusor overactivity (DO) and those with DO. For patients with sensory urgency, without DO, the diary helps to determine at what volume the patient experiences symptoms; and the patient can be taught to void prior to reaching that volume. In addition because many external variables such as caffeine and spicy foods or stress may trigger urinary urgency in these patients, the 24-h bladder

Fig. 11.1 Twenty four-hour OAB bladder diary

a

Uro-Center of New York
Phone: (212) 772-3900 Fax: (212) 772-1919

Name: ______________________________ Date: ______________

Time of Day Diary Started: ___________ AM PM

Time you went to bed __________ Time you got up for the day __________

Time of Urination and /or Incontinence episode	Why did you urinate at this time? (see question # (a) for responses)	Amount of Urination (measure with a cup in cc's, ml's or ounces)	Incontinence (place an X in the box if you were incontinent)
1			
2			
3			
4			
5			
6			
7			
8			
9			
10			
11			
12			
13			
14			
15			

b

Please select the number next to your answer and use it for your response to the above questions.

(a) **Why did you urinate?** (b) **Incontinence grade.**
(0) out of convenience (no urge or desire) **(0)** Grade **0**: no urine loss
(1) because I have a mild urge **(1)** Grade **1**: some drops
(but can delay urination for over **(2)** Grade **2**: moderate loss (wet underpants)
an hour if I have to) **(3)** Grade **3**: extensive loss (wet outer clothes)
(2) because I have a moderate urge
(but can delay urination for more than
10 but less than 60 minutes if I have to)
(3) because I have a severe urge
(but can delay urination for less than 10 minutes)
(4) because I have desperate urge
(must stop what I am doing and go immediately)

OFFICE USE
Total 24 hrs output __________ # of voids ____________ MVV = ______

Day volume _________ # voids Night volume __________ # voids _______ NPI _____

Table 11.1 Case report—before and after BT bladder diaries

	Pre-BT	Post-BT
24 h voided volume (mL)	2,640	1,320
Daytime voided volume (mL)	730	1,080
Nighttime voided volume (mL)	380	240
Total 24 h # voids	11	6
# Daytime voids	8	6
# Night voids	3	1
Maximum voided volume (mL)	250	360
# Incontinent episodes	3	0
# Urgency episodes	4	0

diary in conjunction with records of environmental causes may help determine what these variables might be.

There is data that caffeine is one variable that patients should consider altering as part of their BT regimen. A small study of patients with OAB who were given relatively high doses of caffeine (4.5 mg/kg) and subsequently underwent urodynamics found that caffeine decreased the threshold at first sensation to void [10]. Detrusor overactivity and increased bladder sensory signaling with high doses of caffeine (150 mg/kg) has also been found in animal models of mice [11]. In another study of women with detrusor overactivity, while high caffeine intake (>400 mg day) was correlated to bladder symptoms, moderate and low intake did not significantly affect detrusor overactivity [12]. Anecdotally, some patients have reported worsening OAB symptoms with tobacco use, but there is little good data to confirm this.

Stress and anxiety may also exacerbate OAB symptoms and these should be considered as potentially modifiable variables that may impact symptoms when patients undergo BT. [13–15] Teaching stress reduction techniques should be one component of BT for these patients. Obesity has been strongly linked to both developing OAB symptoms and to the severity of symptoms [16, 17]. Weight loss may aid in alleviating OAB symptoms [18]. Furthermore, BT should also include some evaluation of bowel patterns (e.g., constipation) as these are potentially modifiable variables that also alter OAB symptoms [19–21].

In addition to altering triggers to urination, behavioral modification regimens may also consist of timed voiding in which patients gradually increase the amount that can comfortably be held in the bladder. Upon completing an initial voiding diary to elucidate the frequency of their voiding, patients are instructed to void at a timed interval that is initially more frequent than reported on the diary. After doing this for typically 1–2 weeks, the voiding interval is usually increased by 15–30 min per week and the process repeated once the patient is able to consistently void prior to experiencing the more severe urges that prompted treatment. This process generally takes about 8–12 weeks and although the exact physiological mechanism of timed voiding is not known, data has demonstrated its efficacy [22, 23].

For patients who definitely have or are presumed to have detrusor overactivity (DO), behavioral therapy can either prevent or abort involuntary detrusor contractions. If the bladder diary suggests that symptoms are related to bladder volume, patients are taught to void at a volume before DO is triggered. Patients are also taught to recognize patterns that seem to cause the DO—running water, "key lock and garage door syndrome," etc. If that does not work, the third step is to teach the patient to contract his or her pelvic floor (Kegel maneuver) to prevent or abort involuntary detrusor contractions. Unfortunately, the Kegel maneuver is only effective in aborting the involuntary detrusor contraction in about half of OAB patients. When the patient feels a strong urge to void, she is instructed to contract her pelvic floor in rapid succession for short bursts until the urge subsides. If that does not resolve the urgency, several prolonged contractions for 10 or 15 s may be useful. In either case, she is instructed that once the urge subsides, she should breathe in and out slowly in a relaxed fashion and walk slowly to the bathroom. Rushing or running, we believe, tends to reignite the stimulus for urgency and detrusor overactivity and also may induce sphincteric incontinence.

An additional component to behavioral therapy includes altering patients' reaction to the initial urge to urinate. Patients complaining of OAB will often void preemptively in order to prevent urgency or urge incontinence. This manifests on the bladder diary as UPS voids designated 0–1. By encouraging patients to void only when a stronger urge occurs (UPS score of 2), substantial declines in urinary frequency can occur. In addition to this, a behavioral modification regimen may also look to distraction techniques or even hypnosis to alter urgency perception [24].

The importance of the Urodynamic OAB Classification system and bladder diary cannot be overestimated when behavioral therapy is utilized. The OAB type has a crucial impact on how BT proceeds. For example, patients with Type 2 OAB have involuntary detrusor contractions, but the patient perceives a warning and is able to contract his sphincter, prevent incontinence, and make the detrusor contraction subside so that he can walk to the bathroom in an unhurried fashion. All the behavioral therapist needs to do is incorporate what the patient already is capable of into the BT program. In patients with Type 4 OAB, the patient has no awareness or control of the involuntary detrusor contractions, so a completely different treatment paradigm must be constructed based on the particulars of the patients life style. This type of patient needs to either "relearn" bladder sensations as well as control, or void before the involuntary detrusor contractions occur. The bladder diary provides the metrics by which the initial OAB diagnosis is made and then serves as a monitor of the patient's progress as well as a tool for understanding the behaviors that need to be integrated into the BT process.

Pelvic Floor Muscle Training and Biofeedback

PFMT (often called Kegel exercises) and biofeedback have been used for decades to treat OAB as an alternative and/or adjunct to medications. PFMT, by repeated contractions of the pelvic floor, strengthens the pelvic floor muscles through an unknown neurologic reflex, which shuts off the involuntary detrusor contraction that causes urgency in some patients [25–27].

PFMT can be conducted by the patient after proper instruction from a therapist, with or without biofeedback training. Biofeedback for OAB has two applications: to teach the patient how to control the pelvic floor muscles, and to strengthen those muscles. Biofeedback may be used as an adjunctive technique to PFMT [28] and is particularly effective when combined with behavior modification [29]. The patient is taught how to contract the pelvic floor and to do so whenever an uncomfortable urge to void is felt. By contracting the sphincter, incontinence is prevented during the involuntary bladder contraction; the contraction also activates a neurologic reflex that stops the bladder contraction and provides the patient more time to comfortably find a bathroom.

Biofeedback for OAB is any technique whereby patients are given immediate information about the activity of their pelvic floor thereby allowing patients to better isolate and control its function [30]. Biofeedback is typically done through the use of electromyography (EMG) leads but can also be accomplished with weighted vaginal cones or by sensing the strength of sphincteric contraction by digital palpation. With vaginal cones, when patients feel the cones descending they are instructed to contract their pelvic floor to prevent the cones from falling out. As patients' pelvic floor strength improves, the weight of the vaginal cones can also be increased which allows for a graded approach towards strengthening the sphincter.

We typically use EMG sensors around the vagina or perineum to evaluate the activity of the pelvic floor and use an anal manometer to measure abdominal pressure. Measurement of abdominal pressure allows patients to better isolate their pelvic floor muscles and identify and minimize counterproductive abdominal contractions during exercises. The patients are taught how to contract their pelvic floor, and the strength and duration of each muscle contraction is displayed on a screen as is the abdominal pressure. The sessions are usually scheduled for 30–60 min once a week or every other week. Patients may also purchase or rent a portable unit for use at home and are instructed to continue their PFMT exercise regimen at home. Variables tracked every week include voiding diaries (and 24-h pad tests if patents are incontinent) and changes in the nature (e.g., strength and duration) of contraction that patients were able to generate during the biofeedback session. Based on the progress made each week, an exercise program is planned for the following week.

Although, complications of biofeedback and PFMT are rare, a standardized PFMT and biofeedback regimen has not been accepted. Short-term studies with up to 6-month follow-up have suggested between 54 and 87 % improvement in incontinence [31, 32]. One meta-analysis found biofeedback with pelvic floor exercises to be superior to pelvic floor exercises alone [33]. Although long-term efficacy has not been established in well-designed studies, evidence does suggest it remains effective [4, 29].

Electrical Stimulation

Electrical stimulation of the pelvic floor has been advocated by some for refractory OAB. There are essentially two models of electrical stimulation. The first is high frequency stimulation that is hypothesized to work by using electrodes in or near the vagina, rectum, or perineum to repetitively stimulate the pelvic floor to increase strength and tone of the muscles [34]. The electrodes can either be placed cutaneously or inserted into the rectum or vaginal vault. They cause minimal pain during stimulation and sessions are usually scheduled weekly or at biweekly intervals. In some instances, home stimulation units may be rented. It is hypothesized that repetitive stimulation results will strengthen the muscle, increase its tone, and also, through a negative feedback system, inhibit the bladder from contracting, to much the same effect as biofeedback.

The second type of electrical stimulation utilizes low frequency electrical stimulation to activate inhibitory pathways in the spinal cord and inhibit detrusor contraction. The most common form available is the Percutaneous Tibial Nerve Stimulator (PTNS) which was developed by Marshall Stoller at the University of California in San Francisco and sold as the Stoller Afferent Nerve Stimulator (SANS). PTNS involves placement of a 34 gauge needle cephalad to the medial malleolus to stimulate the posterior tibial nerve with 30 min weekly sessions typically lasting for 12 weeks. Side effects generally are minimal but can include pain and bleeding at the needle insertion site.

Studies are lacking as to the long-term efficacy, but short-term studies, suggest that both local stimulation and PTNS are more efficacious than sham procedures and the addition of AMAs increase their efficacy [35–37]. High frequency (transvaginal) and low frequency stimulation (PTNS) appear to have similar efficacy [38].

Surgical Options

Surgery may also be an option for patients with OAB not secondary to a remediable condition (e.g., pelvic prolapse). Surgery should be considered if they continue to have bothersome symptoms after failing the therapies previously discussed or if the clinician feels that the chance of success is low. These therapies will be discussed elsewhere in the book but include sacral neuromodulation, intravesical Botox, or enterocystoplasty or urinary diversion. Data have demonstrated that neuromodulation can be effective in patients who have failed other treatments [39]. Intravesical Botox has recently been approved by the FDA for OAB treatment and has been shown to be effective in treating patients with refractory OAB for both non-neurogenic detrusor overactivity (DO) and neurogenic DO (particularly multiple sclerosis and spinal cord injury). The RELAX study, a placebo-controlled, double-blind randomized study of 240 women with refractory OAB, found substantial improvement in 24 h voiding frequency (8.3 vs. 9.67), urgency episodes (3.8 vs. 6.67), and episodes of leakage (1.67 vs. 6.0) as compared to placebo. Urinary tract infection (31 %) and urinary retention (16 %) were the most common side effects reported [40]. Multiple other studies have confirmed the utility of Botox in patients with refractory OAB [41–44].

These therapies are discussed in more detail elsewhere in this book.

Finally, enterocystoplasty, ileovesicostomy, or other forms of urinary diversion should be considered when the patient deems symptoms bothersome enough to warrant a major abdominal operation. The success rate of augmentation enterocystoplasty in relieving OAB symptoms, which greatly increases bladder capacity and prevents DO, is in excess of 90 % although, postoperatively, patients may require intermittent self-catheterization [45–47]. For patients with disabilities that make catheterizing through the urethra impractical, a continent abdominal stoma may be created for intermittent catheterization, or an ileovesicostomy or ileal loop may be considered. In patients in whom intermittent catheterization is impractical, a urinary conduit may also relieve the OAB symptoms.

Case Report and Discussion

Patient is a 53-year-old male stock broker who presented with a 20-year history of bothersome urinary frequency, urgency, urge incontinence, and enuresis refractory to treatment with Terazosin 5 mg nightly, prior transurethral microwave therapy, and trials with multiple AMAs.

His exam was consistent with a small (approximately 10 g) prostate without any nodules, normal neurologic exam, and was otherwise normal. Free flow showed a maximum flow rate of 16 mL/s with a voided volume of 251 mL and a residual urine of 50 mL. Cystoscopy demonstrated trilobar prostatic enlargement with an elevated bladder neck, and severe bladder trabeculations and cellules.

VUD can be seen in Figs. 11.2, 11.3, and 11.4. The patient initially demonstrated an involuntary

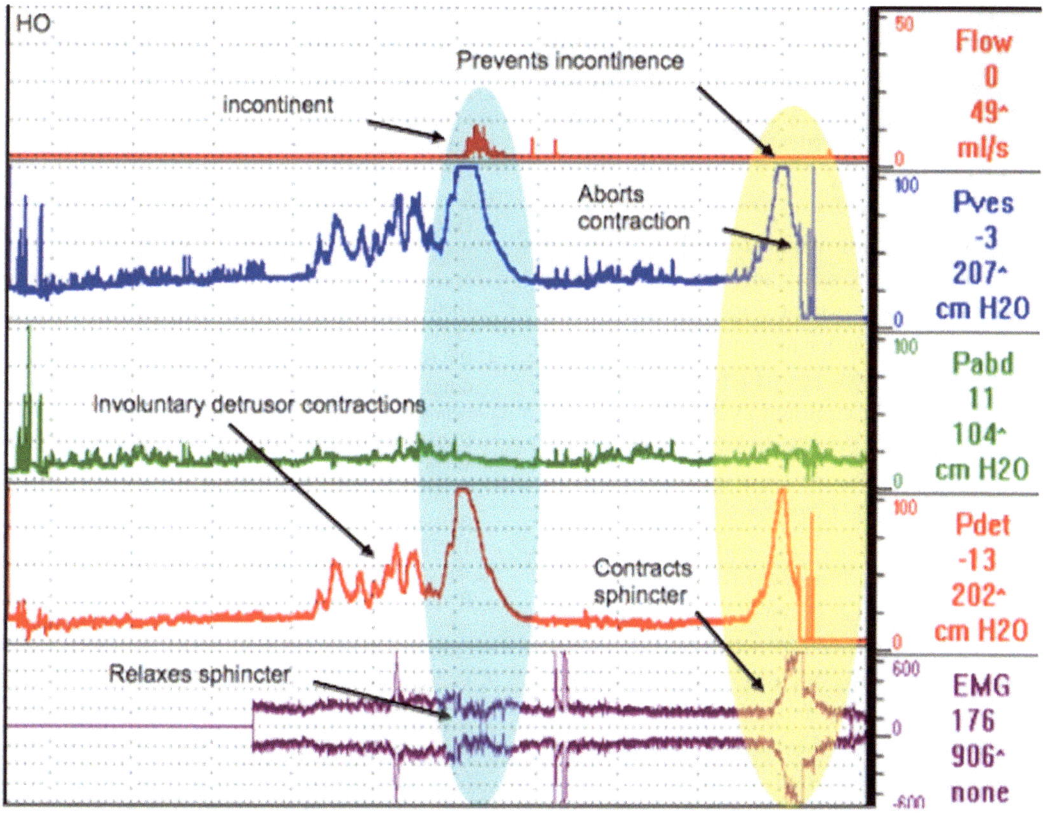

Fig. 11.2 Case report—urodynamic tracing

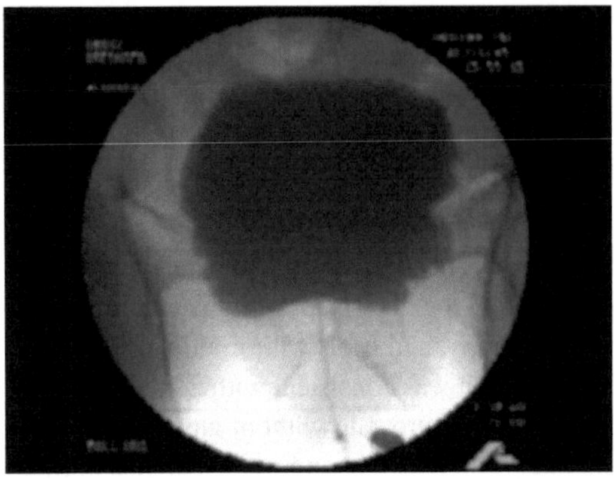

Fig. 11.3 Filling phase

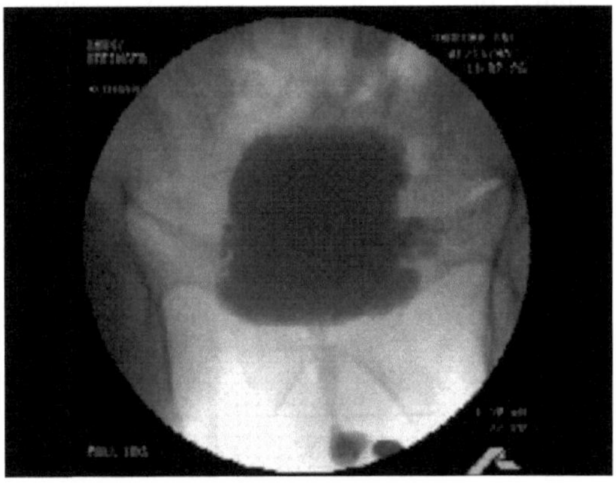

Fig. 11.4 Voiding phase

detrusor contraction which caused incontinence while the patient's sphincter was relaxed. With further filling, the patient was instructed to contract his sphincter when he sensed the involuntary detrusor contraction. The patient was able to successfully abort the contraction and prevent incontinence (Fig. 11.2).

The VUD was also consistent with bladder outlet obstruction. He subsequently underwent an uncomplicated transurethral resection of his prostate (TURP). Postoperatively his flow rate increased to 28 mL/s (from 16 mL/s) on a voided volume of 360 mL and he was noted to have no residual urine. However, his OAB symptoms persisted after his TURP and he underwent a formal course of BT and PFMT. Bladder diaries pre- and post-BT are demonstrated in Table 11.1.

The voiding diaries suggest substantial improvement in his urinary symptoms. The BT emphasized volume restriction. The patient's urge perception score for each void was recorded (not presented) and he was encouraged to contract his sphincter when he developed a mild or moderate urge to void to abort his involuntary detrusor contraction. By doing this, he eliminated his urge incontinence and substantially reduced his voiding frequency.

We typically first address surgically treatable remediable causes of refractory OAB such as prostatic obstruction as we did in this patient. The substantial improvement in his flow rate post-TURP suggests that his diagnosis of bladder outlet obstruction was correct despite a relatively good free flow. If his symptoms were completely cured after this point, the need for BT would have been averted. Because his OAB symptoms remained, BT was started with an excellent outcome.

References

1. Flisser AJ, Walmsley K, Blaivas JG. Urodynamic classification of patients with symptoms of overactive bladder. J Urol. 2003;169:529.
2. Lee UJ, Scott V, Rashid R, Behniwal A, Wein AJ, Maliski SL, Anger JT. Defining and managing overactive bladder: disagreement among the experts. Urology. 2013;81:257.
3. Burgio KL, Goode P, Johnson TM, Hammontree L, Ouslander JG, Markland AD, Colli J, Vaughan CP, Redden DT. Behavioral versus drug treatment for overactive bladder in men: the Male Overactive Bladder Treatment in Veterans (MOTIVE) Trial. J Am Geriatr Soc. 2011;59:2209.
4. Rai BP, Cody J, Alhasso A, Stewart L. Anticholinergic drugs versus non-drug active therapies for non-neurogenic overactive bladder syndrome in adults. Cochrane Database Syst Rev. 2012;12:CD003193.
5. Wyman JF, Klutke C, Burgio K, et al. Effects of combined behavioral intervention and tolterodine on patient-reported outcomes. Can J Urol. 2010; 17:5283.
6. Vaughan CP, Johnson J, Burgio KL, Goode PS, Wolf RA, Johnson II TM. Behavioral therapy to treat urinary incontinence in Parkinson disease. Neurology. 2011;76:1631.
7. Fitzgerald MP, Brubaker L. Variability of 24-hour voiding diary variables among asymptomatic women. J Urol. 2003;169:207.
8. Groutz A, Blaivas JG, Chaikin DC, et al. Noninvasive outcome measures of urinary incontinence and lower urinary tract symptoms: a multicenter study of micturition diary and pad tests. J Urol. 2000;164:698.

9. Blaivas JG, Panagopoulos G, Weiss JP, et al. The urgency perception score: validation and test-retest. J Urol. 2007;177:199.
10. Lohsiriwat S, Hirunsai M, Chaiyaprasithi B. Effect of caffeine on bladder function in patients with overactive bladder symptoms. Urol Ann. 2011;3:14.
11. Kershen R, Mann-Gow T, Yared J, et al. Caffeine ingestion causes detrusor overactivity and afferent nerve excitation in mice. J Urol. 2012;188:1986.
12. Arya LA, Myers DL, Jackson ND. Dietary caffeine intake and the risk for detrusor instability: a case-control study. Obstet Gynecol. 2000;96:85.
13. Zhang C, Hai T, Yu L, et al. Association between occupational stress and risk of overactive bladder and other lower urinary tract symptoms: a cross-sectional study of female nurses in China. Neurourol Urodyn. 2013;32:254.
14. Smith AL, Leung J, Kun S, et al. The effects of acute and chronic psychological stress on bladder function in a rodent model. Urology. 2011;78:967 e1.
15. Knight S, Luft J, Nakagawa S, et al. Comparisons of pelvic floor muscle performance, anxiety, quality of life and life stress in women with dry overactive bladder compared with asymptomatic women. BJU Int. 2012;109:1685.
16. Chancellor MB, Oefelein MG, Vasavada S. Obesity is associated with a more severe overactive bladder disease state that is effectively treated with once-daily administration of trospium chloride extended release. Neurourol Urodyn. 2010;29:551.
17. Lawrence JM, Lukacz ES, Liu IL, et al. Pelvic floor disorders, diabetes, and obesity in women: findings from the Kaiser Permanente Continence Associated Risk Epidemiology Study. Diabetes Care. 2007;30:2536.
18. Greer WJ, Richter HE, Bartolucci AA, et al. Obesity and pelvic floor disorders: a systematic review. Obstet Gynecol. 2008;112:341.
19. Matsumoto S, Hashizume K, Wada N, et al. Relationship between overactive bladder and irritable bowel syndrome: a large-scale internet survey in Japan using the overactive bladder symptom score and Rome III criteria. BJU Int 213;111:4.
20. Akl MN, Jacob K, Klauschie J, et al. The effect of rectal distension on bladder function in patients with overactive bladder. Neurourol Urodyn. 2012;31:541.
21. Panayi DC, Khullar V, Digesu GA, et al. Rectal distension: the effect on bladder function. Neurourol Urodyn. 2011;30:344.
22. Davies JA, Hosker G, Lord J, et al. An evaluation of the efficacy of in-patient bladder retraining. Int Urogynecol J Pelvic Floor Dysfunct. 2000;11:271.
23. Godec C. "Timed voiding"—a useful tool in the treatment of urinary incontinence. Urology. 1984;23:97.
24. Komesu YM, Sapien RE, Rogers RG, et al. Hypnotherapy for treatment of overactive bladder: a randomized controlled trial pilot study. Female Pelvic Med Reconstr Surg. 2011;17:308.
25. Godec C, Cass AS, Ayala GF. Bladder inhibition with functional electrical stimulation. Urology. 1975;6:663.
26. Morrison JF. The excitability of the micturition reflex. Scand J Urol Nephrol Suppl. 1995;175:21.
27. de Groat WC, Fraser MO, Yoshiyama M, et al. Neural control of the urethra. Scand J Urol Nephrol Suppl. 2001;207:35.
28. Wilson PD, Berghmans B, Hagen S, et al. Adult conservative management. http://www.ics.org/Publications/ICI_3/v2.pdf/chap15.pdf.
29. Dannecker C, Wolf V, Raab R, et al. EMG-biofeedback assisted pelvic floor muscle training is an effective therapy of stress urinary or mixed incontinence: a 7-year experience with 390 patients. Arch Gynecol Obstet. 2005;273:93.
30. Smith DA, Newman DK. Basic elements of biofeedback therapy for pelvic muscle rehabilitation. Urol Nurs. 1994;14:130.
31. Susset JG, Galea G, Read L. Biofeedback therapy for female incontinence due to low urethral resistance. J Urol. 1990;143:1205.
32. Burns PA, Pranikoff K, Nochajski T, et al. Treatment of stress incontinence with pelvic floor exercises and biofeedback. J Am Geriatr Soc. 1990;38:341.
33. Weatherall M. Biofeedback or pelvic floor muscle exercises for female genuine stress incontinence: a meta-analysis of trials identified in a systematic review. BJU Int. 1999;83:1015.
34. Bo K. Effect of electrical stimulation on stress and urge urinary incontinence. Clinical outcome and practical recommendations based on randomized controlled trials. Acta Obstet Gynecol Scand Suppl. 1998;168:3.
35. Staskin DR, Peters KM, MacDiarmid S, et al. Percutaneous tibial nerve stimulation: a clinically and cost effective addition to the overactive bladder algorithm of care. Curr Urol Rep. 2012;13:327.
36. Peters KM, Macdiarmid SA, Wooldridge LS, et al. Randomized trial of percutaneous tibial nerve stimulation versus extended-release tolterodine: results from the overactive bladder innovative therapy trial. J Urol. 2009;182:1055.
37. Tellenbach M, Schneider M, Mordasini L, et al. Transcutaneous electrical nerve stimulation: an effective treatment for refractory non-neurogenic overactive bladder syndrome? World J Urol 2013;31:5.
38. Gungor Ugurlucan F, Onal M, Aslan E, et al. Comparison of the effects of electrical stimulation and posterior tibial nerve stimulation in the treatment of overactive bladder syndrome. Gynecol Obstet Invest. 2013;75:46.
39. Kantartzis K, Shepherd J. Sacral neuromodulation and intravesical botulinum toxin for refractory overactive bladder. Curr Opin Obstet Gynecol. 2012; 24:331.
40. Tincello DG, Kenyon S, Abrams KR, et al. Botulinum toxin a versus placebo for refractory detrusor overactivity in women: a randomised blinded placebo-controlled trial of 240 women (the RELAX study). Eur Urol. 2012;62:507.
41. Wefer B, Ehlken B, Bremer J, et al. Treatment outcomes and resource use of patients with neurogenic detrusor overactivity receiving botulinum toxin A

(BOTOX) therapy in Germany. World J Urol. 2010; 28:385.
42. Karsenty G, Denys P, Amarenco G, et al. Botulinum toxin A (Botox) intradetrusor injections in adults with neurogenic detrusor overactivity/neurogenic overactive bladder: a systematic literature review. Eur Urol. 2008;53:275.
43. Dmochowski R, Sand PK. Botulinum toxin A in the overactive bladder: current status and future directions. BJU Int. 2007;99:247.
44. Schmid DM, Sauermann P, Werner M, et al. Experience with 100 cases treated with botulinum-A toxin injections in the detrusor muscle for idiopathic overactive bladder syndrome refractory to anticholinergics. J Urol. 2006;176:177.
45. Flood HD, Malhotra SJ, O'Connell HE, et al. Long-term results and complications using augmentation cystoplasty in reconstructive urology. Neurourol Urodyn. 1995;14:297.
46. Blaivas JG, Weiss JP, Desai P, et al. Long-term followup of augmentation enterocystoplasty and continent diversion in patients with benign disease. J Urol. 2005;173:1631.
47. Herschorn S, Hewitt RJ. Patient perspective of long-term outcome of augmentation cystoplasty for neurogenic bladder. Urology. 1998;52:672.

Part IV

Overactive Bladder

12 Intravesical Therapy for Refractory Overactive Bladder and Detrusor Overactivity in Adults: Botulinum Toxin-A

Arun Sahai, Jai Seth, Muhammed Shamim Khan, and Prokar Dasgupta

It has been 11 years since the first publications on the use of intradetrusor botulinum toxin-A (BTX-A) injections to treat neurogenic detrusor overactivity (NDO) in patients with spinal cord injury (SCI) [1, 2]. OnabotulinumtoxinA (Botox®; Allergan, Ltd., Irvine, USA) has recently been approved for use in the bladder of neurogenic patients with SCI or multiple sclerosis in various parts of the world. In the near future, it is expected that the FDA in the USA and the MHRA in Europe will approve the use of this toxin in idiopathic overactive bladder. Over the last decade, there has been an explosion of publications on the use of this bladder therapy which is primarily used in patients with symptoms of overactive bladder (OAB) and/or detrusor overactivity (DO) who have failed conservative measures and oral medication with antimuscarinics. This is typically due to poor efficacy with antimuscarinics or poor tolerability due to side effects such as dry mouth, dry eyes, blurred vision and constipation. Initially proof of concept/open labelled studies were conducted, whilst later studies focussed on mechanisms of action. From these studies it became apparent that BTX was not simply working by efferent blockade at the neuromuscular junction, as in skeletal muscle, but was likely to have an effect on sensory nerves. Later publications emerged on technique of administration and evidence from level 1 small randomised blinded placebo-controlled trials in both NDO and IDO. Recently drug sponsored phase II and III double-blind randomised placebo-controlled trials have been conducted in both NDO and IDO. These trials are now published with the exception of the phase III data in IDO (at the time of writing this chapter).

OAB is a syndrome characterised by urgency with or without urgency incontinence but usually accompanied by frequency and nocturia [3]. The majority of patients have proven DO but treatment is often instigated without this knowledge by community practitioners based on symptoms alone. Therapeutic options are split into initial treatment and specialised therapy. Initial treatment encompasses lifestyle interventions, 'bladder training' and the use of oral antimuscarnics [4]. Pharmacotherapy in most individuals is still the first-line treatment. In the past, if this failed and symptoms were intractable and had a significant impact on quality of life (QoL) patients were managed with augmentation cystoplasty or urinary diversion. More recently other therapeutic options have been developed and include sacral neuromodulation and BTX injections into the bladder.

A. Sahai, Ph.D., F.R.C.S. (Urol.) (✉) • M.S. Khan, F.R.C.S. (Urol.), F.E.B.U. • P. Dasgupta, M.B.B.S., M.Sc. (Urol.), M.D., D.L.S., F.R.C.S. (Urol.), F.E.B.U.
Department of Urology, Guy's Hospital, MRC Center for Transplantation, King's College London, King's Health Partners, London, UK
e-mail: sonnyroth@yahoo.com

J. Seth, B.Sc., M.Sc., M.R.C.S.
Department of Uro-Neurology, National Hospital for Neurology and Neurosurgery, London, UK

G.H. Badlani (ed.), *Minimally Invasive Therapy for Urinary Incontinence and Pelvic Organ Prolapse*, Current Clinical Urology, DOI 10.1007/978-1-4939-0008-4_12,

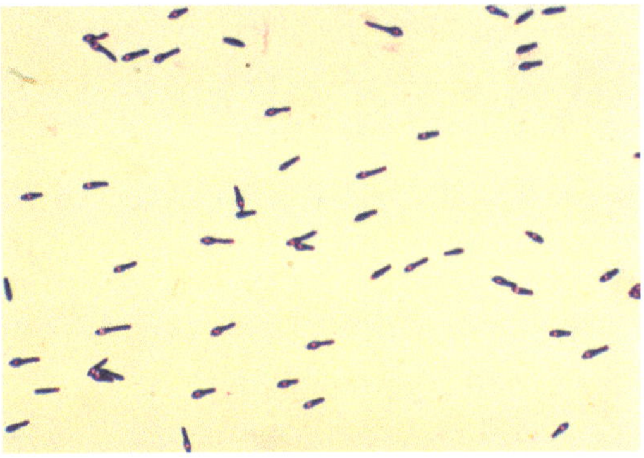

Fig. 12.1 A photomicrograph of *Clostridium botulinum* type A viewed using a Gram stain technique

BTX is a neurotoxin produced by the gram-positive anaerobic spore-producing organism *Clostridium botulinum* (Fig. 12.1). It is one of the most poisonous naturally occurring toxins known to mankind [5]. Its effects range from food poisoning known as 'botulism' to an acute and symmetrical paralysis. The severity of its toxic effects ranges from mild weakness to respiratory failure, coma and death. Seven distinct botulinum neurotoxins isoforms (A-G) have been isolated [6]. Types A and B are presently used in clinical medicine today but some other types are the subject of ongoing research. BTX-A is made up of a heavy and light chain connected by a disulphide bond [7]. Currently several pharmaceutical companies produce and market BTX-A. The two commonest used preparations in the urinary tract are Botox® (Allergan Pharmaceuticals Ltd., USA) and Dysport® (Ipsen Biopharm Ltd., UK). However other preparations are available such as Xeomin® (Merz Pharmaceuticals UK Ltd., Herts, UK), Prosigne® (Lanzhou Biological Products, Lanzhou, China) and PurTox® (Mentor Corporation, Madison, WI, USA). Botulinum toxin type B (BTX-B) is commercially available as Myobloc® in the USA (Elan Pharmaceuticals, Inc.) and Neurobloc® in Europe (Elan Pharma International Ltd.). BTX-A toxicity is measured in mouse units (mU), which is 'the amount fatal to 50 % of a batch of Swiss Webster mice' [8]. One unit of BOTOX® (Allergan, Ltd., USA) is considered equivalent to 3–4 units of DYSPORT® (Ipsen, Ltd., UK). This is an important point to keep in mind when analysing different studies, so as not to inadvertently utilise incorrect doses. In an attempt to prevent dose errors and to recognise the different formulations the FDA has had new terminology recently approved. This is summarised in Table 12.1.

Table 12.1 FDA approved terminology for BTX products

Trade name	Old drug name	New drug name
Botox	Botulinum toxin-A	OnabotulinumtoxinA
Botox cosmetic	Botulinum toxin-A	OnabotulinumtoxinA
Dysport	Botulinum toxin-A	AbobotulinumtoxinA
Xeomin	Botulinum toxin-A	IncobotulinumtoxinA
Myobloc	Botulinum toxin-B	RimabotulinumtoxinB

The use of BTX-A to treat OAB and DO has been recognised by several bodies including the European Association of Urology (EAU) [4] and the National Institute of Clinical Excellence (NICE) [9], to name but a few, and is now featured in their guidelines. In addition the toxin has been given a grade A recommendation by an independent expert European body [10] and in a recent largest of its kind systematic review BTX-A has been recommended in many aspects of lower urinary tract dysfunction [11]. In this chapter we will focus on mechanisms of action of BTX-A in the bladder, its clinical efficacy and safety with emphasis on randomised placebo-controlled trials, review techniques of administration and lastly its cost-effectiveness.

Mechanism of Action

The initial work on mechanisms of action of BTX was studied in skeletal muscle which suggested that the toxin prevented presynaptic vesicular acetylcholine (ACh) release. Four steps are involved in this process: binding, translocation, cleavage and inhibition of transmitter release [7]. Once the neurotoxin is exogenously administered, it diffuses to cholinergic terminals where it binds to the SV2 receptor [12]. Once bound the toxin is internalised inside endocytic vesicles and binds to the lipid bilayer of the vesicle. The heavy chain is thought to play a key role in translocating

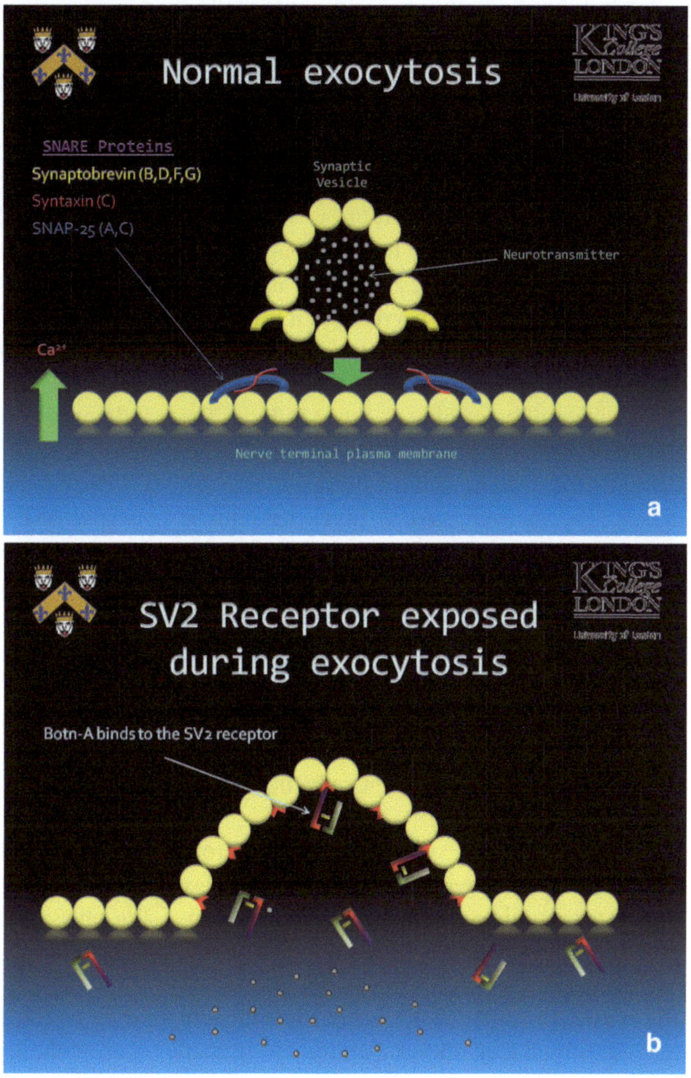

Fig. 12.2 Mechanism of action at the neuromuscular junction (**a**) normal and (**b**) after exogenous BTX-A administration. (From Seth JH, Dowson C, Khan MS, et al. Botulinum toxin-A for the treatment of overactive bladder: UK contributions. J Clin Urol 2013;6:77, copyright 2013 by SAGE. Reprinted by permission of SAGE.)

the light chain into the cytosol, which occurs after the cleavage of the disulphide bond between them [13–15]. The BTX light chain acting like an enzyme is able to cleave SNARE proteins within the nerve terminal [16]. Botulinum toxins B, D, F and G cleave VAMP/Synaptobrevin, A and E cleave SNAP-25 and C cleaves both SNAP-25 and syntaxin [17]. As the SNARE proteins are essential for normal vesicular transport and fusion, botulinum neurotoxins are able to prevent the release of ACh at the pre-synaptic membrane with resultant blockage of synaptic transmission and flaccid paralysis in the target muscle (see Fig. 12.2). This was the rationale for the introduction of this therapy to treat OAB and DO [2]. ATP, a purinergic neurotransmitter is believed to be co-released with ACh from parasympathetic cholinergic nerve terminals [18, 19]. It has been postulated that ATP via purinergic mechanisms contributes a significant amount to unstable contractions in IDO [20, 21]. Studies on guinea pig [19, 22] and rat [19, 22] bladder strips have shown that BTX is able to impair both ACh and ATP release, suggesting that its use in treating patients with DO and symptoms of OAB is well justified. However, it soon became evident that patients were also experiencing a welcome improvement in the sensation of urinary urgency, which is the hallmark of OAB. As a result, scientists and clinicians began investigating the possible effects of BTX on afferent nerves. In recent years there is evidence to suggest that BTX-A modulates sensory neurotransmission, although the exact mechanism remains unclear [23].

The sensation of 'bladder fullness' is provided by the urothelium, which has a strong role in mechanosensation. C-fibres comprise up to two thirds of bladder afferent nerves, and it is thought that these fibres are involved in the reorganisation of the reflex activity seen in OAB. The other predominant afferent fibre is the Aδ fibre. The myelinated Aδ fibres tend to be located within the detrusor muscle and respond to detrusor stretch. The unmyelinated C fibres tend to be dispersed more widely, in the detrusor, suburothelium and adjacent to urothelial cells, providing nociception and are sensitive to changes in temperature and pH. These nerves are thought to be important in the pathogenesis of urgency and OAB [24, 25]. Intrathecal BTX-A injection causes a significant reduction in recordings from c-fibre activity, with a less significant reduction in Aδ fibre activity [26].

Sensory signalling is aided by numerous receptors and sensory peptide substances. These include the capsaicin-sensitive ion channel receptor TRPV1, which has been shown in human and animal studies to have importance in the sensation of noxious stimuli in the bladder. It is thought that the stimulation of urothelium by stretch, inflammation, acidity and temperature causes local release of a variety of neuropeptides, including nerve growth factor (NGF), ATP, substance P (SP), neurokinin A (NKA) and calcitonin gene-related peptide (CGRP) [27]. In a study of dorsal root ganglion (DRG) cells, BTX-A has been shown to reduce the release of SP and disables SNARE-dependent exocytosis of TRPV1 to the plasma membrane [28, 29]. The density of substance P and CGRP immunoreactive nerves was increased by 82 % in patients with IDO, suggesting that there is an increase in these types of afferent neurons in patients with this condition [30]. In an isolated rat bladder model, Rapp et al., investigated the effect of BTX-A on CGRP release [31]. A mixture of capsaicin and ATP was used to evoke CGRP release from the bladder and BTX-A (100 U) was found to significantly reduce this evoked release compared with controls [31]. In a similar model the same group of authors investigated the effect of BTX-A in acute injury (HCL) and chronic inflammation (cyclophosphamide) [32]. They found that both HCL and cyclophosphamide increased substance P neurotransmitter release but only HCL increased CGRP release compared to controls. The administration of BTX-A (10 U) significantly reduced the levels of these neurotransmitters in this inflammatory model to levels consistent with controls [32].

There is growing evidence that the urothelium releases ATP in response to stretch, which in turn activates suburothelial purinergic neurons, which conveys information to the CNS to activate micturition [33]. Urothelial release of evoked ATP is increased in animal models of DO (SCI and cyclophosphamide-induced cystitis) and BTX-A significantly reduces this evoked release compared to controls [34, 35]. Application of ATP in rat bladders in vivo precipitates DO and this is also reduced by BTX-A [36]. By reducing urothelial ACh release, BTX-A may block both excitatory afferent signalling and detrusor parasympathetic transmission during urine storage, similar to oral antimuscarinic medications [23].

Bladder biopsies from patients with either NDO or IDO have shown an increased expression of the capsaicin receptor, TRPV1 and the purinergic receptor, P2X3 compared to controls [37]. BTX-A treatment has been demonstrated to significantly reduce these receptor levels at 4 and 16 weeks post- treatment. The fastest change was in the P2X3 immunoreactivity, which correlated with improvements in urinary urgency at both time points.

NGF is a signalling molecule produced in the urothelium. NGF is necessary for the survival of sympathetic fibres and receptor expression on small sensory fibres. It is thought that ultimately NGF, produced by the urothelium and smooth muscle, plays a role in triggering pathology-induced changes in C-fibre afferent nerve excitability after mechanical stretch, causing increased urinary frequency, reflex bladder activity and unstable bladder contractions [38]. Through immunohistochemistry techniques it has also been demonstrated that the quantities of NGF in human bladder tissue is raised in conditions such as painful inflammatory conditions, OAB, interstitial cystitis, bladder outflow obstruction and chronic prostatitis [38]. It has also been suggested that NGF production in the superficial layers of the bladder may leak into the urine with bladder stretching. Using an enzyme-linked immunosorbent assay (ELISA), the levels of NGF in the urine can be quantified. Significantly higher levels of urinary NGF have been found in OAB compared with healthy controls with no bladder symptoms. Bladder tissue and urinary levels of NGF have been demonstrated to be significantly reduced after BTX-A treatment, which may explain the reduction of nerve sprouting in the urothelium [39, 40].

As afferent mechanisms may be important in the pathophysiology of DO, the excellent therapeutic efficacy of BTX in the bladder may in part be explained by this proposed dual (efferent and afferent) mechanism of action.

Clinical Efficacy and Safety of BTX-A to Treat OAB/DO

Neurogenic Detrusor Overactivity

Level 1 Evidence

In 2005, Schurch et al., reported the first double-blind randomised placebo-controlled trial involving 59 NDO patients, predominantly with spinal cord injury (SCI), who were randomised to receive in a 1:1:1 ratio, 200, 300 U OnabotulinumtoxinA or placebo [41]. The primary end point of urinary incontinence (UI) episodes decreased significantly at all time points except at 12 and 18 weeks in the 200 U group. Interestingly, when compared with placebo, improvements only reached statistical significance in the 300 U group at 2 and 6 weeks and in the 200 U group at 24 weeks. Patients receiving BTX-A at either dose showed significant improvement in QoL as assessed by the incontinence quality of life (I-QOL) questionnaire administered at all follow-up time points. In a subsequent publication the I-QoL scores were broken down into their individual domains of avoidance limiting behaviour, psychosocial impact and social embarrassment and the same improvements were observed at all time points for 300 and 200 U except for psychosocial impact and social embarrassment at 24 weeks [42]. The commonest reported adverse event was UTI in 22 %. The authors concluded that 200 or 300 U was equally efficacious. Surprisingly antimuscarinic use remained similar in the study in contrast to the preliminary pilot study by Schurch et al., in 2000 [1]. The urinary incontinence, urodynamic and I-QOL results are summarised in Table 12.2.

The first double-blind randomised placebo-controlled trial with the use of AbobotulinumtoxinA 500 U in NDO was subsequently published [43]. In this small study 17 patients received AbobotulinumtoxinA and 10 patients placebo. Tolterodine was allowed 1-week post-injection for no or insufficient effect. Tolterodine usage was higher in the placebo group compared with BTX-A over the 26-week study period. UI episodes and MDP were significantly reduced following AbobotulinumtoxinA injections compared to placebo throughout the study and MCC increased significantly except for the end of study time point at 26 weeks. QoL was globally improved in the BTX-A group compared with placebo.

This year a randomised multi-centre double-blinded placebo-controlled study was reported from Canada assessing OnabotulinumtoxinA 300 U compared to placebo in 57 patients [44]. The study demonstrated significant improvements in UI episodes and QoL using the I-QOL questionnaire at 6, 24 and 36 weeks compared to placebo. Urodynamic parameters were generally improved for up to 24 weeks. Antimuscarinics usage at 6 weeks in those that were taking them previously was 67 % and 94 % for OnabotulinumtoxinA and placebo groups, respectively. The commonest adverse event was UTI [44].

Recently in a large phase III double-blind multi-centre placebo-controlled trial 275 patients were randomised to OnabotulinumtoxinA at 200,

Table 12.2 Summary of results from a phase II double-blind randomised placebo-controlled trial of OnabotulinumtoxinA in patients with NDO

Time point (weeks)	300 U ($n=19$)	200 U ($n=19$)	Placebo ($n=21$)
Daily UI episodes			
Baseline	2.8 (1.86)	1.9 (1.78)	3.0 (3.29)
2	−1.3 (1.39)[a]	−1.0 (1.67)[b]	−0.2 (1.02)
6	−1.5 (2.33)[a]	−0.9 (1.84)[b]	−0.2 (1.45)
12	−1.2 (1.66)[b]	−0.9 (2.14)	−0.3 (1.46)
18	−1.2 (1.16)[b]	−0.8 (2.75)	−0.3 (1.59)
24	−0.9 (1.34)[b]	−1.1 (1.92)[a]	−0.1 (1.09)
MCC (mL)			
Baseline	293.6	260.2	254.6
2	479.6 (186.1)[a, b]	482.5 (215.8)[a, b]	282.0 (27.4)
6	462.7 (169.1)[a, b]	448.8 (182.1)[a]	299.6 (45.0)
24	398.2 (92.9)[b]	440.9 (174.2)[a, b]	301.0 (41.6)
RDV (mL)			
Baseline	254.8	169.1	202.4
2	198.1 (8.6)	306.9 (135.3)[b]	206.7 (4.3)
6	268.5 (96.0[b])	234.2 (47.3)	244.6 (42.6)
24	305.4 (72.4)	327.4 (144.6)[a, b]	226.4 (23.5)
MDP (cmH_2O)			
Baseline	92.6	77.0	79.1
2	41.0 (−66.3)[a, b]	31.6 (−52.9)[a, b]	71.4 (−7.7)
6	45.9 (−62.2)	40.1 (−44.4)[a, b]	69.0 (−10.1)
24	55.2 (−35.5)[a, b]	48.8 (−38.7)[a, b]	80.6 (−1.4)
Median I-QOL score			
Baseline	44.3	48.9	42.6
2	72.7[b]	79.5[b]	49.4
6	77.3[b]	84.1[b]	56.3
12	72.7[b]	84.1[b]	45.5
18	69.3[b]	85.2[b]	46.0
24	67.0[b]	86.4[b]	44.3

From Schurch B, de SM, Denys P et al. Botulinum toxin type is a safe and effective treatment for neurogenic urinary incontinence: results of a single treatment, randomised, placebo-controlled 6-month study. *J Urol* 2005;174(1):196-200; and Schurch B, Denys P, Kozma CM, Reese PR, Slaton T, Barron RL. Botulinum toxin A improves the quality of life of patients with neurogenic urinary incontinence. *Eur Urol* 2007;52(3):850-858

Mean values (mean change from baseline) unless indicated

UI urinary incontinence, *MCC* maximum cystometric capacity, *RDV* reflex detrusor volume

[a]Statistically significant within-group changes from baseline and versus placebo

[b]Statistically significant changes versus placebo

300 U and placebo [45]. This is the largest study of its kind and included patients with both multiple sclerosis (MS) and SCI who had ≥14 UI episodes per week. The primary end point of UI episodes at 6 weeks was significantly reduced with OnabotulinumtoxinA at both doses compared with placebo. At this time point fully continent rates were 7.6 %, 38 % and 39.6 % for placebo, 200 U and 300 U, respectively. I-QOL scores were also significantly greater at 6 weeks suggesting improved QoL in those treated with OnabotulinumtoxinA compared with placebo. The urodynamic and UI data is summarised in Table 12.3. The median duration of effect of OnaboutlinumtoxinA was 42.1 weeks in contrast to placebo, which was 13.1 weeks. Seventy-four patients received a second injection with similar benefits. Approximately 50 % were not performing clean intermittent self-catheterisation (CISC) at baseline. The need to instigate CISC was 12 %, 30 % and 42 % in the placebo, 200 U and 300 U groups, respectively. This was at the clinicians' discretion as opposed to a cut-off residual value. No neutralising antibodies were detected in the serum at the exit point of the study. The study concluded 200 U was equivalent to 300 U but with a better safety profile. Although typically open labelled studies utilised 300 U for treating NDO, on the basis of the phase II and III clinical trial data, it is likely the initial recommended dose for this patient population will be 200 U OnabotulinumtoxinA.

Other Relevant Studies and Study Populations

Patient satisfaction is now regarded as an important parameter to assess following treatments especially newer therapies. Using a 5-point scale of very dissatisfied (1) to very satisfied (5) injections of 500 U AbobotulinumtoxinA was shown to improve the satisfaction score from a mean score of 1.6–3.8 in 16 NDO patients [46]. Hori et al., have also recently reported on patients satisfaction in a group of patients with SCI and NDO treated with AbobotulinumtoxinA [47]. Mean satisfaction scores were 6.2/10 and 90 % of

Table 12.3 Summary of results from a phase III double-blind randomised placebo-controlled trial of OnabotulinumtoxinA in patients with NDO

Time point (weeks)	300 U (*n*=91)	200 U (*n*=92)	Placebo (*n*=92)
Weekly UI episodes			
Baseline	31.2 (18.1)	32.5 (18.4)	36.7 (30.7)
2	−15.8 (25.8)[a]	−18.8 (16.7)[b]	−9.7 (17.9)
6	−19.4 (25.7)[a]	−21.8 (18.1)[a]	−13.2 (20.0)
12	−19.8 (18.6)[b]	−20.5 (18.9)[a]	−12.2 (22.2)
MCC (mL)			
Baseline	246.8 (149.1)	247.3 (147.6)	249.4 (139.3)
6	157.2 (185.2)[b]	157.0 (164.8)[b]	6.5 (144.8)
PdetmaxIDC (cmH_2O)			
Baseline	42.1 (33.2)	51.7 (41.0)	41.5 (31.2)
6	−26.9 (33.2)[b]	−28.5 (47.8)[b]	6.4 (41.1)
BC mL/cmH_2O			
Baseline	64.7 (87.6)	54.6 (63.5)	58.1 (76.2)
6	60.9 (147.3)[c]	71.5 (157.1)[c]	2.7 (97.8)
Patients with no IDC %			
6	59.5	64.4	17.4
I-QOL Score			
6	24.3[b]	24.4[b]	11.7
12	25.9[b]	25.1[b]	8.6

From Cruz F, Herscorn S, Aliotta P et al. Efficacy and Safety of OnabotulinumtoxinA in Patients with Urinary Incontinence Due to Neurogenic Detrusor Overactivity: A Randomised, Double-Blind, Placebo-Controlled Trial. Eur Urol. 2011 Oct;60(4):742-50

Mean baseline and change from baseline scores and (standard deviation)

UI urinary incontinence, *MCC* maximum cystometric capacity, *PdetmaxIDC* maximum detrusor pressure during first involuntary detrusor contraction, *BC* bladder compliance

[a] $p<0.01$

[b] $p<0.001$

[c] $p<0.05$ vs. placebo

patients were happy to have AbobotulinumtoxinA treatment as a long-term treatment strategy. Only 15 % would consider a permanent alternative solution such as clam ileocystoplasty.

The majority of studies show improvements in QoL with OnabotulinumtoxinA and AbobotulinumtoxinA injections, however, Kalsi et al., using the UDI-6 and IIQ-7 QoL questionnaires found a statistically significant correlation between improvements in QoL with improvements in frequency, urgency and urge urinary incontinence but not for urodynamic parameters in NDO patients [48].

How quickly do OnabotulinumtoxinA injections begin to change OAB symptoms? In our experience this has been quite variable ranging between 2 days and 2 weeks, although we have had 2 patients who have only experienced a change in symptoms after 4 weeks. Kalsi et al., recently addressed this with a 7-day voiding diary immediately after injection [49]. In the NDO group significant improvements compared to baseline were demonstrated as early as 2 days for urgency, frequency and nocturia with significant improvements with incontinence episodes by day 3.

Grosse et al., recently tried to establish whether any differences could be found when treating NDO with AbobotulinumtoxinA or OnabotulinumtoxinA and whether treatment with increasing doses of AbobotulinumtoxinA would correlate with a dose-dependent effect [50]. Limitations included its retrospective nature and that the OnabotulinumtoxinA group was a matched population of cases. Furthermore doses of AbobotulinumtoxinA varied between 500 and 1,000 U and of OnabotulinumtoxinA between 200 and 400 U. No significant differences were identified between the two formulations apart from continence volume being greater at 3 months in favour of AbobotulinumtoxinA. Furthermore no dose-dependent trend could be seen in clinical and urodynamic parameters at 3 and 9 months between the AbobotulinumtoxinA doses, however, at higher doses of toxin, time between repeat injections appeared longer although this was not statistically significant [50]. Recently a comprehensive systematic review has tried to address this question [11]. A full comprehensive review of the BTX-A literature was conducted and the authors concluded there was good evidence showing the benefits of both OnabotulinumtoxinA and AbobotulinumtoxinA in the treatment of NDO in adults; however, OnabotulinumtoxinA is better studied than abobotulinumtoxinA. Furthermore due to the heterogeneity of study protocols, direct comparisons were not possible. Both formulations improved symptoms, urodynamics and QoL and although interinjection interval and failure rates were quite wide ranging, they were similar between the two toxin formulations [11].

Kuo has also recently conducted a comparative study in patients with NDO with either cerebral vascular accident (CVA) or a suprasacral spinal cord lesion. Both groups were injected with 200 U OnabotulinumtoxinA [51]. Although reflex volume and MCC increased in those with CVA, large post-void residuals were noted with little change in incontinence. Overall, however a successful result (either continence or a subjective improvement in incontinence) was noted in only 50 % in those with CVA compared with 92 % in the SCI group. Further study in this area is required but certainly this study highlights that not all neurogenic bladder responds to BTX-A treatment equally and aetiology maybe significant with regard to outcomes.

Finally, Giannantoni et al., recently reported on 6 patients with NDO and severe Parkinson's disease or Multiple System Atrophy successfully treated with OnabotulinumtoxinA 300 U [52]. Significant improvements in OAB symptoms, urodynamics and QoL as assessed by the I-QoL were observed following treatment at 1 and 3 months post-injection. These authors have also published results on 8 patients treated with OnabotulinumtoxinA 100 U in Parkinson's disease patients alone with similar good results [53].

Repeated Injections

Several authors have published their results of repeated injections of BTX-A in NDO and this has recently been summarised [54]. Studies using OnabotulinumtoxinA [55–60] and AbobotulinumtoxinA [60–64] have both been published and overall the data suggests that repeated injections are equally efficacious as the first with continued benefit with regard to OAB symptoms, urodynamic parameters and QoL improvement [54]. However due to the reporting of these studies (some report on all injections, some report on a set number of patients who have had for example 5 injections), it is difficult to assess true efficacy as all patients who had BTX-A may not have been included. The largest study from Del Popolo et al., assessed Abobotulinum toxin at varying doses of 500–1,000 U in a cohort of 199 SCI patients with NDO [62]. In total 590 injections were performed in 199 patients with 49 patients having at least 5 injections. Statistical analysis was performed for up to 7 injections and significant improvements in maximum cystometric capacity, reflex detrusor volume and bladder compliance were observed. In addition UI rates were significantly reduced as was pad usage. Patient satisfaction improved after each injection compared with baseline and in only 10 % of patients did the effects of the toxin last <6 months [62]. Khan et al., reported on repeated injections in a cohort of 137 patients with multiple sclerosis and NDO treated with OnabotulinumtoxinA 300 U [59]. QoL as assessed by the UDI-6 and IIQ-7 showed considerable improvement 4 weeks after each treatment even when repeated six times. Four weeks after the first treatment, 76 % became completely dry. This efficacy was sustained with repeat injections. The median interval between re-treatments remained constant at 12–13 months. The vast majority were required to perform CISC post-treatment. Finally, Manfred Stoehrer' group have published on their long-term experience using both OnabotulinumtoxinA (200–300 U) and AbobotulinumtoxinA (750–1,000 U) [60, 64]. No significant differences were found in the interval between injections 1–4. Duration of effect for injections 1–4 was approximately 10 months with no difference between the two formulations. Significant improvements in maximum cystometric capacity and reflex detrusor volume were observed. Although bladder compliance improved, this did not reach statistical significance for injections 1–3. Similar outcomes were shown with further follow-up with a mean duration of benefit of 8.7 months [60].

A concern from clinicians is the potential for fibrosis after repeated BTX-A injections, which may lead to reduced bladder compliance and worsening of OAB symptoms. In our repeat BTX-A study, bladder compliance is significantly improved following each repeated injection and no significant difference was demonstrated when comparing compliance following the first and fourth injection [65]. A recent histological study in NDO patients suggested OnabotulinumtoxinA-injected bladders (1–4 injections) had less fibrosis when compared to BTX-A naïve patients [66].

This was based on their own grading scale using a cut-off of 20 %, i.e. mild fibrosis if occupying <20 % of muscle fibres and/or submucosa and important fibrosis if >20 %. No differences in inflammation and oedema were observed in the two groups. Whether fibrosis occurs after 4 injections is yet to be determined but further study is required to assess this, especially as more patients may opt for repeated BTX-A injections over surgical treatment such as augmentation cystoplasty in managing their symptoms. Hafekamp et al., reported on a lack of structural changes before and after BTX injections in patients with NDO [67]. Contrary to reports with striated muscle very little axonal sprouting was observed following treatment. Apostolidis et al., assessed biopsies after one or a limited number of repeat BTX-A treatments and found no significant change in baseline inflammation [68]. Mild fibrosis was seen in 2.2 % of all biopsies which did not alter pre- or post-treatment. No evidence of dysplasia was seen.

Idiopathic Detrusor Overactivity and Bladder Oversensitivity

Level 1 Evidence

Our group reported on the first randomised, double-blind, placebo-controlled trial reporting the efficacy and safety of OnabotulinumtoxinA 200 U in treating patients with IDO [69]. The primary end point of the study, significantly increase in maximum cystometric capacity at 3 months, was achieved following OnabotulinumtoxinA compared with placebo. Overall significant improvements in OAB symptoms, urodynamic parameters and QoL as assessed by UDI-6, IIQ-7 and KHQ were observed in favour of OnabotulinumtoxinA in this small study [69, 70]. In the OnabotulinumtoxinA group, 50 % of patients were continent at follow-up, and the improvement lasted 24 weeks. Urinary frequency normalised in 57 % of patients in the OnabotulinumtoxinA group at 4 weeks and 36 % maintained this benefit at 24 weeks. Until this study the need to instigate CISC was reported typically between 0 and 15 %; however, the incidence in this study was 37.5 %. Since then other level 1 ongoing studies reporting experience with OnabotulinumtoxinA have confirmed that this figure is accurate for 200 U [65, 71]. The other common side effect was UTI, which occurred in 20.5 %, despite the use of prophylactic antibiotics. This is similar to the rate reported in the literature [41, 72].

Since this study was conducted and reported, three other randomised placebo-controlled trials have been published utilising BTX-A in patients with IDO [71, 73, 74]. Brubaker et al., randomised female patients in a 2:1 fashion to OnabotulinumtoxinA 200 U or placebo [71]. An interval analysis suggested high rates of voiding dysfunction, necessitating CISC (43 %), and as a result the trial was halted. However, utilising the Patient Global Impression of Improvement Score (PGI-I), where patient perception is assessed on a 7-point scale, 60 % felt an improvement in the OnabotulinumtoxinA group with mean scores at 2 months better compared with placebo. Significant reduction in UI episodes were also observed in favour of OnabotulinumtoxinA at 1 and 2 months post-injection. Time to failure was longer in those treated with OnabotulinumtoxinA compared with placebo. Incidence of UTI was also high and was more prevalent in those who received OnabotulinumtoxinA and in particular in those performing CISC.

In another trial, OAB patients were recruited and randomised between OnabotulinumtoxinA 300 U, 200 U and placebo [73]. DO was not a prerequisite for inclusion into the study. Only the preliminary results, i.e. 6-week follow-up have been published so far and as the investigators were blinded to the doses, the two OnabotulinumtoxinA groups' data were combined for the purpose of this analysis. Fifteen patients received either OnabotulinumtoxinA 200 or 300 U and 7 patient's placebo. Significant reductions in UI episodes, 24-h pad weights and number of pads per day with improvements in QoL were observed for OnabotulinumtoxinA compared to placebo. However, no significant differences were observed between the two groups when assessing frequency, nocturia, maximum cystomteric capacity or reflex detrusor volume.

Adverse events to note included 18 % with UTI and 27 % in the OnabotulinumtoxinA group had high PVR >200 mL. Despite the latter, only one patient was commenced on CISC.

A recent drug sponsored large phase II dose escalation randomised placebo-controlled study assessing OnabotulinumtoxinA in patients with refractory OAB was recently reported [74]. This multi-centre international study recruited 313 patients and randomised patients to 50, 100, 150, 200, 300 U and placebo. Approximately 75 % had IDO and the rest had bladder oversensitivity (BO), i.e. symptoms of OAB with no DO on urodynamics. At week 12, mean change from baseline in UUI episodes was –17.4, –20.7, –18.4, –23.0, –19.6 and –19.4 for the placebo and OnabotulinumtoxinA dose groups of 50 U, 100 U, 150 U, 200 U and 300 U, respectively. Dry rates were 15.9 %, 29.8 %, 37.0 %, 40.8 %, 30.9 % and 57.1 % in the placebo, and 50 U, 100 U, 150 U, 200 U and 300 U dose groups, respectively. Although a clear placebo effect is seen, there were statistically significant differences between active treatment and placebo at various time points. Using non-parametric analysis and a rank residual score, a dose-dependent effect was observed with minimal additional benefit for this parameter with doses >150 U. The lowest dose of 50 U did not appear to be as effective as doses 100–300 U. Those with IDO or BO had similar benefits. In a separate report assessing urodynamics, all doses were associated with significant increases in maximum cystometric capacity compared to baseline at 6 weeks; however, at 36 weeks this was only the case for 150, 200 and 300 U [75]. Reductions in UUI episodes appeared to be similar regardless of whether DO was present or not. Dose-dependent increases in PVR were observed up to 200 U. The maximal effect of increased PVR was at 2 weeks and thereafter values declined to 36 weeks. Adverse events reported significantly higher in the OnabotulinumtoxinA groups compared with placebo were high PVRs and UTI. The percentage of patients requiring an indwelling catheter or CISC were 0 %, 5.4 %, 10.9 %, 20.0 %, 21.2 % and 16.4 % for placebo, 50 U, 100 U, 150 U, 200 U and 300 U, respectively.

Three other small open labelled studies have also shown symptom benefit in the use of OnabotulinumtoxinA in treating BO [76–78]. However in another randomised double-blind placebo-controlled study, the benefits were less evident [79]. The study utilised 100 U OnabotulinumtoxinA and although the primary end point of increase in maximum cystometric capacity was met in favour of OnabotulinumtoxinA this did not translate into OAB symptom or durable QoL benefit for patients with poor overall response rates.

Other Relevant Studies

Kalsi et al., using the UDI-6 and IIQ-7 questionnaires found a statistically significant correlation between improvements in QoL with improvements in urgency and urge urinary incontinence but not urodynamic parameters in IDO patients treated with OnabotulinumtoxinA 200 U [48]. The same group studied as to when OAB symptoms change following injection of the same dose [49]. The study showed frequency, urgency and UUI was significantly reduced by day 4 following treatment. Nocturia took longer to reduce significantly. Urgency remained significantly reduced after day 4 up until week 4 but frequency and UUI were a little more variable, although by week 4 all OAB symptoms including nocturia were significantly less compared to baseline.

In order to combat the risk of developing high PVR in patients with IDO an interesting and novel study compared bladder injections with bladder and urethral sphincter injections in combination in 44 predominantly female patients [80]. Sphincteric injections were given to those who had a PVR >15 mL at baseline. In total 200–300 U OnabotulinumtoxinA were administered with 50–100 U given in the external sphincter. Improvements in urinary frequency, pad usage and urodynamic parameters were observed. A significant PVR compared to baseline at 4 weeks was seen in those with bladder injection alone (78 mL) compared to combination treatment (28 mL). A potential concern with the technique was the development of de novo stress urinary incontinence in those who received sphincteric injections. Pad usage at 4 weeks was similar in both groups and when assessing questionnaires specific to this aspect, although more patients answered in favour of stress symptoms in the combination group (bladder + sphincter injection), this did not reach statistical significance.

White et al., have recently demonstrated that the use of OnabotulinumtoxinA 200 U appears to be equally efficacious in the elderly population (>75 years of age) [81]. In this study 2/3 of the patients had IDO and 1/3 NDO with 4 patients presenting with mixed incontinence. Approximately 75 % reported >50 % improvement in symptoms following OnabotulinumtoxinA injections at 1 month. Significant reductions were observed for frequency and pad usage per 24 h compared with baseline values. Five patients did not initially respond with two of these five responding after a further injection of OnabotulinumtoxinA. None of the patients interestingly developed high PVR or any other major complications. Mean duration of benefit was approximately 7 months.

In 2007, the first sets of studies using AbobotulinumtoxinA in the management of IDO were published. Ghalayini et al., published on their small series of both NDO and IDO patients treated with 500 U. In the IDO group consisting of 16 patients, significant improvements in OAB symptoms, urodynamic parameters and pad usage were seen at 6 weeks following treatment [46]. Median duration of action was 5 months. One patient developed retention of urine and 3 others required CISC for a short period of time. Another study from the UK utilised 500 U in treating refractory IDO also suggested significant benefit [82]. Sixty-three percent of patients were dry at 1 week and 32 % at 3 and 6 months. Significant reductions in frequency and urgency were seen up to 6 months compared to baseline. Pad usage was significantly less after 6 weeks of treatment. Although trends of improvement were seen in urodynamic parameters only first desire to void was significantly increased in BTX-A treated patients at 3 months. DO seen in 100 % pre-injection had resolved in 40 % by 3 months. Again high rates of voiding dysfunction were seen with 35 % requiring an SPC or CISC at 6 weeks follow-up.

Repeated Injections

We followed up our original cohort of 34 patients involved in the first randomised double-blind placebo-controlled trial in patients with IDO [65]. Twenty patients received a repeat injection and of these nine subsequently received a third and fourth injection. OnabotulinumtoxinA doses of 100–300 U were used. Significant improvements in OAB symptoms and QoL were observed after each injection as compared with baseline. Maximum cystometric capacity and bladder compliance increased with decrease in the maximum detrusor pressure during filling cystometry. When comparing OAB symptoms, QoL and urodynamic parameters 3 months after the first and last injections, no significant differences were found. Nine patients had their BTX-A dose altered, with better outcomes in five. The commonest reported problems were difficulty in emptying the bladder requiring CISC (25 % after the first repeated injection) and UTI. This study is the first to report on OAB symptom outcomes and a dose optimisation strategy following repeated BTX-A injections in an IDO population. This dose optimisation protocol (selected patients had a reduction in dose to try to avoid the need to perform CISC and poor responders to initial treatment had their doses increased) improved outcomes in 5/9 (56 %) patients. Clearly larger scale studies are required with more patients before one can say this is a reasonable and safe approach to employ. In this study 3/4 (75 %) patients who were classified as poor responders had significantly better outcomes with higher doses of the toxin. A subanalysis of our patients series has suggested a high mean MDP (>110 cm H_2O) at baseline was a predictor for a poor response [83]. In these patients OnabotulinumtoxinA 200 U may not be sufficient to improve clinical outcomes and/or patient subjective assessment but with higher doses they are seen to improve both subjectively and objectively. We have also assessed the issue of difficulty emptying the bladder and the need for CISC following OnabotulinumtoxinA treatment with 200 U and have shown that preoperative detrusor contractility variables, calculated from urodynamics, maybe helpful in predicting CISC use.

Khan et al., recently have reported on QoL outcomes following up to six repeated BTX-A injections in IDO patients [84]. In total 129 injections were performed in 81 patients, but <5 patients were assessed after 4 injections. The median inter-interval injection was 14 months. Significant and sustained improvements in QoL were seen using validated questionnaires. The CISC rate was 43 % and UTIs were seen in 15 %.

Finally in our experience few studies report on discontinuation rates and the reasons why. In our recent publication on 207 injections in 100 patients, efficacy was maintained in patients who had 5 injections in terms of OAB symptoms and QoL improvements [85]. The data suggested drop out rates were approximately 25 % for injections 1–2 and then no other patient discontinued beyond the second injection. The commonest reason for discontinuing treatment was poor efficacy (13 %) or dislike of CISC (11 %).

Technique of Injection

The original description of BTX-A injections for the treatment of NDO was through a collagen flexible needle using a rigid cystoscope [1]. Since then the technique has evolved but the way in which the toxin is administered into the bladder has not been standardised and indeed practice varies around the world. In the initial experience with BTX-A and NDO, the trigone was avoided on the assumption that paralysing the trigonal muscle might induce VUR. Since then there has been mounting evidence that BTX may also affect sensory nerves and that afferent mechanisms have an important role in the pathophysiology of DO [27]. Investigators in the USA have advocated injecting the trigone [86], based on the fact that this area of the bladder contains the highest density of nerve fibres, including afferent population. Recently two studies have demonstrated that trigonal injections do not induce VUR, putting to rest the debate frequently contested at international meetings in those involved with injecting [87, 88]. In an OAB population (4 with IDO and 7 with sensory urgency) video urodynamics 6 weeks following BTX-A injections totalling 200 U into the bladder base and trigone suggested no new VUR and in the one patient who had VUR pretreatment this did not worsen [87]. In another study in NDO patients similar results were obtained in a population of 21 patients whose bladders were injected with a total of 300 U OnabotulinumtoxinA of which 50 U were injected in the trigonal area [88]. Again no new cases of VUR were seen.

The 'Dasgupta technique' is a minimally invasive, daycase, local anaesthetic procedure utilising a flexible cystoscope to perform BTX-A injections [89, 90]. Prophylactic antibiotics and 20 mL of 2 % lignocaine intraurethral gel are administered prior to the procedure. The injections are evenly distributed over the dome, posterior, right and left lateral walls of the bladder, avoiding the trigone. The technique has obvious benefits in terms of cost and ease of administration. In addition, the needle length (4 mm) is such that injection beyond the bladder is unlikely. Furthermore as an ultra-fine needle is used the chance of backflow of the toxin after removal of the needle is reduced. The 'Dasgupta technique' is quick; the procedure taking on average 15–20 min to perform and is also well tolerated with pain scores approximately 3–4 out of 10 on a visual analogue scale [91]. This minimally invasive technique has been adopted by some clinicians in the USA to treat patients with refractory OAB using 100 U of OnabotulinumtoxinA [92]. Ten injections are utilised and injected submucosally into the bladder base and trigone only. In their series of 10 patients similar efficacy was reproduced compared with their older rigid cystoscopic technique involving 30 injection sites. The added benefit appears to be that no patient developed urinary retention or an elevated post-void residual with the use of a reduced dose of BTX-A and this modified technique. Another group in the USA also using the 'Dasgupta technique' found the procedure was well tolerated and safe to use in the 'office' (outpatient) setting [93]. In this study mean pain scores in females and males were 3.1 and 1.6 out of 10, respectively. Only 1 patient out of 27 requested sedation if they were to have another BTX injection.

Mehnert et al., conducted a contrast MRI-based study in 6 patients following BTX-A injections + contrast to try and determine where the injection were likely to be placed [94]. As expected the majority of the injections were placed in the detrusor muscle (82 %) but some of the contrast material was seen to reach the perivesical fat tissue outside the detrusor. The technique employed utilised a rigid cystoscope and a 22G needle (0.7 cm) and had a needle length of 8 mm which was inserted into the bladder wall and withdrawn halfway prior to injection. Two injection techniques, 30 or 10 injections, were compared with similar outcomes clinically and in terms of contrast material present within and outside the detrusor.

In an attempt to improve the tolerability of the rigid cystoscopic technique similar to what was initially described by Schurch et al. [1], electromotive drug administration (EMDA) of lignocaine was assessed in a pilot study with good results [95]. Patients were compared with standard lignocaine instillation transurethrally ($n=10$) to lignocaine instillation enhanced by EMDA ($n=28$). The mean pain scores using a 10-point scale were 4 versus 0.5 in the lignocaine and lignocaine EMDA-enhanced groups, respectively. Despite the EMDA, the technique still was cost-effective when compared to spinal or general anaesthesia.

Another topic of debate amongst clinicians is the exact location and ideal depth of injections. As mentioned earlier some believe the bladder base and trigone should be targeted and others feel that a more global bladder approach would be better, particularly in NDO patients. As afferent nerve endings are in the suburothelium, some advocate injecting, ideally, in this layer. In practical terms, experts feel wherever the injection is located, whether the suburothelium or the detrusor, there is likely to be some diffusion of BTX in either direction. In cases of suburothelial injections a 'bleb' is raised and can be readily seen during cystoscopy (Fig. 12.3). Whether these are present or absent appears not to effect efficacy in our opinion and is also a shared view from other clinicians familiar with the technique, suggesting that the therapeutic effect is similar, as long as the bladder is successfully injected and there is no inadvertent injection into the bladder lumen or 'backspill' from the injection into the lumen.

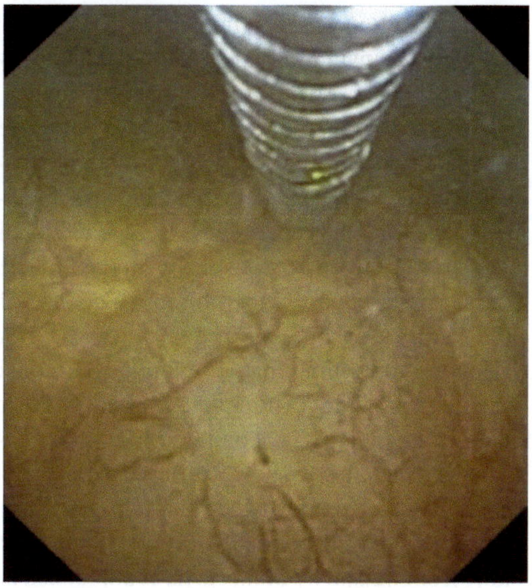

Fig. 12.3 Injection of BTX-A using the Dasgupta technique; Suburothelial bleb seen below sheath

In attempt to address some of these questions, Kuo et al., randomised 45 patients with refractory IDO to detrusor, suburothelial or bladder base injections [96]. Detrusor and suburothelial injections consisted of 40 injections distributed over the bladder avoiding the trigone and the bladder base injections involved only 10 injections into the trigone. In all cases a total of 100 U OnabotulinumtoxinA was administered using a rigid cystoscope. Satisfaction scores at 3 months were best in the suburothelial and detrusor groups with at least 50 % improvement seen in 80 % and 93 % of the groups, respectively, which compared favourably with the bladder base group which achieved the same outcomes in only 67 %. At 6 months this decreased to 47 %, 67 % and 13 % for suburothelial, detrusor and bladder base injections, respectively. Interestingly, no significant differences were observed in OAB symptoms or the urgency severity score at 3 months. Although not statistically significant, difficulty with urination and high post-void residuals were noted in 33 % (detrusor), 47 % (suburothelial) and 13 % in the bladder base. Furthermore acute urinary retention was seen in 13 % in the detrusor and suburothelial groups and in none in the bladder base group. When assessing urodynamics, maximum cystometric capacity and PVR were significantly higher in the detrusor and suburothelial groups compared to bladder base injections at 3 months but conversely functional bladder capacity was statistically higher in the bladder base group. Furthermore no evidence of VUR was seen in any group after BTX-A injections confirming that it is unlikely trigonal injections promote VUR. Lucioni et al., in their study comparing trigonal and non-trigonal injections were not able to show a difference in symptoms or QoL scores between the two groups at any follow-up time point [97]. However, a recent study from Ireland by Manecksha et al., looked at trigone inclusive (20 injections—5 in the trigone and 15 outside the trigone in the bladder) versus trigone sparing (20 injections throughout the bladder) AbobotulinumtoxinA (500 IU total) injections into the bladder to treat refractory OAB [98]. Utilising the overactive bladder symptom score (OABSS), significant reductions were seen in the in overall score and in the urgency subscale in favour of trigone inclusive technique.

Very recently the concept of BTX-A instillation has come to light. Chuang et al., have used liposomes, phospholipid-bilayered vesicles, to potentially facilitate the passage of BTX-A through the urothelium in a rat model [99]. In this unique study baseline cystometrograms were performed and a day later liposomes, BTX-A or lipotoxin (BTX-A + liposomes) were instilled into the bladder for 1 h. On day 8 bladder hyperactivity was induced by instilling acetic acid into the rat bladder and further cystometrograms were recorded. The inter-contraction interval was reduced by 57 %, 56 % and only 21 % following acetic acid administration in the liposome, BTX-A and lipotoxin groups, respectively. This suggests lipotoxin pretreatment suppresses acetic acid-induced bladder hyperactivity. Furthermore lipotoxin pretreated rats had significantly less inflammation in the bladder as assessed by standard immunohistochemistry. Reduced SNAP-25 expression and increased CGRP expression (indicating less release from the suburothelium in response to the acetic acid) was observed in the lipotoxin group when compared to the other groups. This rat-based model is the first to support the use of liposomes to transmit BTX-A to the suburothelium; however, the mechanism by which this is achieved is not yet been established. None the less this promising initial study will hopefully prompt further research into the possibility of BTX-A benefits without the need to perform injections which would most likely translate into better patient tolerability. Since then Khrut et al., have conducted a pilot study using an animal model of DO and compared bladder wall injections and instillations [100]. In the animal study, the average intermicturition and threshold pressures, as well as the number and amplitude of non-voiding bladder contractions decreased significantly in both instillation and injection groups. Micturition pressure decreased significantly only in the intramural injection group. The same authors on this basis decided to conduct a pilot study in 16 patients with refractory IDO. Although the treatment of instillation was well tolerated, 9/16 patients noted no change in symptoms and in those that did derive benefit, the mean duration of action was 6.8 weeks. No significant change in contractility variables were noted either in the human study. This study suggests intravesical instillation alone is not as efficacious as bladder injections, certainly in humans, and any benefit appears short-lived. Whether altered drug delivery with carrier molecules into the suburothelium and detrusor in humans can improve these results is still yet to be determined.

Health Economics and Cost Considerations

There is a limited amount of literature available on the cost-effectiveness of BTX in treating OAB. The current preferred method to assess cost-effectiveness of a new procedure is the cost per quality adjusted life years (QALY) gained [101]. The cost-effectiveness ratio is typically the cost of the new intervention minus the cost of current practice divided by the new intervention QALY minus the current practice QALY. A cost-effectiveness ratio of <£20,000–30,000/QALY is considered cost-effective by NICE [102]. In the UK a cost-effectiveness analysis was conducted. Although a cost per QALY gained calculation was not possible due to the lack of data linking bladder symptoms of DO to utility data needed to calculate QALYs gained, costing of the procedure were calculated based on NHS standard costs and NHS resources used by typical patients [101, 103]. The overall costs of one set of OnabotulinumtoxinA injections including clinic consultation, basic investigations such as urine dipstick and an urodynamic study, the injection procedure with consumables, clinic review in the outpatient clinic post-injection with a further urine dipstick and post-void residual, equated to £826 per patient.

In the USA, a cost-effectiveness model was utilised to assess BTX-A injections in comparison to antimuscarinics in treating urge urinary incontinence [104]. A 2-year time horizon was modelled and this allowed for a repeat injection of BTX-A if necessary. BTX-A treatment was costed at $4392 versus $2563 for anticholinergics but was more effective than anticholinergics. The cost-effectiveness ratio, i.e. the cost per QALY gained was $14,377 (approximately £8830) indicating that the BTX-A treatment was extremely cost-effective.

A more recent multi-centre study in Germany has recently reported outcomes of OnabotulinumtoxinA 300 U in treating NDO and its cost implications [105]. In 136 patients resource data was available 12 months pre- and post-BTX-A injection to make a cost analysis. Significant reductions were observed following treatment in UTIs (68 % to 28 %), incontinence episodes (63 % to 33 %) and incontinence aids (58 % to 28 %). As a result, significant cost savings were possible based on less antibiotic costs to treat UTIs (from approximately €160 to €80/year) and less equipment, e.g. pads, catheter costs used for incontinence (from approximately €2 to €1/day).

Watanabe et al., have assessed the 3-year costs comparing treatment options in patients refractory to anticholinergics, namely sacral neuromodulation, BTX-A injections and augmentation cystoplasty [106]. Their study based from a US tax payers perspective, assessed initial costs for the procedures and follow-up costs for 3 years. Their findings suggested BTX-A was the most cost-effective approach over the study period assessed with the sensitivity analysis suggesting over 3 years, costs included $25,384–$27,357, $4586–$11,476 and $12,315–$16,830, for sacral neuromodulation, BTX-A and augmentation cystoplasty, respectively. Further longer term analysis would be necessary however, as BTX-A injections are likely to be repeated where as neuromodulation and augmentation cystoplasty are more permanent interventions. Furthermore this study and many others do not factor in costs related to adverse events of BTX-A, namely increased UTI rate and the costs related to CISC.

Another study compared OnabotulinumtoxinA 300 U (10 injections over 5 years) and augmentation cystoplasty using a decision analysis model and demonstrated BTX-A treatment was less expensive over 5 years, costing $28,065 and was more cost-effective over 5 years if the effect lasted for >5.1 months. The model was based on a surgical complication rate of 40 % but if this rate fell to <14 %, augmentation cystoplasty was cheaper over the 5 years [107].

Using a Markov analytical model, sacral neuromodulation was compared to BTX-A over 5 years [108]. Success was defined as a 50 % reduction in UI episodes, daytime frequency or pad usage. The cost-effectiveness analysis after a 5-year period showed 4.95 QALYs for neuromodulation compared to 4.72 for BTX. The 5-year costs were €25,780 for SNM and €19,353 for BTX. Sacral neuromodulation only became cost-effective after 4 years. In this analysis it was presumed both procedures were performed under general anaesthesia and OnabotulinumtoxinA 200 U was injected yearly. If the analysis factored in the BTX-A injections under local anaesthesia or when peripheral nerve evaluation or bilateral testing was used for neuromodulation, BTX-A injections were more cost-effective.

Conclusions

Over the last decade, BTX-A has truly established itself as an effective, safe and repeatable option to treat refractory OAB and DO. Significant improvements in symptoms, urodynamic parameters and QoL are achievable. The commonest side effects reported are UTI and voiding dysfunction necessitating CISC. This is less of an issue in the neurogenic population where a considerable amount of patients already will be utilising CISC, however is more relevant to those with IDO and careful counselling with regard to this is essential. The mechanisms of action of the toxin are clearly complex within the bladder and there is significant evidence now which confirms both motor and sensory effects. It is likely following the large phase II and III trials recently published for OnabotulinumtoxinA that doses of 100 U and 200 U will be recommended for IDO and NDO, respectively. In our experience this is generally correct; however, there are some patients who will need dose optimisation and may even require higher doses in order to achieve the required goals (high voiding pressures, symptom control, prevention of voiding dysfunction). Techniques vary around the world and adaptations of the technique can be performed to suit the patient, e.g. trigonal injection may help reduce voiding dysfunction but possibly at the risk of less duration of action. It is expected that FDA and MHRA approval is on the horizon, which can only be a step forward in the right direction, so that the millions of people who suffer with OAB can have better access and be helped by this remarkable toxin.

Acknowledgments A Sahai, MS Khan and P Dasgupta acknowledges financial support from the Department of Health via the National Institute for Health Research (NIHR) comprehensive Biomedical Research Centre award to Guy's & St Thomas' NHS Foundation Trust in partnership with King's College London and King's College Hospital NHS Foundation Trust. They also acknowledge the support of the MRC Centre for Transplantation. Christopher Dowson for his assistance with the figures in the chapter.

References

1. Schurch B, Stohrer M, Kramer G, Schmid DM, Gaul G, Hauri D. Botulinum-A toxin for treating detrusor hyperreflexia in spinal cord injured patients: a new alternative to anticholinergic drugs? Preliminary results. J Urol. 2000;164(3 Pt 1):692–7.
2. Schurch B, Schmid DM, Stohrer M. Treatment of neurogenic incontinence with botulinum toxin A. N Engl J Med. 2000;342(9):665.
3. Abrams P, Cardozo L, Fall M, et al. The standardisation of terminology of lower urinary tract function: report from the Standardisation Sub-committee of the International Continence Society. Neurourol Urodyn. 2002;21(2):167–78.
4. Thuroff JW, Abrams P, Andersson KE, et al. EAU guidelines on urinary incontinence. Eur Urol. 2011; 59(3):387–400.
5. Gill DM. Bacterial toxins: a table of lethal amounts. Microbiol Rev. 1982;46(1):86–94.
6. Simpson LL. Molecular pharmacology of botulinum toxin and tetanus toxin. Annu Rev Pharmacol Toxicol. 1986;26:427–53.
7. Dolly JO, Aoki KR. The structure and mode of action of different botulinum toxins. Eur J Neurol. 2006;13 Suppl 4:1–9.
8. Harper M, Fowler CJ, Dasgupta P. Botulinum toxin and its applications in the lower urinary tract. BJU Int. 2004;93(6):702–6.
9. NICE. Urinary incontinence. The management of urinary incontinence in women. Report No.: NICE Clinical Guideline 40;2006.
10. Apostolidis A, Dasgupta P, Denys P, et al. Recommendations on the use of Botulinum toxin in the treatment of lower urinary tract disorders and pelvic floor dysfunctions: a European Consensus Report. Eur Urol. 2009;55(1):100–19.
11. Mangera A, Andersson K-E, Apostolidis A, et al. Contemporary management of lower urinary tract disease with Botulinum toxin A: a systematic review of Botox (OnabotulinumtoxinA) and Dysport (AbobotulinumtoxinA). Eur Urol. 2011;60(4):784–95.
12. Dong M, Yeh F, Tepp WH, et al. SV2 is the protein receptor for botulinum neurotoxin A. Science. 2006;312(5773):592–6.
13. Black JD, Dolly JO. Interaction of 125I-labeled botulinum neurotoxins with nerve terminals. I. Ultrastructural autoradiographic localization and quantitation of distinct membrane acceptors for types A and B on motor nerves. J Cell Biol. 1986;103(2):521–34.
14. Black JD, Dolly JO. Interaction of 125I-labeled botulinum neurotoxins with nerve terminals. II. Autoradiographic evidence for its uptake into motor nerves by acceptor-mediated endocytosis. J Cell Biol. 1986;103(2):535–44.

15. Dolly JO, Black J, Williams RS, Melling J. Acceptors for botulinum neurotoxin reside on motor nerve terminals and mediate its internalization. Nature. 1984;307(5950):457–60.
16. Herreros J, Lalli G, Montecucco G, Schiavo G. Pathophysiological properties of clostridial neurotoxins in The comprehensive sourcebook of bacterial protein toxins. London: Academic; 2006.
17. Schiavo G, Matteoli M, Montecucco C. Neurotoxins affecting neuroexocytosis. Physiol Rev. 2000; 80(2):717–66.
18. Burnstock G. Purinergic nerves. Pharmacol Rev. 1972;24(3):509–81.
19. Mackenzie I, Burnstock G, Dolly JO. The effects of purified botulinum neurotoxin type A on cholinergic, adrenergic and non-adrenergic, atropine-resistant autonomic neuromuscular transmission. Neuroscience. 1982;7(4):997–1006.
20. Bayliss M, Wu C, Newgreen D, Mundy AR, Fry CH. A quantitative study of atropine-resistant contractile responses in human detrusor smooth muscle, from stable, unstable and obstructed bladders. J Urol. 1999;162(5):1833–9.
21. O'Reilly BA, Kosaka AH, Knight GF, et al. P2X receptors and their role in female idiopathic detrusor instability. J Urol. 2002;167(1):157–64.
22. Smith CP, Franks ME, McNeil BK, et al. Effect of botulinum toxin A on the autonomic nervous system of the rat lower urinary tract. J Urol. 2003; 169(5):1896–900.
23. Kanai A, Wyndaele JJ, Andersson KE, et al. Researching bladder afferents-determining the effects of beta(3) -adrenergic receptor agonists and botulinum toxin type-A. Neurourol Urodyn. 2011;30(5):684–91.
24. de Groat WC, Yoshimura N. Plasticity in reflex pathways to the lower urinary tract following spinal cord injury. Exp Neurol. 2012;235(1):123–32.
25. Michel MC, Chapple CR. Basic mechanisms of urgency: roles and benefits of pharmacotherapy. World J Urol. 2009;27(6):705–9.
26. Duggan MJ, Quinn CP, Chaddock JA, et al. Inhibition of release of neurotransmitters from rat dorsal root ganglia by a novel conjugate of a Clostridium botulinum toxin A endopeptidase fragment and Erythrina cristagalli lectin. J Biol Chem. 2002;277(38): 34846–52.
27. Apostolidis A, Dasgupta P, Fowler CJ. Proposed mechanism for the efficacy of injected botulinum toxin in the treatment of human detrusor overactivity. Eur Urol. 2006;49(4):644–50.
28. Morenilla-Palao C, Planells-Cases R, Garcia-Sanz N, Ferrer-Montiel A. Regulated exocytosis contributes to protein kinase C potentiation of vanilloid receptor activity. J Biol Chem. 2004;279(24): 25665–72.
29. Welch MJ, Purkiss JR, Foster KA. Sensitivity of embryonic rat dorsal root ganglia neurons to Clostridium botulinum neurotoxins. Toxicon. 2000; 38(2):245–58.
30. Smet PJ, Moore KH, Jonavicius J. Distribution and colocalization of calcitonin gene-related peptide, tachykinins, and vasoactive intestinal peptide in normal and idiopathic unstable human urinary bladder. Lab Invest. 1997;77(1):37–49.
31. Rapp DE, Turk KW, Bales GT, Cook SP. Botulinum toxin type a inhibits calcitonin gene-related peptide release from isolated rat bladder. J Urol. 2006;175(3 Pt 1):1138–42.
32. Lucioni A, Bales GT, Lotan TL, McGehee DS, Cook SP, Rapp DE. Botulinum toxin type A inhibits sensory neuropeptide release in rat bladder models of acute injury and chronic inflammation. BJU Int. 2008;101(3):366–70.
33. Burnstock G. Therapeutic potential of purinergic signalling for diseases of the urinary tract. BJU Int. 2011;107(2):192–204.
34. Khera M, Somogyi GT, Kiss S, Boone TB, Smith CP. Botulinum toxin A inhibits ATP release from bladder urothelium after chronic spinal cord injury. Neurochem Int. 2004;45(7):987–93.
35. Smith CP, Vemulakonda VM, Kiss S, Boone TB, Somogyi GT. Enhanced ATP release from rat bladder urothelium during chronic bladder inflammation: effect of botulinum toxin A. Neurochem Int. 2005;47(4):291–7.
36. Atiemo H, Wynes J, Chuo J, Nipkow L, Sklar GN, Chai TC. Effect of botulinum toxin on detrusor overactivity induced by intravesical adenosine triphosphate and capsaicin in a rat model. Urology. 2005; 65(3):622–6.
37. Apostolidis A, Popat R, Yiangou Y, et al. Decreased sensory receptors P2X3 and TRPV1 in suburothelial nerve fibers following intradetrusor injections of botulinum toxin for human detrusor overactivity. J Urol. 2005;174(3):977–82.
38. Kuo HC, Liu HT, Chancellor MB. Can urinary nerve growth factor be a biomarker for overactive bladder? Rev Urol. 2010;12(2–3):e69–77.
39. Giannantoni A, Di Stasi SM, Nardicchi V, et al. Botulinum-A toxin injections into the detrusor muscle decrease nerve growth factor bladder tissue levels in patients with neurogenic detrusor overactivity. J Urol. 2006;175(6):2341–4.
40. Liu HT, Chancellor MB, Kuo HC. Urinary nerve growth factor levels are elevated in patients with detrusor overactivity and decreased in responders to detrusor botulinum toxin-A injection. Eur Urol. 2009;56(4):700–6.
41. Schurch B, de SM, Denys P, et al. Botulinum toxin type a is a safe and effective treatment for neurogenic urinary incontinence: results of a single treatment, randomized, placebo controlled 6-month study. J Urol. 2005;174(1):196–200.
42. Schurch B, Denys P, Kozma CM, Reese PR, Slaton T, Barron RL. Botulinum toxin A improves the quality

of life of patients with neurogenic urinary incontinence. Eur Urol. 2007;52(3):850–8.
43. Ehren I, Volz D, Farrelly E, et al. Efficacy and impact of botulinum toxin A on quality of life in patients with neurogenic detrusor overactivity: a randomised, placebo-controlled, double-blind study. Scand J Urol Nephrol. 2007;41(4):335–40.
44. Herschorn S, Gajewski J, Ethans K, et al. Efficacy of botulinum toxin A injection for neurogenic detrusor overactivity and urinary incontinence: a randomized, double-blind trial. J Urol. 2011;185(6):2229–35.
45. Cruz F, Herschorn S, Aliotta P, et al. Efficacy and safety of onabotulinumtoxinA in patients with urinary incontinence due to neurogenic detrusor overactivity: a randomised, double-blind, placebo-controlled trial. Eur Urol. 2011;60(4):742–50.
46. Ghalayini IF, Al-Ghazo MA. Intradetrusor injection of botulinum-A toxin in patients with idiopathic and neurogenic detrusor overactivity: urodynamic outcome and patient satisfaction. Neurourol Urodyn. 2007;26(4):531–6.
47. Hori S, Patki P, Attar KH, Ismail S, Vasconcelos JC, Shah PJ. Patients' perspective of botulinum toxin-A as a long-term treatment option for neurogenic detrusor overactivity secondary to spinal cord injury. BJU Int. 2009;104(2):216–20.
48. Kalsi V, Apostolidis A, Popat R, Gonzales G, Fowler CJ, Dasgupta P. Quality of life changes in patients with neurogenic versus idiopathic detrusor overactivity after intradetrusor injections of botulinum neurotoxin type A and correlations with lower urinary tract symptoms and urodynamic changes. Eur Urol. 2006;49(3):528–35.
49. Kalsi V, Apostolidis A, Gonzales G, Elneil S, Dasgupta P, Fowler CJ. Early effect on the overactive bladder symptoms following botulinum neurotoxin type A injections for detrusor overactivity. Eur Urol. 2008;54(1):181–7.
50. Grosse J, Kramer G, Jakse G. Comparing two types of botulinum-A toxin detrusor injections in patients with severe neurogenic detrusor overactivity: a case-control study. BJU Int. 2009;104(5):651–6.
51. Kuo HC. Therapeutic effects of suburothelial injection of botulinum a toxin for neurogenic detrusor overactivity due to chronic cerebrovascular accident and spinal cord lesions. Urology. 2006;67(2):232–6.
52. Giannantoni A, Rossi A, Mearini E, Zingaro MD, Porena M, Berardelli A. Botulinum toxin A for overactive bladder and detrusor muscle overactivity in patients with Parkinson's disease and multiple system atrophy. J Urol. 2009;182(4):1453–7.
53. Giannantoni A, Conte A, Proietti S, et al. Botulinum toxin type A in patients with Parkinson's disease and refractory overactive bladder. J Urol. 2011; 186(3):960–4.
54. Dowson C, Khan MS, Dasgupta P, Sahai A. Repeat botulinum toxin-A injections for treatment of adult detrusor overactivity. Nat Rev Urol. 2010;7(12): 661–7.
55. Giannantoni A, Mearini E, Del ZM, Porena M. Six-year follow-up of botulinum toxin A intradetrusorial injections in patients with refractory neurogenic detrusor overactivity: clinical and urodynamic results. Eur Urol. 2009;55(3):705–11.
56. Kalsi V, Gonzales G, Popat R, et al. Botulinum injections for the treatment of bladder symptoms of multiple sclerosis. Ann Neurol. 2007;62(5):452–7.
57. Karsenty G, Reitz A, Lindemann G, Boy S, Schurch B. Persistence of therapeutic effect after repeated injections of botulinum toxin type A to treat incontinence due to neurogenic detrusor overactivity. Urology. 2006;68(6):1193–7.
58. Pannek J, Gocking K, Bersch U. Long-term effects of repeated intradetrusor botulinum neurotoxin A injections on detrusor function in patients with neurogenic bladder dysfunction. BJU Int. 2009; 104(9):1246–50.
59. Khan S, Game X, Kalsi V, et al. Long-term effect on quality of life of repeat detrusor injections of botulinum neurotoxin-A for detrusor overactivity in patients with multiple sclerosis. J Urol. 2011;185(4):1344–9.
60. Stoehrer M, Wolff A, Kramer G, et al. Treatment of neurogenic detrusor overactivity with botulinum toxin A: the first seven years. Urol Int. 2009; 83(4):379–85.
61. Akbar M, Abel R, Seyler TM, et al. Repeated botulinum-A toxin injections in the treatment of myelodysplastic children and patients with spinal cord injuries with neurogenic bladder dysfunction. BJU Int. 2007;100(3):639–45.
62. Del PG, Filocamo MT, Li Marzi V, et al. Neurogenic detrusor overactivity treated with english botulinum toxin a: 8-year experience of one single centre. Eur Urol. 2008;53(5):1013–20.
63. Ghalayini IF, Al-Ghazo MA, Elnasser ZA. Is efficacy of repeated intradetrusor botulinum toxin type A (Dysport((R))) injections dose dependent? Clinical and urodynamic results after four injections in patients with drug-resistant neurogenic detrusor overactivity. Int Urol Nephrol. 2009;41(4):805–13.
64. Grosse J, Kramer G, Stohrer M. Success of repeat detrusor injections of botulinum a toxin in patients with severe neurogenic detrusor overactivity and incontinence. Eur Urol. 2005;47(5):653–9.
65. Sahai A, Dowson C, Khan MS, Dasgupta P. Repeated injections of botulinum toxin-A for idiopathic detrusor overactivity. Urology. 2010;75(3):552–8.
66. Comperat E, Reitz A, Delcourt A, Capron F, Denys P, Chartier-Kastler E. Histologic features in the urinary bladder wall affected from neurogenic overactivity—a comparison of inflammation, oedema and fibrosis with and without injection of botulinum toxin type A. Eur Urol. 2006;50(5):1058–64.
67. Haferkamp A, Schurch B, Reitz A, et al. Lack of ultrastructural detrusor changes following endoscopic injection of botulinum toxin type a in overactive neurogenic bladder. Eur Urol. 2004; 46(6):784–91.
68. Apostolidis A, Jacques TS, Freeman A, et al. Histological changes in the urothelium and suburothelium of human overactive bladder following intradetrusor injections of botulinum neurotoxin type A for

the treatment of neurogenic or idiopathic detrusor overactivity. Eur Urol. 2008;53(6):1245–53.
69. Sahai A, Khan MS, Dasgupta P. Efficacy of botulinum toxin-A for treating idiopathic detrusor overactivity: results from a single center, randomized, double-blind, placebo controlled trial. J Urol. 2007;177(6):2231–6.
70. Sahai A, Dowson C, Khan MS, Dasgupta P. Improvement in quality of life after botulinum toxin-A injections for idiopathic detrusor overactivity: results from a randomized double-blind placebo-controlled trial. BJU Int. 2009;103(11):1509–15.
71. Brubaker L, Richter HE, Visco A, et al. Refractory idiopathic urge urinary incontinence and botulinum A injection. J Urol. 2008;180(1):217–22.
72. Werner M, Schmid DM, Schussler B. Efficacy of botulinum-A toxin in the treatment of detrusor overactivity incontinence: a prospective nonrandomized study. Am J Obstet Gynecol. 2005;192(5):1735–40.
73. Flynn MK, Amundsen CL, Perevich M, Liu F, Webster GD. Outcome of a randomized, double-blind, placebo controlled trial of botulinum A toxin for refractory overactive bladder. J Urol. 2009;181(6):2608–15.
74. Dmochowski R, Chapple C, Nitti VW, et al. Efficacy and safety of onabotulinumtoxinA for idiopathic overactive bladder: a double-blind, placebo controlled, randomized, dose ranging trial. J Urol. 2010;184(6):2416–22.
75. Rovner E, Kennelly M, Schulte-Baukloh H, Zhou J, Haag-Molkenteller C, Dasgupta P. Urodynamic results and clinical outcomes with intradetrusor injections of onabotulinumtoxinA in a randomized, placebo-controlled dose-finding study in idiopathic overactive bladder. Neurourol Urodyn. 2011;30(4): 556–62.
76. Kanagarajah P, Ayyathurai R, Caruso DJ, Gomez C, Gousse AE. Role of botulinum toxin-A in refractory idiopathic overactive bladder patients without detrusor overactivity. Int Urol Nephrol. 2012; 44(1):91–7.
77. Schulte-Baukloh H, Weiss C, Stolze T, Sturzebecher B, Knispel HH. Botulinum-A toxin for treatment of overactive bladder without detrusor overactivity: urodynamic outcome and patient satisfaction. Urology. 2005;66(1):82–7.
78. Schmid DM, Sauermann P, Werner M, et al. Experience with 100 cases treated with botulinum-A toxin injections in the detrusor muscle for idiopathic overactive bladder syndrome refractory to anticholinergics. J Urol. 2006;176(1):177–85.
79. Dowson C, Sahai A, Watkins J, Dasgupta P, Khan MS. The safety and efficacy of botulinum toxin-A in the management of bladder oversensitivity: a randomised double-blind placebo-controlled trial. Int J Clin Pract. 2011;65(6):698–704.
80. Schulte-Baukloh H, Weiss C, Stolze T, et al. Botulinum-A toxin detrusor and sphincter injection in treatment of overactive bladder syndrome: objective outcome and patient satisfaction. Eur Urol. 2005;48(6):984–90.
81. White WM, Pickens RB, Doggweiler R, Klein FA. Short-term efficacy of botulinum toxin a for refractory overactive bladder in the elderly population. J Urol. 2008;180(6):2522–6.
82. Jeffery S, Fynes M, Lee F, Wang K, Williams L, Morley R. Efficacy and complications of intradetrusor injection with botulinum toxin A in patients with refractory idiopathic detrusor overactivity. BJU Int. 2007;100(6):1302–6.
83. Sahai A, Khan MS, Le GN, Dasgupta P. Urodynamic assessment of poor responders after botulinum toxin-A treatment for overactive bladder. Urology. 2008;71(3):455–9.
84. Khan S, Kessler TM, Apostolidis A, et al. What a patient with refractory idiopathic detrusor overactivity should know about botulinum neurotoxin type a injection. J Urol. 2009;181(4):1773–8.
85. Dowson C, Watkins J, Khan MS, Dasgupta P, Sahai A. Repeated botulinum toxin type A injections for refractory overactive bladder: medium-term outcomes, safety profile, and discontinuation rates. Eur Urol. 2012;61(4):834–9.
86. Smith CP, Nishiguchi J, O'Leary M, Yoshimura N, Chancellor MB. Single-institution experience in 110 patients with botulinum toxin A injection into bladder or urethra. Urology. 2005;65(1):37–41.
87. Karsenty G, Elzayat E, Delapparent T, St-Denis B, Lemieux MC, Corcos J. Botulinum toxin type a injections into the trigone to treat idiopathic overactive bladder do not induce vesicoureteral reflux. J Urol. 2007;177(3):1011–4.
88. Mascarenhas F, Cocuzza M, Gomes CM, Leao N. Trigonal injection of botulinum toxin-A does not cause vesicoureteral reflux in neurogenic patients. Neurourol Urodyn. 2008;27(4):311–4.
89. Harper M, Popat RB, Dasgupta R, Fowler CJ, Dasgupta P. A minimally invasive technique for outpatient local anaesthetic administration of intradetrusor botulinum toxin in intractable detrusor overactivity. BJU Int. 2003;92(3):325–6.
90. Sahai A, Kalsi V, Khan MS, Fowler CJ. Techniques for the intradetrusor administration of botulinum toxin. BJU Int. 2006;97(4):675–8.
91. Popat R, Apostolidis A, Kalsi V, Gonzales G, Fowler CJ, Dasgupta P. A comparison between the response of patients with idiopathic detrusor overactivity and neurogenic detrusor overactivity to the first intradetrusor injection of botulinum-A toxin. J Urol. 2005; 174(3):984–9.
92. Smith CP, Chancellor MB. Simplified bladder botulinum-toxin delivery technique using flexible cystoscope and 10 sites of injection. J Endourol. 2005;19(7):880–2.
93. Cohen BL, Rivera R, Barboglio P, Gousse A. Safety and tolerability of sedation-free flexible cystoscopy for intradetrusor botulinum toxin-A injection. J Urol. 2007;177(3):1006–10.
94. Mehnert U, Boy S, Schmid M, et al. A morphological evaluation of botulinum neurotoxin A injections into the detrusor muscle using magnetic resonance imaging. World J Urol. 2009;27(3):397–403.

95. Schurch B, Reitz A, Tenti G. Electromotive drug administration of lidocaine to anesthetize the bladder before botulinum-A toxin injections into the detrusor. Spinal Cord. 2004;42(6):338–41.
96. Kuo HC. Comparison of effectiveness of detrusor, suburothelial and bladder base injections of botulinum toxin a for idiopathic detrusor overactivity. J Urol. 2007;178(4 Pt 1):1359–63.
97. Lucioni A, Rapp DE, Gong EM, Fedunok P, Bales GT. Intravesical botulinum type A toxin injection in patients with overactive bladder: Trigone versus trigone-sparing injection. Can J Urol. 2006; 13(5):3291–5.
98. Manecksha RP, Cullen IM, Ahmad S, et al. Prospective randomised controlled trial comparing trigone-sparing versus trigone-including intradetrusor injection of abobotulinumtoxinA for refractory idiopathic detrusor overactivity. Eur Urol. 2012; 61(5):928–35.
99. Chuang YC, Tyagi P, Huang CC, et al. Urodynamic and immunohistochemical evaluation of intravesical botulinum toxin A delivery using liposomes. J Urol. 2009;182(2):786–92.
100. Krhut J, Zvara P. Intravesical instillation of botulinum toxin A: an in vivo murine study and pilot clinical trial. Int Urol Nephrol. 2011;43(2):337–43.
101. Sangster P, Kalsi V. Health economics and intradetrusor injections of botulinum for the treatment of detrusor overactivity. BJU Int. 2008;102 Suppl 1:17–9.
102. Devlin N, Parkin D. Does NICE have a cost-effectiveness threshold and what other factors influence its decisions? A binary choice analysis. Health Econ. 2004;13(5):437–52.
103. Kalsi V, Popat RB, Apostolidis A, et al. Cost-consequence analysis evaluating the use of botulinum neurotoxin-A in patients with detrusor overactivity based on clinical outcomes observed at a single UK centre. Eur Urol. 2006;49(3):519–27.
104. Wu JM, Siddiqui NY, Amundsen CL, Myers ER, Havrilesky LJ, Visco AG. Cost-effectiveness of botulinum toxin a versus anticholinergic medications for idiopathic urge incontinence. J Urol. 2009; 181(5):2181–6.
105. Wefer B, Ehlken B, Bremer J, et al. Treatment outcomes and resource use of patients with neurogenic detrusor overactivity receiving botulinum toxin A (BOTOX((R))) therapy in Germany. World J Urol. 2010;28(3):385–90.
106. Watanabe JH, Campbell JD, Ravelo A, Chancellor MB, Kowalski J, Sullivan SD. Cost analysis of interventions for antimuscarinic refractory patients with overactive bladder. Urology. 2010;76(4):835–40.
107. Padmanabhan P, Scarpero HM, Milam DF, Dmochowski RR, Penson DF. Five-year cost analysis of intra-detrusor injection of botulinum toxin type A and augmentation cystoplasty for refractory neurogenic detrusor overactivity. World J Urol. 2011;29(1):51–7.
108. Leong RK, de Wachter SG, Joore MA, van Kerrebroeck PE. Cost-effectiveness analysis of sacral neuromodulation and botulinum toxin A treatment for patients with idiopathic overactive bladder. BJU Int. 2011;108(4):558–64.

Part V

Neuromodulation

13 Sacral Neurostimulation: InterStim

Ravi Kacker and Anurag K. Das

Urinary frequency, urgency, and urge incontinence represent common problems in the urologist's practice. The term overactive bladder (OAB) is defined by the International Continence Society as "urgency or frequency with or without urge incontinence in the absence of other pathological or metabolic conditions to explain these symptoms" [1]. Although pharmaceutical management and pelvic floor rehabilitation combined with behavioral modification provide relief to many patients with symptoms of OAB, many patients have insufficient improvement or are unable to tolerate pharmacologic therapy [2]. By some estimates, up to 40 % of patients either are refractory to primary management or have an unsatisfactory response. In such cases, sacral neuromodulation (SNS) is a minimally invasive and reversible treatment with a high rate of success that is an attractive option before consideration of more invasive and permanent treatment modalities.

Neuromodulation therapy for OAB symptoms represents a recent step in the long history of the use of electrical stimulation for medical purposes. Early medical applications of electrical stimulation in the nineteenth century were aimed at a broad range of disorders including depression and excess libido. Over the next half century, pioneering applications in urology applied electrical stimulation to the bladder, pelvic floor, or sacral roots for neurogenic urinary retention or neurogenic overactivity. Advances in cardiac pacing and miniaturization of electrical instruments led to a resurgence of interest in neuromodulation of bladder function. The Department of Urology at the University of California, San Francisco led by Drs. Richard Schmidt and Emil Tanagho was instrumental in performing some of the early work and laying the foundation for the use of SNS for the treatment of refractory voiding dysfunction. Drs. Craggs and Fowler in London [3] and Drs. DeGroat and Chancellor [4] at the University of Pittsburgh have performed further work on the mechanism of action of SNS.

Initial large-scale trials were funded by Medtronic (Minneapolis, MN, USA) in the mid-1990s and led to approval from the United States Food and Drug Administration of InterStim for SNS for urge incontinence in 1997 and for urgency/frequency and nonobstructive urinary retention in 1999. Since then, over 25,000 patients have undergone SNS [5]. A systematic literature review by Brazelli [6] demonstrated evidence for safety and efficacy of SNS for neuromodulation in both randomized controlled trials (RCTs) and case series. For the RCTs,

R. Kacker, M.D. (✉)
Division of Urology, Department of Surgery, Beth Israel Deaconess Medical Center, 330 Brookline Avenue, Rabb 440, Boston, MA 02115, USA
e-mail: rkacker@bidmc.harvard.edu

A.K. Das, M.D., F.A.C.S.
Department of Urology, Center for Neuro-urology and Continence, Beth Israel Deaconess Medical Center, Boston, MA, USA

G.H. Badlani (ed.), *Minimally Invasive Therapy for Urinary Incontinence and Pelvic Organ Prolapse*, Current Clinical Urology, DOI 10.1007/978-1-4939-0008-4_13,

80 % of patients achieved either 90 % continence or a 50 % improvement in their urge incontinence symptoms after SNS.

Mechanism of Action

The exact mechanism of action of SNS is unknown, but it may restore the balance of inhibitory and excitatory influences on bladder and sphincter function controlled by spino-bulbo-spinal pathways. Bladder afferents project to the pontine micturition center which then modulate micturition reflexes. In this theory, sensory somatic input from the pelvic floor acts to inhibit bladder afferents and may be deficient in the OAB syndrome [7]. SNS acts by somehow restoring these inhibitory pathways at the level of S2–4 which provide the primary autonomic (pelvic nerve) and somatic (pudendal nerve) innervation for the bladder, urethra, and pelvic floor. Studies on the latency of the motor response to SNS after chronic treatment have suggested that somatic afferents, in particular, are activated [8].

Cortical sensory changes are also observed during SNS. EEG studies show activity that best correlates with the sensory cortex and combined PET/MRI (magnetic resonance imaging) studies do not show activation of the areas associated with bladder filling sensation and micturition. These findings support the theory that SNS modulates somatic sensory pathways rather than directly influencing bladder and sphincter function. Neural plasticity may also play a role over the course of SNS and PET studies show an initial activation of areas associated with motor learning, followed by activation of motor areas associated with pelvic floor and abdominal musculature [9].

Such PET findings may relate to another theory that the mechanism of action of SNS lies in efferent-mediated augmentation of the guarding reflex [10]. Indeed, in animal models, chronic SNS leads to hypertrophy of striated external sphincter muscle fibers and increased urethral closure pressures [11]. It is, however, unclear if these changes are secondary to modulation of somatic afferents or direct stimulation of motor pathways via Onuf's nucleus. Recent studies have also investigated the neurotransmitters that mediate the effect of SNS and found that both non-NMDA and vanilloid receptors play a role [3].

Case Studies

Here we present two illustrative cases of patients with refractory OAB symptoms treated with SNS.

Case 1

A 35-year-old G2P2 white female presents with a 5-year history of urinary frequency and urgency. She denies hematuria or significant pain component and has never had urge incontinence. She voids every 45 min to hourly during the day and has nocturia about twice a night. She dates her urinary symptoms as starting soon after undergoing hysterectomy for fibroids. Medical and surgical history otherwise is remarkable only for constipation and appendectomy. There are no culture-proven urinary tract infections, but the patient has tried several courses of antibiotics without significant improvement. She has tried anticholinergics without any significant improvement of her urinary symptoms and worsening of her constipation. Physical examination is unremarkable and pelvic examination shows normal external genitalia without significant prolapse or estrogenized introitus. Neurological examination including perianal sensation and rectal sphincter tone is normal.

Voiding diary reveals a functional capacity of 220 mL with an average void of 125 mL. There are 16 and 18 voids on two 24-h diaries. Urodynamics reveals first sensation at 40 mL, with a strong desire at 75 mL and a capacity of 130 mL. Emptying is normal, but there is some Valsalva augmentation during voiding. There is no evidence of detrusor overactivity. Cystoscopy is unremarkable and essentially normal except for hypersensitivity and limited capacity.

Case 2

A 55-year-old white female presents with complaints of inability to make it to the bathroom in time. She has accidents where she loses large amounts of urine 2–3 times weekly, but more commonly (3–4 times daily), she will lose up to three tablespoons as she is entering the bathroom or trying to undress. The urge incontinence has been present for 5–6 years but the large volume incontinence is new. She denies any bowel incontinence, has mild constipation, and denies any neurologic disease. She is otherwise healthy, with mild hypertension, and is G3P3 (all deliveries were performed with Caesarean section); she denies any stress incontinence or fecal incontinence.

Her examination essentially is unremarkable, with no evidence for any prolapse and a normal abdominal and neurological examination. Urine is clear with no hematuria or pyuria. Cystoscopy is normal and urodynamics reveals terminal detrusor overactivity with inability to inhibit the detrusor contraction. Anticholinergic medications are of minimal help.

Indications

SNS is indicated for the treatment of refractory urge incontinence and refractory urinary frequency/urgency syndromes, or refractory OAB, depending on one's terminology. Generally, patients who have failed or could not tolerate more conservative therapy, such as behavioral modification, pelvic floor rehabilitation (including pelvic floor biofeedback/muscular vaginal electrical stimulation), and anticholinergic/antimuscarinic medications, are given a trial of SNS. Some physicians exhaust all possible options, including high-dose combinations of antimuscarinics and tricyclic antidepressants, before considering neuromodulation as an option; others will move to SNS earlier.

In 2009, the International Consortium on Incontinence published an algorithm for the management of patient with OAB [12]. SNS is the only minimally invasive treatment option for refractory OAB to be granted a level A recommendation (high level of evidence) by the International Consortium on Incontinence. These recommendations are based on RCTs of SNS for urgency/frequency and urge incontinence demonstrating safety and efficacy along with subsequent follow-up studies demonstrating a durable response. These studies are reviewed later in this chapter.

In the United States, the current approval is for the treatment of refractory urinary frequency/urgency syndromes, urinary urge incontinence, and nonobstructive urinary retention of a non-neurogenic etiology. However, since the introduction of SNS for OAB, there has been growing recognition of the potential benefit of SNS for a broader range of pelvic disorders that may involve some OAB symptoms. Although these applications are investigational, research is ongoing into the potential use of SNS for interstitial cystitis/painful bladder syndrome and neurogenic voiding dysfunction among others.

It is important to remember that patients with neurologic disease were excluded from the initial industry-sponsored trials and subsequent follow-up studies. There is some evidence for patients benefiting from SNS, particularly for early intervention for patients with spinal cord injury, but SNS has not been studied in a systematic fashion for these applications [13]. One major practical limitation of SNS for neurologic disorders is the need of many of these patients to undergo MRI studies.

Terminology is evolving for the condition known as interstitial cystitis/painful bladder syndrome, and the diagnosis is certainly applied to many patients with severe urgency and frequency and minimal pelvic pain. Urinary symptoms in these patients may respond better to SNS than do pain symptoms [14]. Multiple small series have demonstrated short-term efficacy. The highest response rates were reported by Comiter for carefully selected patients who underwent a successful period of test stimulation [15]. In this study, only 27 of 39 patients progressed from test stimulation to permanent implantation, but the rate of success was 94 % among those patients undergoing permanent implantation. A recent series by

Powell with an average of 59.9-month follow-up had a low rate of loss of benefit over time for patients who underwent a test stimulation before implantation. However, 50 % of patients underwent explantation due to technical reasons, infection, battery depletion, or pain at the implantation site [16].

Psychological Considerations

A history of psychological disorders is common among candidates for SNS therapy and can pose a challenge for the clinician. While many patients will have substantial physical and psychological benefit from successful therapy, a history of psychiatric disorders may influence the rate and duration of a successful response to SNS therapy.

Weil et al. found that patients with a history of psychological dysfunction were more likely to fail implantation after a successful test procedure than patients without such a history (82 % versus 28 %). Among patients with an initially successful implantation, the duration of the therapeutic effect was shorter for patients with a history of psychological disorders (12 versus 36 months) [17]. Other publications also have speculated that psychological disorders may interfere with the patient's voiding symptoms and, ultimately, the patient's response to therapy.

Conversely, voiding symptoms impose a clear burden on quality of life and may contribute to the presence or severity of psychological or mental disorders. The MDT-103 trial demonstrated a clear benefit in terms of depression and health-related quality of life after SNS therapy. Of the 89 patients in the trial, 73 % had some degree of depression at baseline. Patients assigned to direct implantation showed significant improvement in the Beck Depression Index after SNS therapy at 3, 6, and 12 months after starting therapy, while patients in the delayed group showed a slight worsening of depression symptoms [18].

These data suggest that significant psychological benefit may be gained from successful SNS therapy. However, in some cases, such as when there is concern that preexisting psychological disorders may interfere with response to therapy, a psychiatric evaluation may be warranted.

Test Procedure

A test procedure provides a short-term trial of SNS and is important to patient selection before permanent implantation of an implantable pulse generator (IPG). The response during the test period can be used to select the optimal lead position (left versus right, S3 versus S4) and establish patient expectations for symptomatic improvement. The test procedure can be performed in the office, ambulatory-surgery unit, or operating room, and lets the patient and physician decide whether the benefits of permanent implantation are worth the risk and costs of the therapy.

The patient performs a 2- to 3-day voiding diary before the test procedure. In the test procedure one or more leads are placed into the sacral foramina based on the appropriate neural response (discussed later). When planning for a "one-stage" SNS placement, temporary insulated wires are placed in the office setting. In the "two-stage" procedure, permanent quadripolar tined leads are placed in the ambulatory-surgery unit or the operating room. The test period lasts for a few days up to 1 week for temporary and 2 weeks for permanent leads. In both cases, the wires are attached to an external stimulator. The patient maintains stimulation at a comfortable level (it should not be painful) and completes a voiding diary in order to provide objective data while undergoing neuromodulation. Based on the patient's subjective experience and the objective data obtained through the voiding diary, a final decision is made to proceed or not proceed with permanent implantation. Usually, the patient needs to exhibit significant subjective improvement, and the voiding diary should show at least 50 % improvement in voiding parameters to warrant proceeding to implantation of the IPG.

Test Procedure with Temporary Leads

The office-based test procedure sometimes is referred to as percutaneous nerve evaluation (PNE). While the pioneers of SNS performed this test procedure without fluoroscopy, most practitioners perform it under straight local anesthesia under fluoroscopic guidance. The patient is placed in the prone position with one or two pillows under the lower abdomen to improve the sacral approach. The sacrum is prepped with antiseptic solution and the sacral notches and coccygeal drop-off are identified by palpation or fluoroscopy. S3 usually is located 1.5–2 cm lateral to the midline at the level of the sacral notches, or about 9 cm above the coccygeal drop-off. Local anesthesia is achieved from S2 to S4 over the underlying skin and subcutaneous tissue, making certain not to enter the foramen.

Utilizing the previously mentioned landmarks and fluoroscopic guidance, primarily with lateral imaging, insulated foramen needles are placed percutaneously in the S3 and S4 foramen, and the sensory and motor responses are identified. Once the appropriate responses have been obtained, an insulated wire is placed through the 18-gauge needle in the foramen and the needle is removed. These temporary wires are inexpensive and easy to place. For patients without a clear optimal site of lead placement, two or more such wires can be taped in place and attached to an external stimulator. The patient is taught how to adjust for optimal results and can try out left and right sides or S3 and S4 and decide on the best response. Bilateral test stimulation may be helpful for some patients who fail an initial trial with unilateral placement [19].

Test Procedure with Permanent Leads for Two-Stage SNS

In equivocal cases, or if the insulated wires move, a trial can be carried out with a quadripolar tined lead. The initial procedure is similar to the test stimulation described but cannot be performed in the office setting. Broad spectrum antibiotics are given, and adequate monitored anesthesia care is obtained. Once the needles have been placed in the appropriate foramen and the motor and sensory responses have been obtained, a decision is made to use the best responses. The needle's stylet is removed, a guide wire is inserted, and the tract is dilated over the guide wire under fluoroscopic guidance once the needle has been removed. The sheath from the dilating apparatus is then left in place; the tined lead (so called as it has tines that hold it in place) is inserted and the position optimized by checking for neural responses. The sheath then is removed, and the tines hold the lead in place. The tined lead now is tunneled to the location of the eventual IPG, where it is connected to an externalizing wire, and then another tunnel is created to externalize the connection and to prevent infection.

Neural Response

Intraoperative motor and sensory neural responses guide lead positioning during the test stimulation. Sensory responses generally include a tingling, pulling, or vibratory sensation in the vagina and rectum in women and in the scrotum, phallus, and rectum in men. Motor responses include levator tightening (bellows response) and plantar flexion of the big toe. Sometimes at S3, a plantar flexion of the entire foot is noted. In such cases, S4 may be the more appropriate foramen, as most patients are significantly bothered by such a foot response.

An intraoperative motor response during the test procedure generally is considered to be more predictive of success after IPG implantation than a sensory response. Cohen et al. followed 35 patients, of which 21 progressed to permanent IPG implantation after a test procedure using quadripolar tined leads. A positive motor response was observed in 95 % of those progressing to permanent implantation versus only 21.4 % of patients who failed the test procedure. Patients with a positive sensory response in the absence of a motor response had only a 4.7 % chance of having a positive result after implantation [20]. Another recent study examined the role of sensory testing in patients with both OAB and pain symptoms, a group that might be expected to benefit from sensory testing. There was no difference in the rate of symptomatic improvement or explantation for patients who did or did not have sensory testing [21].

While intraoperative motor responses are the primary neural responses used to locate the ideal site of electrode implantation, neuromodulation is usually applied at a level below that needed to stimulate a motor response. The patient may use sensory perception to stimulation as an indicator of continued neuromodulation. Loss of sensory perception after implantation may herald a loss in benefit from neurostimulation.

Permanent Versus Temporary-Lead Test Procedure

Before the development of a test procedure with permanent quadripolar leads, use of a temporary lead was the only means for patient selection for SNS. The test procedure itself is considered safe, and complications at the pre-implantation stage are rare. However, lead migration and the risk of infection limit the trial period to about 1 week. Lead migration often presents with pain and decreased efficacy and occurs at a rate of about 10–15 %. In a series by Siegel et al. the rate of temporary-lead migration was 11.8 % of 918 test stimulations. Other complications reported were pain in 2.1 % and technical problems in 2.6 % [22]. Short-term failure rates of up to 27 % have been reported for IPG implantation after successful temporary-lead placement [23]. It is not clear if these failures are due to lead migration, an inadequate test period, or other reasons.

Since the introduction of permanent quadripolar tined leads for test stimulation in 1997, multiple groups have published on the successful use of these leads. Today, most physicians in the United States perform a test procedure with these leads. One advantage of the quadripolar-lead test procedure is that the same responses should be obtained once the external neurostimulator is replaced by the permanent IPG because the lead–nerve interface does not change. The tined lead rarely migrates, and thus a 1- to 2-week or longer trial can easily be done.

A prospective trial by Everaert et al. [24] randomized 41 patients who had a successful trial procedure with temporary leads to either direct (one-stage) IPG implantation or undergo a test procedure with tined leads before implantation (two-stage). Patients in the two-stage group worse an external pulse generator for 3–5 weeks until there was a greater than 50 % improvement in urinary symptoms. All patients in this group progressed to IPG implantation. At 24 months of follow-up, patients who underwent a two-stage procedure had a lower rate of failure compared to the patients who had undergone a single-stage procedure (14 % versus 33 %). This study suggests that temporary-lead test stimulation may have a significant false-positive rate, although it is interesting to note that all patients in the two-stage group eventually progressed to IPG implantation.

There is some evidence that there also may be a significant false-negative rate with a temporary-lead test procedure. Temporary leads are likely to migrate during such a long test procedure and only quadripolar tined leads can be used for a longer test period. Van Voskuilen et al. reported an 80 % rate for a successful test procedure with quadripolar leads, which is considerably higher than published rates for successful test procedures with temporary leads [25]. There may be a significant number of false-negative test procedures with temporary leads due to undetected lead migration or insufficient length of the test period. Kessler et al. demonstrated the predictive benefit of a prolonged testing period. In a retrospective study of 20 patients (13 with urgency/frequency or urge incontinence), an increase in the testing period from 4 to 7 days to a minimum of 14 days increased the rate of eligibility for IPG implantation from 50 to 80 % ($p=0.031$) [24].

While a longer test period may increase patient eligibility for neurostimulation, patients screened by either method have similar long-term outcomes. Hundred patients underwent either temporary or permanent lead placement and proceeded to implantation only after a 50 % reduction in symptoms during the test period. The rate of progression to implantation was higher for patients who had permanent leads placed (69 % versus 47 %). However, there was no difference in the rate of failure after implementation. Patients who were screened using either test procedure had about a 2 % rate of failure over 2-year follow-up [26]. While this study included both patients with OAB symptoms and urinary retention, it suggests that the method of test stimulation does not affect long-term outcomes after implantation.

Rarely, lead migration may occur with tined leads for particularly thin patients, either before or after IPG implantation. Overall, lead migration after implantation occurred for 16 % of patients in Brazelli's [6] review of SNS trials. Hijaz and Vasavada suggested that the risk of lead migration after IPG implantation may be reduced but not eliminated when tined leads are used during the test procedure [27]. Infection is an additional risk of longer trial periods with tined leads due to the percutaneous passage of an extension wire to an external neurostimulator. Huyler et al. performed a microbiologic examination of explanted tined leads from 20 patients who underwent an unsuccessful test period for 2 weeks or longer and identified *Staphylococcus* species growth in four patients. However, these bacteria were susceptible to perioperative antibiotics and only one of these patients had clinical signs of infection [28]. Similarly, a review of complications in series of 44 patients undergoing a test procedure for at least 14 days identified one case of lead migration, one patient who required revision for pain, and no cases of infection [29]. Overall, these reports suggest a complication rate for a prolonged testing period comparable to a shorter period with temporary leads.

Implantation Procedure

After successful test stimulation, patients may be considered for IPG implantation after being counseled on the risks and benefits. The foreseeable need for an MRI is a contraindication to IPG implantation. The risks of the neurostimulator to a fetus are unknown and patients who are or may become pregnant should consider delaying therapy or choosing alternative therapies. The currently available neurostimulator is the InterStim® device manufactured by Medtronic, Inc. with a battery life of 6–10 years depending on the settings. Medtronic recently introduced the InterStim II, which received regulatory approval in both the United States and Europe in 2006. The new version is smaller in volume and lighter and does not require an extension cable to connect to the tined leads [30]. The implantation procedure itself is for the most part unchanged.

The procedure is performed under general anesthesia using short-acting or nonparalytic anesthetic agents. Perioperative prophylactic broad-spectrum antibiotics are provided and strict antiseptic precautions are maintained. The patient is positioned prone and prepped with multiple layers of providone-iodine, and a midline sacral incision is made. The incision is carried down to the level of the lumbodorsal fascia and this is opened sharply about 1.5 cm from the midline. The underlying paravertebral muscles are separated or divided, and the sacral periosteum is identified. The sacral foramen can be palpated as dimples or a marbling effect on the sacral surface. An insulated needle is placed into the appropriate foramen as determined during the test period. Neural responses are evaluated as discussed earlier until the appropriate foramen is located.

A quadripolar tined lead is placed in the foramen and secured in place by suturing the fixed collar on the lead to the periosteum. Neural motor responses are again tested and excellent motor responses in the form of levator bellows and big toe movement should be obtained in at least three of the four leads. A second incision is then made over the upper buttock 3–5 cm below with superior posterior iliac crest. This position should be planned so as to minimize the risk of discomfort with sitting and daily activities. For the original InterStim® model, a tunneling tool is used to transfer the free end of the lead to the buttock incision. Using a short 10-cm connecting lead, the appropriate connections are now made between the extension lead and the stimulating quadripolar lead and between the connecting lead and the IPG. In the InterStim II® model, the neurostimulator is directly connected to the tined lead. For both models, the incisions are closed in layers generally without drain placement. A confirmatory radiograph is obtained. The patient is discharged home usually within 23 h and returns 1 week later for activation of the neurostimulator.

In some cases, buttock placement of the IPG is not possible due to previous infection, sacral wounds, or other reasons. Alternatively, the IPG can be placed in the anterior abdomen either subcutaneously or under the rectus for very thin patients. While this procedure is similar, a much longer 50-cm extension lead is used. The technique is described in detail by Siegel et al. [31]. The neurostimulator may be controlled using an external programmer allowing adjustment of the amplitude of stimulation within a defined range. The patient should set the amplitude to a comfortable level. Periodic adjustments can be performed as needed.

Most physicians use this implantation procedure with only small variations in technique, but some variations such as bilateral SNS and the use of guarded cuff electrodes deserve further attention. Guarded cuff electrodes have the potential to maintain a fixed distance between electrode and nerve root and prevent any lead movement. Because implantation requires a sacral laminectomy and there is limited availability of guarded cuff electrodes this procedure is rarely done in the United States.

In some patients, bilateral temporary leads as part of a test procedure may be helpful in identifying the lead placement with the optimal response, particularly for patients who fail a unilateral test procedure [32]. However, the value of continued bilateral stimulation and bilateral IPG implantation remains unclear. Kaufmann et al. studied the value of bilateral stimulation in a porcine model of OAB by inducing detrusor hyperactivity using formalin. Bilateral stimulation in this model appeared to increase the chance of stimulating the relevant fibers over a unilateral approach [33]. The clinical relevance of this study is unclear and there is little clinical evidence of any advantage to bilateral over unilateral IPG placement.

The IPG produces a square waveform and can be set to various pulse rates (2.1–130 Hz), amplitudes (0.005–10.55 V), and pulse widths (60–450 μs). An initial pulse rate can be determined during the test period and adjusted after implantation to obtain the appropriate response. Urethral closure pressure studies suggest an initial pulse rate of 10 and 16 Hz [34]. Natural stimuli of C fibers, Aδ fibers, and Aβ fibers occur at different pulse rates, suggesting that different pulse rates may lead to different clinical outcomes [35]. While a study of pulse rate changes did not result in better clinical outcomes on average for a cohort of patients with suboptimal responses to SNS, individual patients did benefit from changes in pulse rate [36].

Cost Considerations

SNS is associated with high initial treatment costs due to device costs, costs related to the test procedure, and operating room and anesthesia costs for implantation. A recent study by Wantanabe and colleagues estimated that these initial costs amounted $22,226 [37]. Treatment failures, while uncommon, involve additional cost for explantation, usually done in the operating room under local or general anesthesia. These high costs, particularly in the current economic environment, require that both patient and provider carefully consider the costs of treatment before proceeding.

One important question is whether the increased costs of the use of permanent leads, in the so-called two-stage procedure, justify the potentially lower risk of treatment failure after implantation. While permanent leads cost about $2,000 each, the cumulative difference in cost between a test procedure with permanent and temporary leads also depends heavily on operative costs, which vary in different health care environments. In the randomized trial by Everaert et al. costs per patient were about €2,000 higher for patients undergoing a two-stage versus a one-stage procedure [25]. To our knowledge, no cost–benefit analysis has yet demonstrated an advantage for a two-stage procedure due to a lower rate of treatment failure.

A few studies have examined the costs of SNS versus comparable treatments for anticholinergic refractory OAB symptoms. Not surprisingly, the initial costs of SNS exceed initial costs for intra-detrussor botox and augmentation cystoplasty. In the cost-analysis by Wantanabe et al. SNS therapy remained the most expensive form of therapy after 3 years with cumulative costs of

$26,269 versus $7,651 for intra-detrussor Botox and $14,377 for augmentation cystoplasty.

Leong et al. developed a Markov decision model with either SNS or botox therapy as treatment options to determine cost-effectiveness of each therapy. In the model where both procedures are done under general anesthesia, SNS achieved cost-effectiveness (defined as under €40,000 per QALY) over botox after 4 years. Interestingly, SNS was no longer cost-effective if a test procedure or two-stage procedure was used [38]. In a similar Markov model using the US cost data, the societal costs of SNS over botox exceeded $100,000 per QALY at 2 years of therapy [39]. These studies have significant limitations including the lack of long-term efficacy data for both therapies, but overall these studies suggest that SNS must have excellent long-term efficacy in order to justify high initial costs.

Outcomes

A recent review of the initial RCTs of SNS for urgency/frequency and urge incontinence and multiple subsequent observational studies reported an initial response rate of between 64 and 88 % of all patients [38]. A similar repose rate of 80 % was found in a review by Brazelli et al. defined by either 90 % continence or a 50 % improvement in their urge incontinence symptoms after SNS [6]. Recent follow-up data demonstrate a durable response. These data for 121 patients showed a persistent response at 5 years after initial 1-year success for 84 % of patient with urge incontinence and 71 % with urgency/frequency [40]. A successful clinical response is defined as a greater than 50 % response in urgency, frequency (or normalization), or urge incontinence.

Three prospective randomized trials of SNS for urgency/frequency or urge incontinence merit mention. A study by Schmidt et al. enrolled 155 patients from 16 international centers with urge incontinence refractory to medications and without pelvic pain or known neurologic conditions. All patients underwent a test period of 3–7 days and 98 patients had a greater than 50 % improvement in their symptoms. These patients were randomized to undergo either immediate IPG implantation or delayed implantation after 6 months of medical therapy. After 6 months of SNS for the immediate implantation group, 47 % of patients were completely dry and 29 % had a greater than 50 % reduction in incontinence with efficacy retained at 18 months of follow-up. Urodynamic parameters improved for the immediate versus delayed implantation group at 6 months with a higher percentage demonstrating stable detrusor function (56 % versus 16 %; $p=0.014$). For all patients, 32.5 % underwent surgical revision for generator or implant site pain or lead migration [10].

A second trial on SNS for urge incontinence randomized 44 patients to SNS or medical management with an average reduction of 88 % in episodes of incontinence and 90 % in leakage severity. 56 % of implant patients versus 4 % of controls had complete resolution of incontinence and urodynamics demonstrated by roughly quadrupling the volume at first contraction. Based on long-term follow-up, the 3-year actuarial estimate for treatment failure was 32.4 % [41].

The effectiveness of SNS for urgency/frequency was evaluated in a later multicenter trial that randomized 51 patients after a successful test stimulation to immediate InterStim® implantation or a control group. In the treatment group, 56 % of patients achieved either a 50 % reduction in symptoms or less than 7 voids per day. Eight percentage of patients had no improvement in voiding symptoms at all. After 6 months, voiding diary, quality of life, and urodynamic parameters were significantly improved on average in the implant group versus no improvement in the control group. After 6 months of therapy the neurostimulator was turned off and symptoms returned to baseline [42].

A few studies have attempted to identify factors that predict success or failure of SNS. Amundsen et al. prospectively evaluated patients with medication refractory urge incontinence who underwent SNS with a mean follow-up of 29 months. Cure, as defined by no resolution of daily incontinence, was associated with age less than 55 and lack of comorbidities. Patients above

75 years of age had less than a 30 % cure compared to over 80 % of patients under 45. No patients with three or more comorbidities were cured. However, it should be noted that some patients in the study had known neurologic comorbidities, unlike the patients in the previously mentioned clinical trials [43]. Along these lines, another study of patients who failed sacral neuromodulation found that many such patients had some degree of pudendal neuropathy [44].

Algorithm for Management of OAB with SNS

There are multiple acceptable algorithms for management of patients considered for management of OAB. Optimal management is patient specific. We present our standard algorithm here.

All patients considered for SNS must have a complete history and physical examination, including a genital, rectal, and neurological examination. These patients should perform accurate voiding diaries and undergo urodynamic studies to confirm the diagnosis and ascertain whether they are suitable candidates. These patients should have failed or could not tolerate more conservative therapies such as behavioral modification or appropriate medication.

All patients initially undergo a test stimulation with temporary leads placed in the office. Temporary wires are tested bilaterally at S3 or at S3 and S4 (if there is significant foot flexion at S3) looking for the best sensory and motor responses as described earlier. The temporary lead is left in at least two separate foramina and sometimes more; it is rare for us to leave only one wire. A voiding diary is kept for 3–5 days. Patients with a 50 % improvement in symptoms or normalization are considered successful and progress to a one-stage procedure. As discussed above, the permanent quadripolar lead and the IPG then are implanted in the same setting.

If the results of the test are equivocal or if there is suspicion of lead migration during the test procedure, we proceed to a two-stage procedure. A quadripolar lead is implanted in the operating room in the first stage and the patient will wear an external generator and maintain a voiding diary for 2 weeks. At this point, if there is greater than 50 % improvement in symptoms, we proceed to IPG implantation.

Patients may return with recurrent symptoms. In this case, reprogramming of the device is the first step in troubleshooting the generator. First, we cycle through each of the setting levels to see if the patient regains the target sensation. Next, pulse width and amplitude are varied. If there is no success, the patient may need revision with repeat lead placement in the operating room.

Case Study

Returning to the case study presented earlier, the first patient presented with urgency and frequency and had hypersensitivity and low capacity. She underwent a test placement of temporary leads in the office. Under local anesthesia and fluoroscopic guidance, wires were placed at the left and right S3 foramen. Sensory responses were obtained toward the vagina and rectum, and there was a good levator response with very slight toe flexion. Voiding diary during the 5-day test stimulation showed improvement in voided volume to 220 mL, with the number of voids decreasing to 10 or 11. The patient slept through the night with a functional capacity of 320 mL. The patient had an overall better response on the left side and was implanted on the left with continued improvement. At 6 months, voiding function was essentially normal, with voided volume per void of 250 mL and 8–10 voids daily. The patient also thought her constipation was improved, although this was just an observation.

The second patient presented with urge incontinence not helped with anticholinergics and had terminal detrusor overactivity on urodynamics. She underwent a trial of office-based test stimulation. At the S3 level, bilaterally, there is not only a levator response but also a strong foot response involving all toes. She feels the response primarily in the perineum. At S4, she has a levator response with no foot or toe response and feels the response primarily in the rectum and perineum. Wires are left at left S3 and S4 and she responds at both leads, although at S3, the foot movement is bothersome for her. She has no large volume leakage and has a decrease in small volume leakage to 1–2 times daily. She is implanted at left S4, and, at 6 months postprocedure, had no large volume leakage and rare episodes (2–3 times weekly) of a few drops of leakage.

These cases represent good results obtained with SNS with an office-based test procedure followed by permanent lead placement and IPG implantation in one stage in the operating room. Certainly, there are many patients who either do not respond during a test stimulation with either temporary or permanent leads, or have a loss of efficacy after a successful test stimulation. Nonetheless, in this difficult population with limited therapeutic choices, SNS is a promising therapeutic option once behavior treatments and pharmacotherapy have failed.

Conclusions

Since approval of SNS for OAB symptoms, the procedure has grown in popularity, with multiple case series and RCTs demonstrating safety and efficacy of the procedure. Given the high cost of the procedure, the selection of patients most likely to have a sustained benefit is important. At this time, few studies have determined factors that predict a response to SNS for OAB symptoms. In some cases, the etiology of urinary symptoms may not be known. The response rate to SNS is unclear for patients with a neurogenic or pain component to their symptoms. Previous studies on SNS outcomes have focused on patients without known neurologic deficits and current approval is for urgency/frequency and urge incontinence of a nonneurogenic etiology.

A test procedure is helpful in determining the optimum site of lead placement in addition to screening patients before implantation. Only patients who have a successful response with test stimulation should progress to implantation of the neurostimulator. A test procedure may be performed either with temporary leads placed in the office or with permanent leads placed in the OR. There are advantages and disadvantages to either approach. The placement of permanent tined leads allows a longer test period but is substantially more costly. There is some evidence that a longer test period may improve patient selection. However, patients who proceed to implantation after either test stimulation seem to have similar long-term outcomes. Further study is needed to determine if permanent lead placement is cost-effective.

Overall, the rate of successful resolution of urgency/frequency and urge incontinence is high with SNS, in terms of patient symptoms, satisfaction, and urodynamic parameters. Technologic advances have led to leads that are less likely to change position and smaller neurostimulators. Future advancement may better define pulse rate and other stimulation parameters that are tailored to address an expanding set of indications.

Disclosure Dr. Anurag Das has received compensation for teaching courses, proctoring, and developing teaching materials for Medtronic, Inc.

References

1. Abrams P, Cardozo L, Fall M, et al. The standardization of terminology of lower tract function: report from the Standardization Sub-committee of the International Continence Society. Neurourol Urodyn. 2002;21:167–78.
2. Basra RK, Wagg A, Chapple C, et al. A review of adherence to drug therapy in patients with overactive bladder. BJU Int. 2008;102:774–7.
3. Yoshimura N, Seki S, Chancellor MB, de Groat WC, Ueda T. Targeting afferent hyperexcitability for therapy of the painful bladder syndrome. Urology. 2002;59(5 Suppl):61–7.
4. Fowler CJ, Swinn MJ, Goodwin RJ, Oliver S, Craggs M. Studies of the latency of pelvic floor contraction during peripheral nerve stimulation show that the muscle is reflexly mediated. J Urol. 2000;163:881–3.
5. Oerlemans DJ, van Kerrebroeck PE. Sacral nerve stimulation for neuromodulation of the lower urinary tract. Neurourol Urodyn. 2008;27:28–33.
6. Brazzelli M, Murray A, Fraser C. Efficacy and safety of sacral nerve stimulation for urinary urge incontinence: a systematic review. J Urol. 2006;175:835–41.
7. Fall M, Lindstrom S. Electrical stimulation. A physiologic approach to the treatment of urinary incontinence. Urol Clin North Am. 1991;18:393–407.
8. Malaguti S, Spinelli M, Lazzeri M, Giardiello G. Evaluation of afferent pathway modulation in patients implanted with sacral neuromodulation for lower

urinary tract symptoms (LUTS). Eu Urol. 2003;1 Suppl 2:143.
9. van der Pal F, Heesakkers JPFA, Bemelmans BLH. Current opinion on the working mechanisms of neuromodulation in the treatment of lower urinary tract dysfunction. Curr Opin Urol. 2006;16:261–7.
10. Schmidt RA, Jonas U, Oleson KA, et al. Sacral nerve stimulation for the treatment of refractory urinary urge incontinence. Sacral Nerve Stimulation Study Group. J Urol. 1999;162:352–7.
11. Bazeed MA, Thuroff JW, Schmidt RA, et al. Effect of chronic electrostimulation of the sacral roots on the striated urethral sphincter. J Urol. 1982;128: 1357–62.
12. Abrams P, Andersson KE, Birder I, Brubaker I, Cardozo I, Chapple C, et al. 4th International Consultation on Incontinence: recommendations of the International Scientific Committee: evaluation and treatment of urinary incontinence, pelvic organ prolapse and fecal incontinence. Neurourol Urodyn. 2009;29(1):213–40.
13. Sievert KD, Amend B, Gakis G, et al. Early sacral neuromodulation prevents urinary incontinence after complete spinal cord injury. Ann Neurol. 2010;67: 74–84.
14. Zabihi N, Mourtzinos A, Maher MG, et al. Short-term results of bilateral S2-S4 sacral neuromodulation for the treatment of refractory interstitial cystitis, painful bladder syndrome, and chronic pelvic pain. Int Urogynecol J Pelvic Floor Dysfunct. 2008;19:553–7.
15. Comiter CV. Sacral neuromodulation for the symptomatic treatment of refractory interstitial cystitis: a prospective study. J Urol. 2003;169:1369–73.
16. Powell CR, Kreder KJ. Long-term outcomes of urgency-frequency syndrome due to painful bladder syndrome treated with sacral neuromodulation and analysis of failures. J Urol. 2010;183:173–6.
17. Weil EH, Ruiz-Cerdá JL, Eerdmans PH, et al. Clinical results of sacral neuromodulation for chronic voiding dysfunction using unilateral sacral foramen electrodes. World J Urol. 1998;16:313–21.
18. Das AK, Carlson AM, Hull M; U.S. MDT-103 Study Group. Improvement in depression and health-related quality of life after sacral nerve stimulation therapy for treatment of voiding dysfunction. Urology. 2004;64:62–8.
19. Marcelissen TA, Leong RK, Serroyen J, van Kerrekroeck PE, De Wachter SG. The use of bilateral sacral nerve stimulation in patients with loss of unilateral treatment efficacy. J Urol. 2011;185(3):976–80.
20. Cohen BL, Tunuguntla HS, Gousse A. Predictors of success for first stage neuromodulation: motor versus sensory response. J Urol. 2006;175:2178–81.
21. Peters KM, Killinger KA, Boura JA. Is sensory testing during lead placement crucial for achieving positive outcomes after sacral neuromodulation? Neurourol Urodyn. 2011;30(8):1489–92.
22. Siegel SW, Catanzaro F, Dijkema HE, et al. Long-term results of a multicenter study on sacral nerve stimulation for treatment of urinary urge incontinence, urgency-frequency, and retention. Urology. 2000;56(6 Suppl 1):87–91.
23. Koldewijn EL, Rosier PF, Meuleman EJ, et al. Predictors of success with neuromodulation in lower urinary tract dysfunction: results of trial stimulation in 100 patients. J Urol. 1994;152:2071–5.
24. Everaert K, Kerckhaert W, Caluwaerts H, et al. A prospective randomized trial comparing the 1-stage with the 2-stage implantation of a pulse generator in patients with pelvic floor dysfunction selected for sacral nerve stimulation. Eur Urol. 2004;45:649–54.
25. Van Voskuilen AC, Oerlemans DJ, Weil EH, et al. Medium-term experience of sacral neuromodulation by tined lead implantation. BJU Int. 2007;99:107–10.
26. Kessler TM, Madersbacher H, Kiss G. Prolonged sacral neuromodulation testing using permanent leads: a more reliable patient selection method. Eur Urol. 2005;47:660–5.
27. Hijaz A, Vasavada S. Complications and troubleshooting of sacral neuromodulation therapy. Urol Clin North Am. 2005;32:65–9.
28. Leong RK, DeWachter SG, Nieman FH, deBie RA, van Kerrebroeck PE. PNE versus 1st stage tined lead procedure: a direct comparison to select the most sensitive test method to identify patients suitable for sacral neuromodulation therapy. Neurourol Urodyn. 2011;30(7):1249–52.
29. Huwyler M, Kiss G, Burkhard FC, Madersbacher H, Kessler TM. Microbiological tined-lead examination: does prolonged sacral neuromodulation testing induce infection? BJU Int. 2009;104:646–50.
30. Kessler TM, Burkhard FC, Madersbacher H, Kofler A, Poewe W, Kiss G. Safety of prolonged sacral neuromodulation tined lead testing. Curr Med Res Opin. 2008;24(2):343–7.
31. Spinelli M, Sievert K-D. Latest technologic and surgical developments in using InterStim Therapy for sacral neuromodulation: impact on treatment success and safety. Eur Urol. 2008;54:1287–96.
32. Siegel SW. Management of voiding dysfunction with an implantable neuroprosthesis. Urol Clin North Am. 1992;19:163–70.
33. Scheepens WA, de Bie RA, Weil EH, van Kerrebroeck PE. Unilateral versus bilateral sacral neuromodulation in patients with chronic voiding dysfunction. J Urol. 2002;168(5):2046–50.
34. Kauffman S, Naumann CM, Mamann MF, Seif C, Braun PM, Junemann KP, et al. Unilateral vs bilateral sacral neuromodulation in pigs with formalin-induced detrusor hyperactivity. BJU Int. 2009;103:230–63.
35. Thon WF, Baskin LS, Jonas U, et al. Neuromodulation of voiding dysfunction and pelvic pain. World J Urol. 1991;9:138.
36. Koga L, Furue H, Rashid MH, et al. Selective activation of primary afferent fibers evaluated by sincewave electrical stimulation. Mol Pain. 2005;1:13.
37. Wantanabe JH, Campbell JD, Ravelo A, et al. Cost analysis of intervention of antimuscarinic refractory

patients with overactive bladder. Urology. 2010; 76(4):835–40.
38. Leong RK, de Wachter SG, Joore MA, der Kerrebroeck PE. Cost-effectiveness analysis of sacral neuromodulation and botulinum toxin A treatment for patients with idiopathic overactive bladder. BJU Int. 2011;108(4):558–64.
39. Siddiqui NY, Amundsen CL, Visco AG, Myers ER, Wu JM. Cost-effectiveness of sacral neuromodulation versus intravesical botulinum A toxin for treatment of refractory urge incontinence. J Urol. 2009;162(6):2799–804.
40. van Kerrebroeck PE, van Voskuilen AC, Heesakkers JP, et al. Results of sacral neuromodulation therapy for urinary voiding dysfunction: outcomes of a prospective, worldwide clinical study. J Urol. 2007;178:2029–34.
41. Weil EH, Ruiz-Cerda JL, Eerdmans PH, Janknegt RA, Bemelmans BL, van Kerrebroek PE. Sacral root neuromodulation in the treatment of refractory urinary urge incontinence: a prospective randomized controlled clinical trial. Eur Urol. 2000;37(2):161.
42. Hassouna MM, Siegel SW, Lycklama A, Nyeholt AAB, Elhilali MM, van Kerrebroeck PEV, Das AK, Gajewski JB, Janknegt RA, Rivas DA, Dijkema H, Milam DF, Oleson KA, Schmidt RA. Sacral neuromodulation in the treatment of urgency frequency symptoms: a multicenter study of efficacy and safety. J Urol. 2000;163:1849–54.
43. Amundsen CL, Romero AA, Jamison MG, Webser GD. Sacral neuromodulation for intractable urge incontinence: are there factors associated with cure? Urology. 2005;66(4):746.
44. Antolak Jr SJ, Antolak CM. Failed sacral neuromodulation: simple tests demonstrate pudendal neuropathy. A case series. J Pelvic Med Surg. 2006;12:3.

14 Neuromodulation: PTNS

Gaspar Msangi and Kenneth M. Peters

The International Continence Society (ICS) defines OAB syndrome as urinary urgency with or without urge incontinence usually with increased daytime frequency and nocturia in the absence of a pathologic or metabolic condition [1]. Using this definition, recent surveys estimate the prevalence of OAB to be 18.6 %, being higher in women (26.1 %) than in men (10.7 %). This corresponds to 42.2 million adults in the USA having OAB. The societal cost of OAB among community dwelling adults is estimated to be at least 24.9 billion per year [2].

OAB has a negative impact on quality of life, with patients reporting the lowest levels of quality of life and work productivity and the highest levels of anxiety and depression [3]. Many patients have impaired mobility, disturbed sleep, impaired domestic function, social isolation, and decreased sexual enjoyment [4].

Treatment of OAB

Behavioral therapy should be the first-line treatment for OAB. Patients are instructed to limit fluid intake, eliminate foods like caffeine, alcohol, and medications like diuretics that could exacerbate symptoms. Other measures include timed voiding and pelvic floor physical therapy. Antimuscarinics are the mainstay of pharmacologic therapy. These drugs are effective in blocking muscarinic receptors but their action is not bladder-specific. Within 12 months, the majority of patients discontinue their antimuscarinic drug due to their cost, insufficient symptom relief, and significant side effects [5]. If behavioral and pharmacologic methods fail to resolve the OAB symptoms, neuromodulation is the next logical step.

Neuromodulation

Concept of Neuromodulation

Neuromodulation is the electrical or chemical modulation of a nerve to influence the physiologic behavior of an organ. Tanagho et al. in 1989 pioneered the initial investigations into electrical stimulation for neuromodulation [6]. Neuromodulation has become an important tool in the treatment of bladder dysfunction. Neuromodulation has been avidly embraced for the treatment of OAB primarily when noninvasive therapies such as behavioral modification, pelvic floor rehabilitation, and pharmacological therapy have failed. In the past once these noninvasive therapies were exhausted surgical procedures such as augmentation enterocystoplasty, detrusor myomectomy, bladder denervation, and urinary diversion were often employed to treat

G. Msangi, M.D. • K.M. Peters, M.D. (✉)
Department of Urology, Oakland University, William Beaumont School of Medicine, 3535 West 13 Mile Road, 438, Royal Oak, MI 48073, USA
e-mail: kmpeters@beaumont.edu

G.H. Badlani (ed.), *Minimally Invasive Therapy for Urinary Incontinence and Pelvic Organ Prolapse*, Current Clinical Urology, DOI 10.1007/978-1-4939-0008-4_14,

OAB and resulted in significant perioperative and long-term morbidity [7]. Neuromodulation offers a minimally invasive, nonsurgical and reversible means to treat voiding dysfunction. Sacral neuromodulation has been FDA approved for over 13 years to treat urinary urgency, frequency, urge incontinence, and non-obstructive urinary retention.

Neuromodulation of the Posterior Tibial Nerve

The posterior tibial nerve is a peripheral mixed sensory–motor nerve that originates from spinal roots L4 through S3, which also contribute directly to sensory and motor control of the urinary bladder and pelvic floor. Stimulation of the posterior tibial nerve was pioneered by Stoller and colleagues with the introduction of the stoller afferent nerve stimulator (SANS) which delivers electrical stimulation to the posterior tibial nerve via a 34-gauge needle just cephalad to the medial malleolus [8]. Multiple studies have demonstrated that posterior tibial nerve stimulation shows some efficacy in treating symptoms of OAB and altering urodynamic findings in patients with OAB [9, 10]. Stimulation of the nerve inhibits bladder activity by depolarizing somatic sacral and lumbar afferent fibers. Afferent stimulation provides central inhibition of the preganglionic bladder motor neurons through a direct route in the sacral cord [11].

Tibial nerve stimulation was first described in 1983. McGuire and colleagues showed efficacy in the treatment of a variety of voiding dysfunctions related to detrusor overactivity (DO) by electrical stimulation of the tibial nerve. His group reported on 16 patients with involuntary bladder contractions of varying etiology who were treated with common peroneal or posterior tibial nerve patch electrode stimulation. Twelve patients initially were dry, three were improved, and one was "possibly improved." Okada and coworkers reported a positive experience with transcutaneous stimulation of the thigh muscle in 19 patients with detrusor overactivity; the maximal cystometric capacity was increased by 57 % in 11 of 19 patients [12, 13]. Vereecker and associates [14], however, were unable to suppress hyperactivity by this method in patients with suprasacral spinal cord injury or disease [14].

More recently, Vandoninck et al. in 2004 reported on their outcomes in 39 patients with chronic voiding dysfunction who were treated with tibial nerve stimulation. All patients had detrusor overactivity with elevated post-void residual urine or complete urinary retention; each patient performed self-catheterization. Each patient underwent 12 weekly tibial nerve stimulations at the medial malleolus for 30 min. The primary outcome was measured as total voided volume along with total catheterized volume. In 41 % of the patients, 24-h catheterized volume was reduced by 50 %. An additional 26 % noted 25–50 % reduction in their residuals. After the study, 59 % chose to continue treatment. Urodynamic testing was also performed. While patients' cystometric capacity remained the same, detrusor pressure at maximum flow increased from 25 to 33 cm H_2O, a statistically significant difference. In addition, both the bladder contractility index ($BCI = P_{det} \times Q_{max} + 5 \times Q_{max}$) as well as the bladder voiding efficiency ($BVE = 100 \times$ (voided volume/total bladder capacity)) showed statistically significant increases. Detrusor overactivity did exist in five patients at baseline. After stimulation, DO continued in three patients, disappeared in two and appeared de novo in seven patients. No significant side effects were reported [15].

Van Balken et al. reported on their treatment of patients with bladder overactivity as well as idiopathic urinary retention. In 37 patients with overactive bladder, 22 reported subjective improvement and requested continuation of therapy. However, all 37 showed significant improvement in day and night voiding frequency. In 30 urge incontinent patients, all 30 showed reduction in their incontinent episodes, pad use, and severity of leakage. Finally, for 12 patients with idiopathic urinary retention, a decrease in number and volume of catheterization was reported, but this did not reach statistical significance. They concluded that percutaneous tibial nerve stimulation is a promising, cost-effective, and easily applicable treatment for lower urinary tract dysfunction [10].

Ruiz and colleagues from Spain reported on 51 patients treated over 3 years for similar symptom complexes. Twenty-six patients described the frequency–urgency syndrome, 22 described urge incontinence and 3 carried a diagnosis of interstitial cystitis. Patients underwent 10, 30-min sessions wherein the tibial nerve was stimulated using a similar technique as in prior articles. Mean follow up was 21 months. Across the entire patient population, they reported statistically significant improvement in all seven categories measured: daytime frequency, daytime voided volume, daytime leakage episodes, nighttime frequency, nighttime leakage episodes, nighttime voided volume, and hypogastric/suprapubic pain [16].

Posterior tibial nerve stimulation was also evaluated in the acute setting by Amarenco et al. in 2003 [11]. They studied 44 patients with irritative lower urinary tract symptoms, including uninhibited detrusor contractions as seen on filling cystometrogram. The etiology was demonstrable in 37 patients, including multiple sclerosis, spinal cord injury, brain injury, and Parkinson's disease; the remaining seven patients had idiopathic detrusor overactivity. Cystometry was performed at a rate of 50 cc/min using an 8 french catheter. Patients were filled until they experienced uninhibited bladder contractions, leakage was observed or if they achieved a volume of 400 cc. CMG was performed again after posterior tibial nerve stimulation was initiated. A positive test consisted of an increase in the bladder volume at which a contraction occurred of 100 cc or greater, or if that involuntary contraction occurred at a bladder volume that was 50 % greater than baseline. Twenty-two of 44 (50 %) cases tested positive. Further urodynamic data was collected. Mean bladder volume that the first involuntary contraction occurred was 162 cc at baseline, and increased to 232 cc after stimulation. Maximum cystometric capacity was 221 cc at baseline and increased to 277 cc after stimulation.

Finally, posterior tibial nerve stimulation has been applied to the interstitial cystitis population, a subset of patients with voiding dysfunction. Zhao and Nordling applied posterior tibial nerve stimulation to 14 patients diagnosed with IC. Patients were treated during a total of 10, 30-min sessions. One patient withdrew from the study, leaving 13 patients who completed the course of therapy. The results did not meet clinical significance in pain, voided volume, and quality of life scores [17].

The lure of the tibial nerve is that it is easily accessible without requiring an operating room or an anesthetic. As with all novel techniques, the data was initially anecdotal and non-randomized. Studies with modest numbers have shown efficacy. One of the most significant studies was the OrBIT trial comparing PTNS versus tolterodine. This was a multicenter study where a total of 100 adult patients with OAB symptoms were randomized 1:1 to either PTNS or tolterodine therapy. PTNS arm patients received 30 min weekly treatments for 12 consecutive weeks while the pharmacotherapy patient arm received 4 mg Tolterodine-ER daily (decreased to 2 mg if intolerability was experienced) for 12 weeks. Two-day voiding diaries were collected at baseline and at study end. The primary end point was to compare whether PTNS was better than tolterodine at reducing the frequency of urinary voids per day after 12 weeks of therapy. Secondary endpoints included change in urge incontinence episodes per 24 h, number of voids causing waking, volume voided per day as well as number of urgency episodes per day. Subject and investigator ratings of improvement in OAB symptoms were assessed. Adverse reactions were also monitored.

Results

79.5 % of PTNS patients compared to 54.8 % of tolterodine patients considered themselves improved or cured. This was paralleled to investigator assessment showing improvement or cure in 79.5 % of PTNS patients versus 60.5 % of tolterodine patients. Each group showed significant improvement in all OAB symptoms from baseline to 12 weeks but when compared between groups, there was no significant difference. The improvements were seen in more PTNS patients than in tolterodine patients even though there was no statistical significance [18].

Effects of PTNS are long term. In the phase II OrBIT trial which looked at long-term effects of PTNS, study subjects continued to receive periodic PTNS treatments. At 6 and 12 months, there was still significant improvement in urinary frequency, urge incontinence, nocturia, and voided volume. Both patients and investigators classified OAB symptoms as improved. Treatment intervals were tapered during this long-term follow-up period with a mean of 21 days between treatments. PTNS treatment frequency can be individualized according to patients' response which would allow for better compliance [19].

Sham-Controlled Data

The placebo effect on patients with OAB cannot be ignored, with placebo-controlled drug trials showing a placebo effect as high as 64 % for some incontinence symptoms [20]. Effects of PTNS have been shown to be not due to placebo effect. First a sham was designed and validated [21] and then subsequently used in a multicenter, double-blind, randomized trial that provided level one evidence to the safety and efficacy of PTNS. The SumiT trial had 220 adults with OAB randomized 1:1–12 weeks of treatment with weekly PTNS or sham. In this study 54.5 % of the PTNS subjects showed moderately or markedly improvement in bladder symptoms compared to 20.9 % of the sham which was statistically different. Urinary frequency, nighttime voids, moderate to severe urgency, and urge incontinence episodes all improved significantly compared to sham [22]. A smaller prospective double-blind placebo-controlled trial had 35 female patients 17 receiving PTNS while 18 had a sham. Seventy-one percentage of the PTNS showed greater than 50 % reduction in urge incontinence episodes while 0 in the placebo group responded [23].

PTNS offers a significant new modality for management of this debilitating condition; it provides an option for patients who are refractory to drugs, is less invasive and costly than SNS, and is clinically and cost-effective when considering the alternatives within the current algorithm of practice.

Patient Selection

Patients with bothersome symptoms of OAB who have not responded or could not tolerate behavioral or pharmacologic therapy should be considered for PTNS. Baseline voiding diaries evaluating urinary urgency, frequency, voided volume, and urge incontinent episodes should be completed. Urodynamic evaluation would be at the discretion of the clinician.

Technique

Patients are placed in the sitting position with their leg elevated (Fig. 14.1). The medial aspect of the foot is inspected. The needle insertion site is palpated about 5 cm cephalad to the medial malleolus between the posterior margin of the tibia and the soleus muscle (Fig. 14.2). A 34-gauge needle electrode is inserted at a 60° angle cephalad, about 3–4 cm deep to the tibial nerve (Fig. 14.3). A self-adhesive grounding pad is placed on the lower foot and the grounding pad and hook electrode are connected to the stimulator (Urgent® PC, Uroplasty, Minneapolis MN). The hook electrode is attached to the needle (Fig. 14.4). Current is slowly increased from 0 to 10 mA while assessing sensory and motor responses. If the needle is correctly placed, patient will experience flexion of the toes and sensory stimulation of the bottom of the foot. If this does

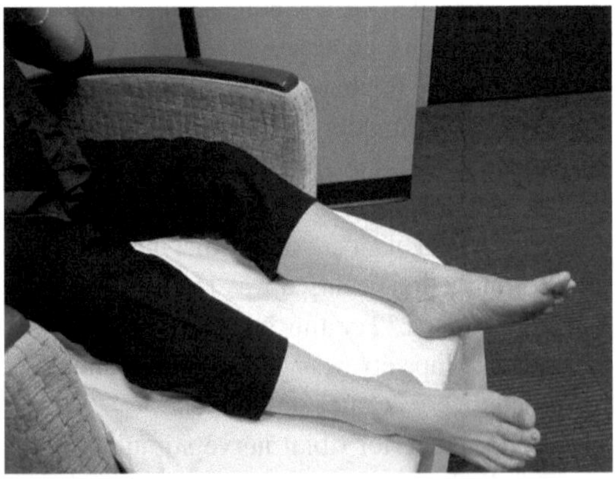

Fig. 14.1 Patient positioning

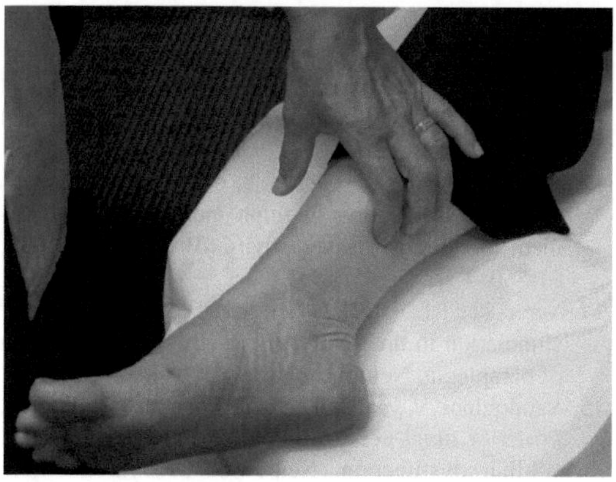

Fig. 14.2 Palpation of needle insertion site

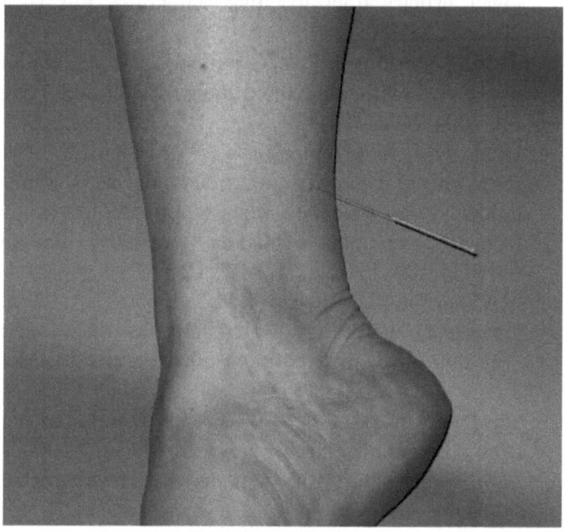

Fig. 14.3 Needle positioning

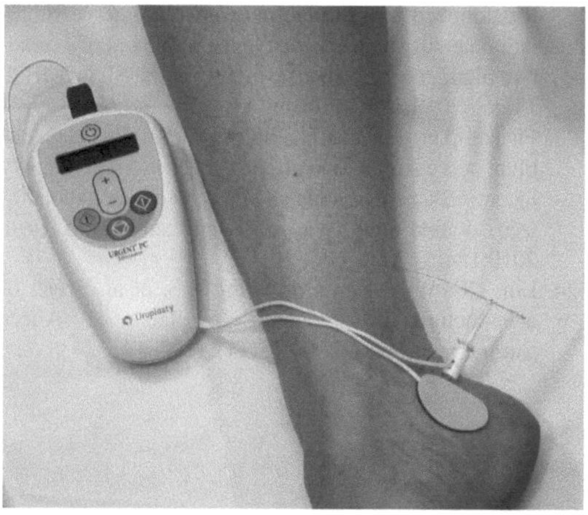

Fig. 14.4 Connection of the stimulator

not happen, the needle is advanced or withdrawn until it is confirmed to be in the correct position. The electrical current is set at an intensity that is well tolerated. A 30-min stimulation session is given at 20 Hz with a 200 μs fixed pulse width. After treatment, the needle and grounding pad are removed and disposed.

Treatment Interval

Patients return weekly for 12 weeks to obtain a 30-min treatment session. If at the end of 12 treatments there has been a documented significant improvement in symptoms, the patient returns once per month for a maintenance treatment. The treatment interval can be tailored to the patient's clinical response.

Contraindication and Complications of Tibial Nerve Stimulation

Tibial nerve stimulation is very safe. A few patients may complain of pain at the needle puncture site, mild bruising or bleeding, but no serious adverse events have been reported. Safety of PTNS has not been studied in pregnant women and should therefore not be used in this population. The stimulation point (acupuncture point SP6) is associated with ripening of the cervix and induction of labor [24]. As with any neuromodulation device, there is a relative contraindication in patients with a cardiac pacemaker.

Conclusions

OAB is a syndrome characterized by urinary urgency with or without urge incontinence. OAB has significant economic impact, with first-line therapies showing poor compliance due to significant side effects, treatment failures, and high costs. Surgical interventions for OAB result in significant perioperative and long-term morbidity. PTNS offers a minimally invasive, non-ablative, and reversible means to treat OAB with minimal side effects. Stimulation of the nerve inhibits bladder activity by depolarizing somatic sacral and lumbar afferents with central nervous system effects. Through prospective double-blind and sham-controlled studies, there is ample data to show efficacy of PTNS on OAB. No significant side effects have been reported.

References

1. Wein AJ, Rovner ES. Definition and epidemiology of overactive bladder. Urology. 2002;60(5 Suppl 1):7–12.
2. Onukwugha E, Zuckerman IH, McNally D, et al. The total economic burden of overactive bladder in the United States: a disease specific approach. Am J Manag Care. 2009;15:S90–7.
3. Coyne KS, Sexton CC, Kopp ZS, et al. The impact of overactive bladder on mental health, work productivity and health-related quality of life in the UK and Sweden: results from EpiLUTS. BJU Int. 2011;108(9): 1459–71.
4. Abrahams P, Kelleher CJ, Kerr LA, et al. Overactive bladder significantly affects quality of life. Am J Manag Care. 2000;6(11 Suppl):S580–90.
5. Pelletier EM, Vats V, Clemens Q. Pharmacotherapy adherence and costs versus nonpharmacologic management in overactive bladder. Am J Manag Care. 2009;15:S108.
6. Tanagho EA, Schmidt RA, Orvis BR. Neural stimulation for control of voiding dysfunction: a preliminary report in 22 patients with serious neuropathic voiding disorders. J Urol. 1989;142:340–5.
7. Sherman ND, Amundsen CL. Current and future techniques of neuromodulation for bladder dysfunction. Curr Urol Rep. 2007;8:448–54.
8. Cooperberg MR, Stoller ML. Percutaneous neuromodulation. Urol Clin North Am. 2005;32:71–8.
9. Govier F, Litwiller S, Nitti V, et al. Percutaneous afferent modulation for the refractory over active bladder: results of a multicenter study. J Urol. 2001; 165:1193–8.
10. Van Balken MR, Vandoninck V, Gisolf K, et al. Posterior tibial nerve stimulation as neuromodulatory treatment of lower urinary tract dysfunction. J Urol. 2001;166:914–8.
11. Amarenco G, Ismael SS, Even-Schneider A, et al. Urodynamic effect of acute transcutaneous posterior tibial nerve stimulation in overactive bladder. J Urol. 2003;169(6):2210–5.
12. McGuire EJ, Shi-Chun Z, Horwinski ER. Treatment for motor and sensory detrusor instability by electrical stimulation. J Urol. 1983;129:78–84.
13. Okada N, Igawa Y, Ogawa Y, et al. Transcutaneous electrical stimulation of thigh muscles in the treatment of detrusor overactivity. Br J Urol. 1998; 81:560–4.
14. Vereecker RL, Das RJ, Grisar P. Electrical sphincter stimulation in the treatment of detrusor hyperreflexia of paraplegia. Neurourol Urodyn. 1984;3:145–9.
15. Vandoninck V, van Balken MR, Finazzi Agro E, et al. Posterior tibial nerve stimulation in the treatment of voiding dysfunction. Neurourol Urodyn. 2004;23: 246–51.
16. Ruiz BC, Outeirino PXM, Martinez CP, et al. Peripheral afferent nerve stimulation for treatment of lower urinary tract irritative symptoms. Eur Urol. 2004;45:65–9.
17. Zhao J, Nordling J. Posterior tibial nerve stimulation in patients with intractable interstitial cystitis. BJU Int. 2004;94(1):101–4.
18. Peters KM, MacDiarmid SA, Wooldridge LS, et al. Randomized trial of percutaneous tibial nerve stimulation versus extended release tolterodine: results from the overactive bladder innovative therapy (OrBIT) trial. J Urol. 2009;182:1055.
19. MacDiarmid SA, Peters KM, Shobeiri SA, et al. Long-term durability of percutaneous tibial nerve stimulation for the treatment of overactive bladder. J Urol. 2010;183(1):234–40.
20. van Leeuwen JH, Castro R, Busse M, et al. The placebo effect in the pharmacologic treatment of patients with lower urinary tract symptoms. Eur Urol. 2006; 50(3):440–52.
21. Peters K, Carrico D, Burks F. Validation of a sham for percutaneous tibial nerve stimulation. Neurourol Urodyn. 2009;29:177.
22. Peters KM, Carrico DJ, Perez-Marrero RA, et al. Randomized trial of percutaneous tibial nerve stimulation versus sham efficacy in the treatment of overactive bladder syndrome: results from the SUmiT trial. J Urol. 2010;183:1438–43.
23. Finazzi-Agro E, Petta F, Sciobica F, et al. Percutaneous tibial nerve stimulation effects on detrusor overactivity incontinence are not due to a placebo effect: a randomized, double-blind, placebo controlled trial. J Urol. 2010;184(5):2001–6.
24. Lim CE, Wilkinson JM, Wong WS, et al. Effect of acupuncture on induction of labor. J Altern Complement Med. 2009;15(11):1209–14.

15 Pudendal Nerve Stimulation

Philip E.V. van Kerrebroeck and Martijn A.C. Smits

Sacral neurostimulation (SNS) is a minimally invasive treatment option for symptoms of overactive bladder (OAB) when non-invasive therapies such as behavioural modification, pelvic floor rehabilitation and pharmacological therapy have failed. The efficacy of SNS in patients with idiopathic OAB has been shown in clinical trials, with a reported long-term success rate of approximately 70 % [1, 2] and a 5-year patient satisfaction of up to 90 % [3]. The largest systematic review evaluating SNS for neurogenic lower urinary tract dysfunction calculated an overall success rate of 68 % [4]. It follows from these data that in spite of its potential, SNS still offers no solution to the problems of a considerable number of patients with symptoms of (neurogenic) OAB.

Sacral neuromodulation consists of implantation of a tined electrode in the S3 sacral foramen with subsequent connection to an implantable pulse generator. The working mechanism of SNS is unclear, but it is indicated that electrical stimulation of the S3 sacral nerve root leads to modulation of the afferent signals and micturition reflex pathways in the central nervous system [5]. One limitation of the selection of S3 is that only one of the pathways inducing the inhibitory reflex is stimulated.

The pudendal nerve (PN) originates from S2, S3 and S4 sacral nerve roots. Therefore selection of the pudendal nerve, as a site for stimulation, provides afferent stimulation of S2, S3 and S4 nerve roots. Since more afferents are stimulated with direct pudendal nerve stimulation (PNS) than with SNS, chronic PNS may be an alternative option in patients in whom SNS fails [6].

The Pudendal Nerve

The pudendal nerve (PN) is a peripheral nerve, and consists mainly of afferent sensory fibres from sacral nerve roots S1, S2 and S3. Human cadaveric studies have shown that 50 % of the pudendal nerves contain nerve fibres originating from the roots S2, S3 and S4, 40 % only from S2 and S3 and 10 % from S3 and S4 only [7]. Consequently, the PN is a major contributor to bladder afferent regulation and hence bladder function. Pudendal nerve entrapment often leads to significant voiding dysfunction, including urinary incontinence and detrusor overactivity [8–10].

Anatomy of the Pudendal Nerve

The PN originates in the sacral plexus and derives its fibres from the ventral rami of second, third and fourth sacral nerves (S2, S3 and S4).

P.E.V. van Kerrebroeck, M.D., Ph.D., M.M.Sc. (✉)
M.A.C. Smits, M.D.
Department of Urology, Maastricht University Medical Centre, P. Debyelaan 25, Maastricht 6229 HX, The Netherlands
e-mail: urolmaas@hotmail.com

G.H. Badlani (ed.), *Minimally Invasive Therapy for Urinary Incontinence and Pelvic Organ Prolapse*, Current Clinical Urology, DOI 10.1007/978-1-4939-0008-4_15,

The nerve also gets contributions from the adjacent roots of S1 and S5 [7]. The pudendal nerve roots emerge from the anterior sacral foramina containing both somatic and autonomic fibres. The PN together with the internal pudendal artery exits the pelvis through the greater sciatic foramen, travelling anterior to the piriformis muscle and posterior to the coccygeal muscle and the sacrospinous ligament. At this point the PN winds posteriorly around the ischial spine, medial to the pudendal vessels and deep to the sacrotuberous ligament in the biligamentary tunnel. It swings anteriorly through the lesser sciatic foramen and the Alcock's canal to enter the perineum. Here the PN terminally branches into the dorsal genital nerve (DGN), the inferior rectal nerve and the perineal nerve [7, 11]. The DGN eventually runs through the suspensory ligament to the dorsum of the penis or clitoris. The inferior rectal nerve extends motor branches to the levator ani muscle and the external anal sphincter, and sensory branches to the perianal region and the scrotum. Alongside these branches to the scrotum runs the scrotal branch of the perineal nerve into the common scrotal branch, which innervates the scrotal skin. The other branches of the perineal nerve, the bulbocavernosus branch and the medial urethral sphincter branch, run down to the striated urethral sphincter [11, 12].

Pudendal Nerve Stimulation

Stimulation of nerve fibres can be achieved by implanting an electrode close to the nerve. The initial nerve localisation and implanting techniques used were initially complex and have recently been replaced by minimally invasive, percutaneous approaches. The percutaneous procedures can be performed with use of the quadripolar tined lead that is also used for SNS, connected to an implantable pulse generator. Using the combination of this tined lead and an implantable pulse generator gives the opportunity for a staged implant procedure. During the first stage the lead is implanted adjacent to the PN and connected to external stimulator. If during the testing period the stimulation is successful, the second stage consists of implanting an implantable pulse generator.

An alternative to this 'electrode' system is a lead-less mini-neurostimulator with integrated electrodes, which can be implanted at its target location (Alcock's canal) [6].

Surgical Access to the Pudendal Nerve

The anatomy of the PN and its branches enables the implantation of an electrode at several sites. At the ischial spine, the PN is a relatively isolated structure and stimulation at this site theoretically diminishes the risk of unwanted activation of S2 motor fibres to sciatic nerve [13]. The PN can be accessed percutaneously for stimulation at the ischial spine by a posterior or perineal approach for insertion of the electrode. With the perineal approach the PN can also be reached at the Alcock's canal [14].

When implanting an electrode by the posterior approach at the ischial spine, the ischial spine can be located by palpating the lower margin of the sacrotuberous ligament where it forms an angle with the ischial tuberosity [14–16]. The electrode can also be inserted perpendicularly at the intersection of a horizontal line from the greater trochanter and a vertical line from the ischial tuberosity tip (using fluoroscopy) [13, 14].

The perineal approach is performed by insertion of the electrode perpendicularly to the perineum between the ischial tuberosity and the anus. A finger is placed into the rectum or the vagina to prevent puncturing the bowel or vagina and then used to guide the needle to the ischial spine or Alcock's canal [6, 17, 18].

EMG Recordings for Ensuring Correct Electrode Placement

Since the outcome of PNS depends on the proximity of the electrode to the nerve [19], it has been suggested at the time of the development of the percutaneous placement techniques that placement of the electrode needs electrophysiological confirmation. Anal sphincter electromyography (EMG) and measurement of amplitude and latency during acute stimulation have been used [17]. In practice, the positioning of the electrode based on EMG recordings appears to be difficult. A recent study combining clinical results with cadaver studies has shown that the electrode can also be positioned satisfactorily without EMG confirmation. The authors conclude that lead placement can be based on evidence of visible and palpable sphincter contraction [13].

Dorsal Genital Nerve Stimulation

As an alternative method to direct stimulation of the PN, stimulation of nerve branches originating from the PN can be used. For this purpose, the DGN has been used as a peripheral stimulation site of the PN. The DGN can be accessed either using surface electrodes, as part of the DGN is localised superficially to the skin outside the pelvis, or with an electrode inserted more proximal along the tract of the DGN. In addition to using sensory function of the nerve to locate the stimulus in the glans penis or the clitoris, electrodes can be positioned near the DGN using the genito-anal reflex [20].

Mechanism of Action

Stimulation of the PN is different from SNS, as it provides afferent stimulation not only of the S3 sacral nerve root but also of the S2 and S4 roots. Both forms of stimulation, however, seem to rely on the same neurophysiological mechanisms. The working mechanism of stimulation of sacral nerve roots is not fully understood. In OAB, neurostimulation is supposed to act by inhibiting bladder afferent activity through its action on somatic afferent pathways, and hence blocking abnormal sensory input to spinal cord and brain. Neurostimulation may also block interneuron transmission of bladder sensory input and can directly inhibit bladder preganglionic neurons of bladder efferent pathways as well [5, 21].

Experimental Studies

The modulatory effects of PNS have been studied in normal and spinal animals, and important aspects of the spinal mechanism of action have been identified. These mechanisms rely on spinal interaction between somatic afferent fibres of the pudendal nerve and autonomic pathways controlling the bladder and bladder neck [22–26]. Projection of pudendal pathways into spinal sympathetic and sacral parasympathetic systems has been found in several animal experiments but also in humans [27–29].

Clinical Results

The number of published studies and the experience with PNS are limited compared to SNS. In SNS, in a single blinded crossover trial 30 patients randomly received a test with SNS and PNS (both tined quadripolar lead) by the perineal approach for OAB and urinary retention (10 %). The overall reduction in symptoms was 63 % for PNS and 46 % for SNS. PNS was chosen as a superior lead in 79.2 % of patients [16]. Another study evaluating the success of PNS with a percutaneous nerve evaluation test included 14 female patients with idiopathic OAB. Six patients (42 %) responded positively (>50 % improvement in urodynamic parameters) and received permanent PNS with a lead-less mini-neurostimulator [6]. One of the first relevant clinical studies on the effect of PNS with use of intermittent (weekly) needle stimulation was performed in a heterogeneous group of patients with idiopathic and neurogenic detrusor overactivity ($n=29$). These authors succeeded in showing a significant increase in functional bladder capacity in all patients and a 30 % decrease of frequency in 11 patients [18]. There is only one other study that has evaluated the effect of PNS in patients with neurogenic OAB. In this study test stimulation has been performed with a tined quadripolar lead in 15 patients. Eight patients regained continence during the test phase and two patients improved by more than 88 %. Two patients reduced the number of incontinence episodes by 50 % and three patients had no improvement [17].

Clinical Experience with DGN

Studies using stimulation of the DGN have been performed in acute and experimental settings, without long-term chronic trials. Only one larger study using continuous stimulation during 1 week is available. Of 21 female patients with urgency incontinence 55 % showed an increase in cystometric capacity and 47 % experienced a greater than 50 % reduction in incontinence episodes [30].

Other Indications

As with SNS, the effect of PNS has also been evaluated for other (urological) indications. In a small (21 patients) prospective, single blind, randomised crossover trial of SNS versus PNS for bladder pain syndrome, 77 % of patients had a significant improvement in the outcome of pain questionnaires and received a permanent implant. PNS was chosen as the better method of stimulation in 77 % [31]. In one study the effect of PNS on non-obstructive urinary retention was evaluated in three patients as part of a study mixed with patients suffering from OAB [16]. Faecal incontinence is currently being evaluated as a novel indication for PNS. One study showed a success rate of 70 %, considering a more than 50 % symptom reduction as success [13]. This indicates that patients suffering from OAB in combination with faecal incontinence, not responding to SNS for both problems, could be candidates for PNS.

Conclusions

PNS is considered an interesting alternative form of electrical stimulation for the treatment of OAB when non-invasive therapies have failed. As the pudendal nerve (PN) contains afferent fibres of S2, S3 and S4 nerve roots, more afferents are stimulated with PNS than with sacral nerve stimulation (SNS), and therefore may be an alternative option in patients in whom SNS fails. Anatomically the PN can be approached in different ways and clinical research indicates better overall results with PNS than with SNS. However only a limited number of permanent implantations have been performed and long-term results are lacking. Therefore further research has to clarify the exact place of PNS in the treatment of lower urinary tract dysfunction.

References

1. van Kerrebroeck PE, van Voskuilen AC, Heesakkers JP, Lycklama a Nijholt AA, Siegel S, Jonas U, et al. Results of sacral neuromodulation therapy for urinary voiding dysfunction: outcomes of a prospective, worldwide clinical study. J Urol. 2007;178(5):2029–34. Epub 2007 Sep 18.
2. Marcelissen TA, Leong RK, de Bie RA, van Kerrebroeck PE, de Wachter SG. Long-term results of sacral neuromodulation with the tined lead procedure. J Urol. 2010;184(5):1997–2000. Epub 2010 Sep 21.
3. Leong RK, Marcelissen TA, Nieman FH, De Bie RA, Van Kerrebroeck PE, De Wachter SG. Satisfaction and patient experience with sacral neuromodulation: results of a single center sample survey. J Urol. 2011;185(2):588–92. Epub 2010 Dec 21.
4. Kessler TM, La Framboise D, Trelle S, Fowler CJ, Kiss G, Pannek J, et al. Sacral neuromodulation for neurogenic lower urinary tract dysfunction: systematic review and meta-analysis. Eur Urol. 2010;58(6):865–74. Epub 2010 Oct 12.
5. Blok BF, Groen J, Bosch JL, Veltman DJ, Lammertsma AA. Different brain effects during chronic and acute sacral neuromodulation in urge incontinent patients with implanted neurostimulators. BJU Int. 2006;98(6):1238–43. Epub 2006 Oct 13.
6. Groen J, Amiel C, Bosch JL. Chronic pudendal nerve neuromodulation in women with idiopathic refractory detrusor overactivity incontinence: results of a pilot study with a novel minimally invasive implantable mini-stimulator. Neurourol Urodyn. 2005;24(3):226–30. Epub 2005 Apr 13.
7. Mahakkanukrauh P, Surin P, Vaidhayakarn P. Anatomical study of the pudendal nerve adjacent to the sacrospinous ligament. Clin Anat. 2005;18(3):200–5. Epub 2005 Mar 16.
8. Popeney C, Ansell V, Renney K. Pudendal entrapment as an etiology of chronic perineal pain: diagnosis and treatment. Neurourol Urodyn. 2007;26(6):820–7. Epub 2007 May 8.
9. Beco J, Climov D, Bex M. Pudendal nerve decompression in perineology: a case series. BMC Surg. 2004;4:15. Epub 2004 Nov 2.
10. Burks FN, Bui DT, Peters KM. Neuromodulation and the neurogenic bladder. Urol Clin North Am. 2010;37(4):559–65. Epub 2010 Oct 20.

11. Schraffordt SE, Tjandra JJ, Eizenberg N, Dwyer PL. Anatomy of the pudendal nerve and its terminal branches: a cadaver study. ANZ J Surg. 2004;74(1–2): 23–6. Epub 2004 Jan 17.
12. Shafik A, Doss S. Surgical anatomy of the somatic terminal innervation to the anal and urethral sphincters: role in anal and urethral surgery. J Urol. 1999;161(1):85–9. Epub 1999 Feb 26.
13. George AT, Dudding TC, Nicholls RJ, Vaizey CJ. A new minimally invasive technique for pudendal nerve stimulation. Colorectal Dis. 2012;14(1):98–103. Epub 2010 Nov 9.
14. Martens FM, Heesakkers JP, Rijkhoff NJ. Surgical access for electrical stimulation of the pudendal and dorsal genital nerves in the overactive bladder: a review. J Urol. 2011;186(3):798–804. Epub 2011 Jul 27.
15. Schmidt RA. Technique of pudendal nerve localization for block or stimulation. J Urol. 1989;142(6):1528–31. Epub 1989 Dec 1.
16. Peters KM, Feber KM, Bennett RC. Sacral versus pudendal nerve stimulation for voiding dysfunction: a prospective, single-blinded, randomized, crossover trial. Neurourol Urodyn. 2005;24(7):643–7. Epub 2005 Sep 24.
17. Spinelli M, Malaguti S, Giardiello G, Lazzeri M, Tarantola J, Van Den Hombergh U. A new minimally invasive procedure for pudendal nerve stimulation to treat neurogenic bladder: description of the method and preliminary data. Neurourol Urodyn. 2005;24(4):305–9. Epub 2005 Jun 25.
18. Ohlsson BL, Fall M, Frankenberg-Sommar S. Effects of external and direct pudendal nerve maximal electrical stimulation in the treatment of the uninhibited overactive bladder. Br J Urol. 1989;64(4):374–80. Epub 1989 Oct 1.
19. Ranck Jr JB. Which elements are excited in electrical stimulation of mammalian central nervous system: a review. Brain Res. 1975;98(3):417–40. Epub 1975 Dec 1.
20. Martens FM, Heesakkers JP, Rijkhoff NJ. Minimal invasive electrode implantation for conditional stimulation of the dorsal genital nerve in neurogenic detrusor overactivity. Spinal Cord. 2011;49(4):566–72. Epub 2010 Oct 6.
21. Elkelini MS, Abuzgaya A, Hassouna MM. Mechanisms of action of sacral neuromodulation. Int Urogynecol J. 2010;21 Suppl 2:S439–46. Epub 2010 Oct 26.
22. Boggs JW, Wenzel BJ, Gustafson KJ, Grill WM. Frequency-dependent selection of reflexes by pudendal afferents in the cat. J Physiol. 2006;577(Pt 1):115–26. Epub 2006 Sep 2.
23. Boggs JW, Wenzel BJ, Gustafson KJ, Grill WM. Bladder emptying by intermittent electrical stimulation of the pudendal nerve. J Neural Eng. 2006;3(1):43–51. Epub 2006 Mar 3.
24. Tai C, Wang J, Chancellor MB, Roppolo JR, de Groat WC. Influence of temperature on pudendal nerve block induced by high frequency biphasic electrical current. J Urol. 2008;180(3):1173–8. Epub 2008 Jul 22.
25. Yoo PB, Woock JP, Grill WM. Bladder activation by selective stimulation of pudendal nerve afferents in the cat. Exp Neurol. 2008;212(1):218–25. Epub 2008 May 27.
26. Woock JP, Yoo PB, Grill WM. Mechanisms of reflex bladder activation by pudendal afferents. Am J Physiol Regul Integr Comp Physiol. 2011;300(2): R398–407. Epub 2010 Nov 12.
27. Reitz A, Schmid DM, Curt A, Knapp PA, Schurch B. Afferent fibres of the pudendal nerve modulate sympathetic neurons controlling the bladder neck. Neurourol Urodyn. 2003;22(6):597–601. Epub 2003 Sep 3.
28. Reitz A, Gobeaux N, Mozer P, Delmas V, Richard F, Chartier-Kastler E. Topographic anatomy of a new posterior approach to the pudendal nerve for stimulation. Eur Urol. 2007;51(5):1350–5; discussion 5–6. Epub 2006 Oct 31.
29. Yoo PB, Klein SM, Grafstein NH, Horvath EE, Amundsen CL, Webster GD, et al. Pudendal nerve stimulation evokes reflex bladder contractions in persons with chronic spinal cord injury. Neurourol Urodyn. 2007;26(7):1020–3. Epub 2007 May 8.
30. Goldman HB, Amundsen CL, Mangel J, Grill J, Bennett M, Gustafson KJ, et al. Dorsal genital nerve stimulation for the treatment of overactive bladder symptoms. Neurourol Urodyn. 2008;27(6):499–503. Epub 2007 Dec 20.
31. Peters KM, Feber KM, Bennett RC. A prospective, single-blind, randomized crossover trial of sacral vs pudendal nerve stimulation for interstitial cystitis. BJU Int. 2007;100(4):835–9. Epub 2007 Sep 8.

Part VI

Pelvic Organ Prolapse

Pelvic Organ Prolapse: Planning for Surgery—Indications, Decision, Special Instruments, and Controversies

16

Dominic Lee and Philippe Zimmern

Back to Basics?

Time has not been kind to the management of pelvic organ prolapse (POP). In an era of vast progress in other fields, prolapse repair it seems has stood relatively still. Despite our intense efforts to improve outcomes and to benefit patients, we are still rooted in traditional approaches where the operative techniques have changed very little for the past 100 years, and the results have been underwhelming to say the very least or is it?

From the beginning, most of what has been done in prolapse repair is not evidence based and few have challenged the prevailing concepts. Over a century ago, the Manchester repair came into existence, and along with the anterior colporrhaphy, both became the surgical standard for prolapse repair for apical and anterior defects but where was the data to support its efficacy? Similarly the posterior repair came into being as a form of repair for episiotomy tears and quickly became the most prevalent surgery for posterior defect repair without any anatomical understanding. Gradually more elaborate concepts came to bear, and from the 1950s and 1960s we saw the emergence of vault suspension techniques including sacrospinous ligament fixation popularized by Randall and Nichols and later by Miyazaki, and abdominal sacrocolpopexy (SCP) by Lane, which restored vaginal axis and vaginal capacity but with the risk of bowel complications and bleeding.

Still there were issues. Prolapse recurrence was not uncommon and the anterior compartment was the most affected with failure rates of up to 70 % within the first postoperative year [1]. DeLancey brought greater understanding of the pelvic anatomy highlighting the various levels of pelvic organ support [2]. Basic research started to flourish and confirmed the intuition that connective tissue defects with reduction in collagen and proteoglycan synthesis may have a pivotal role in prolapse development [3]. Translational research slowed but the race was on to find a suitable graft material to augment the repairs. Biologic grafts were advocated but the outcomes were disappointing [4]. Encouraged by the utility of synthetic material in abdominal hernia repairs and inspired by the success of tension-free vaginal tape (TVT) sling, we entered into the era of transvaginal synthetic mesh, and momentarily it offered a glimpse of hope. Anatomical outcomes were superior in a few short-term studies, and before we knew it the die was cast [5, 6]. Transvaginal mesh and its various kit transformations were championed by the medical device industry and promoted extensively amongst physicians. Not surprisingly, the new surgical concept also led to new complications; viscus perforation

D. Lee, M.B.B.S. (Hon.), F.R.A.C.S. (Australia) (✉) • P. Zimmern, M.D.
Department of Urology, University of Texas Southwestern Medical Center, 5323 Harry Hines Boulevard, Dallas, TX 75390-9110, USA
e-mail: domi_2020@yahoo.com.au

G.H. Badlani (ed.), *Minimally Invasive Therapy for Urinary Incontinence and Pelvic Organ Prolapse*, Current Clinical Urology, DOI 10.1007/978-1-4939-0008-4_16,

not recognized at the time of surgery. Mesh erosions and contractions surfaced, presenting often at times beyond the duration of the trial protocols [7]. The need for scientific reevaluation beckoned but regrettably, there was more effort spent marketing these devices rather than allowing for sufficient data to accumulate supporting their use. Clearly, there was inadequate understanding of the effects of synthetic material on delicate and atrophied vaginal tissues. The US Food and Drug Administration (FDA) intervened [8, 9], and as it stands we are entering the dominion of "meshology"; an evolving field of sub-specialization dedicated to a growing population of incapacitated women with scarred vaginas, extruded meshes, and chronic pain from vaginal mesh placement seeking relief and rallying for change.

To confuse matters further, outcome measures for success seem to be moving targets themselves. Previous successes were judged on anatomical correction, but now this seems inadequate, as 50 % of women were found asymptomatic despite recurring anatomical defects [10]. Symptom relief and sexual satisfaction became incorporated into our reporting, and yet there is no consensus on the true definition of success in prolapse surgery.

As we stare into the eyes of our patients with limited evidence to guide our approaches, we ask ourselves: Where did it all go wrong? What can be done? The answer seems logical—we need a scientific pipeline in POP, from basic sciences to clinical trials; a cultivation of sound scientific and clinical data based on a systematic approach. It may be time to go back to basics.

Planning for Surgery

Vaginal prolapse is rarely a life threatening condition. Most prolapses will progress with time and can only be corrected with intravaginal pessary or restorative surgery. Indications for surgical management are largely directed by the patient's presenting symptoms, and on rare occasions resultant complications associated with vaginal prolapse such as urinary retention or obstructive uropathy. Patient factors are important to consider as it can impact on the approach and outcome to management. As in other surgeries, the primary attempt at corrective surgery is the most likely to succeed, thus the most important. Therefore, a pelvic reconstructive surgeon should have expertise in several repair procedures for POP, including vaginal, laparoscopic/robotic, and open surgical techniques. The overall goal is to restore vaginal anatomy and improve symptoms and organ function.

For this chapter, we will take for granted that the patient has been fully worked up and a diagnosis has been reached confirming the presence of a bothersome prolapse condition for which surgery is indicated. The patient expectation can be simple (correction of a bothersome bulge) or more complex involving other domains such as restoration of sexual function, or correction of associated urinary or bowel symptoms. This needs to be addressed thoroughly to prevent postoperative disappointments but the setting of realistic expectations is beyond the reach of this chapter and is limited at present by few available tools to explore this important domain. For clarification, this chapter will exclude patients unfit for surgery, unwilling to undergo surgery, or those preferring a nonsurgical alternative such as a pessary. We will also exclude from our discussion patients who are not sexually active and can only undergo a short obliterative procedure such as a colpocleisis because of age and anesthesia risks for example. So, in summary, we will discuss the index patient who has a bothersome POP, wishes surgical repair (indication), and can be amenable to all currently available surgical approaches (decision).

Indications for Surgery

Vaginal prolapse can affect several compartments and demands astute clinical judgement from the surgeon in balancing between the patient's operative risks and chances for success. Consideration needs to be given to the following when deciding on surgical repair: (1) thorough assessment of prolapse symptom(s) and organ dysfunction(s), (2) the absence or presence of urinary incontinence, (3) patient comorbidities, (4) examination findings, (5) additional testing, (6) patient expectations, and (7) surgeon expertise.

Patient Factors

Patients that are at high risk for recurrence including those who had failed previous surgical repairs and those with predisposing comorbidities for poor healing should be identified. Overall medical condition such as patients with diabetes mellitus or on chemotherapy and/or steroids should seek medical clearance prior to proceeding with repair. Patient with chronic cough inducing respiratory conditions such as COPD and asthma should be medically optimized. Poorly estrogenized tissues should be treated with hormone cream for a minimum of 3 months if possible prior to procedure. Bowel evaluation may be needed in case of chronic constipation to avoid the risk of tearing a native tissue repair.

Lifestyle activities may be an issue and heavy physical duties may have to be curtailed in the perioperative period to ensure adequate healing and not jeopardizing repair. Sexual function is important in the indication as it sometimes eliminates a vaginal approach by fear of inducing vaginal pain, narrowing, and/or shortening. The presence or absence of uterus, and patient's interest to retain or remove this organ may need to be explored; and post-hysterectomy patients will need their ovarian status reviewed if they had elected to keep their ovaries thus far. Transvaginal mesh may be beneficial when used in the appropriate setting with "at risk for recurrence" individuals following thorough patient counseling by an adequately trained surgeon.

Finally patients with one compartment defect may need a different surgery than those with dual prolapse (anterior and apex, or apex and posterior, including enterocele and/or rectocele) or triple compartment prolapse. Furthermore, the presence of occult or urodynamic stress urinary incontinence (SUI) on testing needs to be factored into the final operative management.

Surgeon Factors

Aside from surgical repertoire and training issues, several factors may persuade the surgeon either to adopt an abdominal approach or to consider minimally invasive techniques such as laparoscopy/robotic-assisted laparoscopy or a vaginal approach. Overweight patients are not well suited for open, robotic, or laparoscopic techniques due to higher rates of perioperative complications. Patients with prior abdominal surgeries, hernia repairs (inguinal or midline), and colon issues (diverticulitis) need specific attention. Similarly, the need for an adjunct procedure such as a concomitant oophorectomy can affect the approach undertaken.

Decisions for Surgery

We will highlight three cases that illustrate our treatment choices and decision process taken in recent patients. In each case of prolapse the treatment should be individualized to the patient with considerations given to symptoms of bother, primary versus secondary presentation, associated comorbidities, sexual function, and past surgical history. In addition, the impact of prolapse on quality of life (QOL) as well as a thorough physical assessment documenting the anatomic defects in tandem with radiological or functional testing should be defined. Full disclosure of risks and benefits of operative approach to patient based on a comprehensive evaluation ensues, i.e., vaginal versus abdominal approach (laparoscopic/robotic or open), uterine conservation or not, mesh or no mesh, and with or without concomitant anti-incontinence procedure.

Case 1

A 53-year-old woman presents with a symptomatic cystocele following total vaginal hysterectomy 3 years ago for uterine prolapse. She reports mixed urinary incontinence (stress greater than urge) and wears two pads per day. She denies dyspareunia and reports no sexual activity secondary to partner's erectile dysfunction. Previous surgical history includes laparoscopic cholecystectomy and an appendectomy. Exam shows stage 2 cystocele and stage 1 vault prolapse. POP-Q Staging: Aa −2, Ba +1, C point −4, Ap −3, Bp −2. She desires treatment.

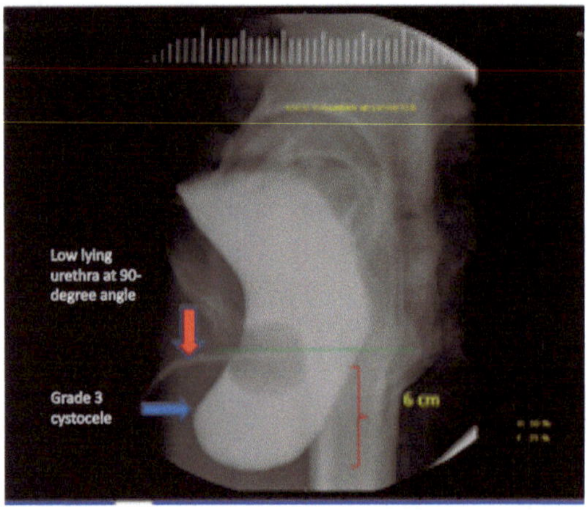

Fig. 16.1 Lateral view on VCUG showing a Grade 3 cystocele and a poorly supported, low-lying urethra

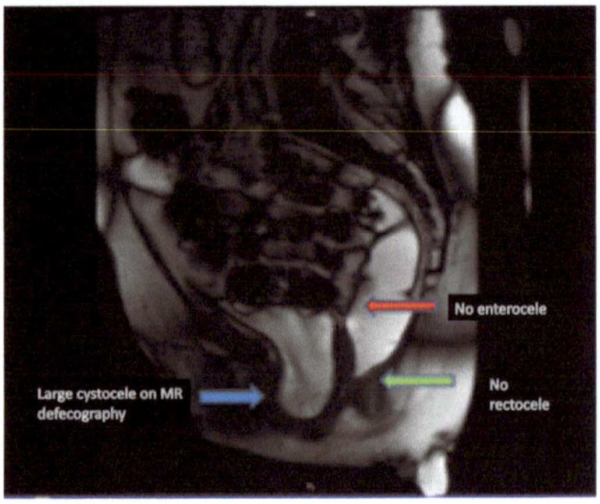

Fig. 16.2 MR defecography (T2) confirming anterior compartment defect

This lady presents interesting diagnostic and therapeutic considerations with dual complaints of symptomatic prolapse and urinary incontinence. Validated questionnaires are recommended to quantify these complaints and to establish baseline as a comparison for treatment success. Further testing was obtained to address her leakage mechanism and degree of urethral mobility with multichannel urodynamic studies (UDS) incorporating prolapse reduction with vaginal packing [11] and a standing voiding cystourethrogram (VCUG) with lateral views at rest and with straining. Prolapse evaluation with magnetic resonance imaging (MRI) defecography was suggested to evaluate apical support and assess for the presence of an enterocele that could impact on surgical approach.

Her evaluation returned with the following testing information:

VCUG: maximum cystometric capacity (MCC) at 450 mL. Grade 3 cystocele with the lower part of the bladder at 6 cm below the lower edge of the pubic symphysis on straining views. Low-lying urethra at a 90° angle, with normal urethral views during voiding, and a moderate post-void residual confirming her clinical impression of incomplete bladder emptying (Fig. 16.1).

MRI revealed a minimal vault descent and no posterior compartment defect, specifically no enterocele or rectocele (Fig. 16.2). No SUI with or without packing, or detrusor overactivity (DO) was evidenced during UDS. During pressure-flow study, a prolonged flow curve with low maximum flow at 10 mL/s along with Valsalva efforts was noted, with normal range voiding pressures.

Given the predominant cystocele defect on VCUG and MRI with minimal apical involvement, we planned for a transvaginal repair of her cystocele with an anterior vaginal wall suspension technique to repair the cystocele defect and provide support to the bladder neck area at the same setting [12]. A concurrent anti-incontinence procedure was not offered (see controversies), as patient had no demonstrable occult SUI (OSUI) on clinical exam or on UDS. Secondary incontinence (sphincteric deficiency and/or bladder overactivity) may occur, but is unlikely given her current findings. In the absence of vaginal vault weakness and/or posterior compartment defect, a mesh repair with an abdominal SCP was not recommended but could be considered if despite this thorough evaluation, her vault support fails secondarily.

Case 2

A 65-year-old woman presents with a 1-year history of symptomatic recurrent prolapse following failed trial of pessary. She is status post laparoscopic-assisted vaginal hysterectomy (LAVH) for uterine prolapse and a cystocele repair performed 2 years ago. She reports no SUI. She denies any pain or bowel symptoms. She is G4P3 with all vaginal deliveries. Patient is sexually active and intends to remain active. Examination confirms no leak with cough or strain. No anterior vaginal wall compartment defect is noted (Fig. 16.3), but a large posterior compartment defect is appreciated with POP-Q: Aa −3, TVL −9, C +1, Ap at +1. Vaginal trophicity is adequate with no evidence of ulcerations.

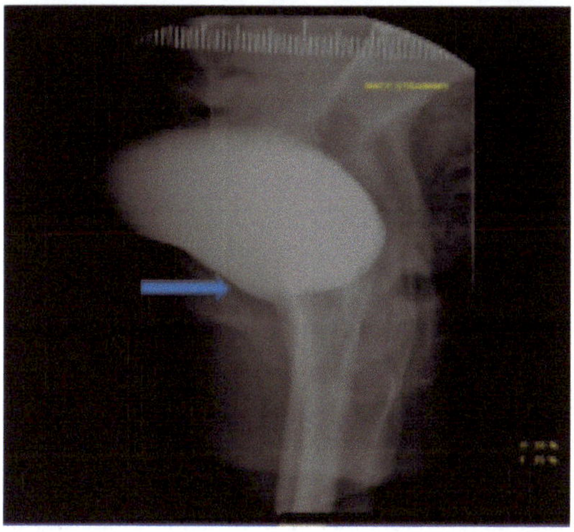

Fig. 16.3 Well supported urethra and bladder base during straining on lateral standing VCUG

The impression was that she had a secondary vault prolapse with an associated rectocele and suspicion of enterocele. MR defecography, ordered to determine if this was a large rectocele alone or with an associated enterocele, demonstrated widening of the levator hiatus and anorectal junction with descent of the anorectal junction during defecation. Aside from a large distal rectocele during defecation, a small enterocele was noted (Fig. 16.4a, b).

In counseling this patient we took into consideration her previous surgical history and her desire for maintenance of sexual activity. We discussed the risk and benefits of a transvaginal posterior repair with a potential 15–20 % rate of dyspareunia versus a laparoscopic/robotic-assisted abdominal mesh SCP (RA-SCP) with restoration of vaginal capacity and axis at the expense of mesh erosion risks around 5 %, mesh infection (<2 %), and secondary bowel obstruction (<5 %). Finally the patient opted for a robotic repair to preserve vaginal size and length. The intraoperative findings revealed a larger enterocele defect than estimated on MR defecography (Fig. 16.5).

This is a case in point that imaging in supine position has a degree of false negative rate and clinical suspicion is still paramount, as it would have impacted on intraoperative management and outcome if a posterior repair had been pursued.

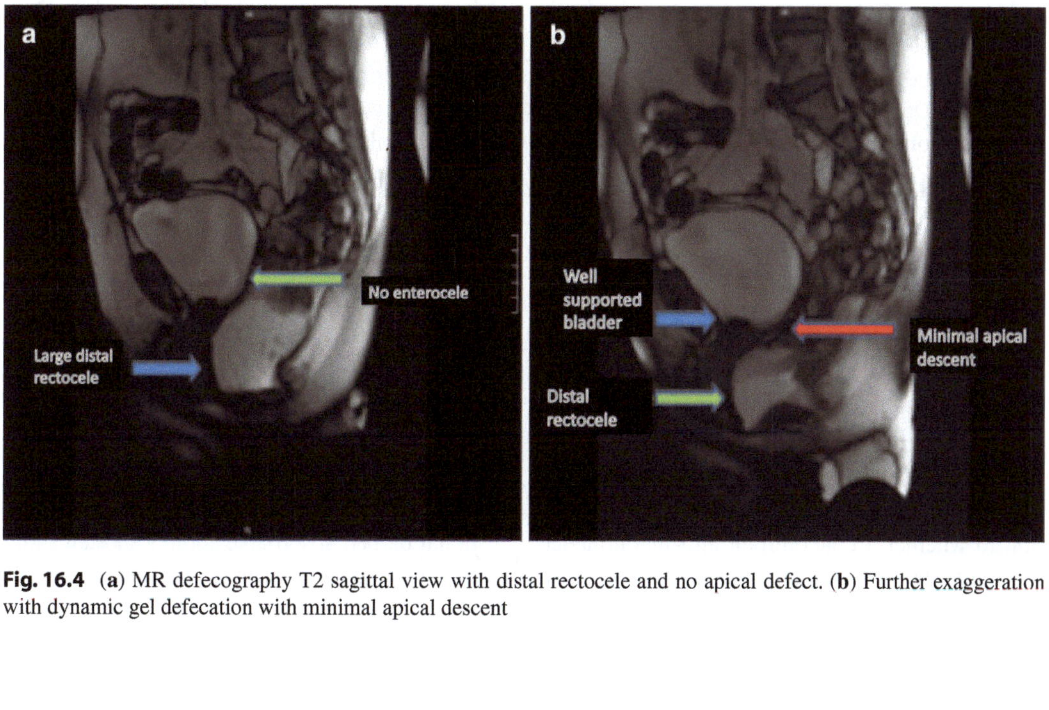

Fig. 16.4 (**a**) MR defecography T2 sagittal view with distal rectocele and no apical defect. (**b**) Further exaggeration with dynamic gel defecation with minimal apical descent

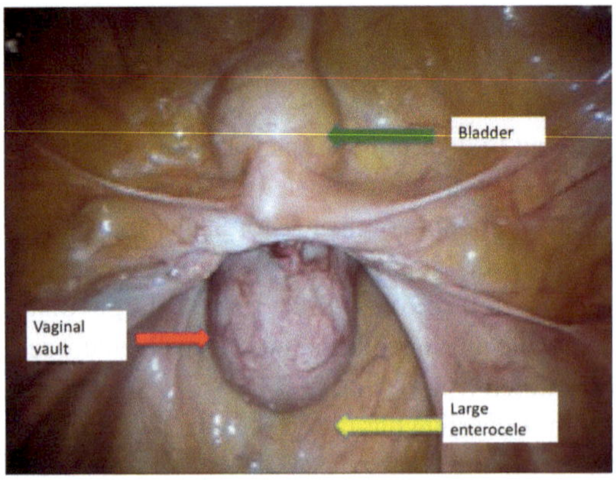

Fig. 16.5 Intraoperative view of large enterocele defect at robotic surgery

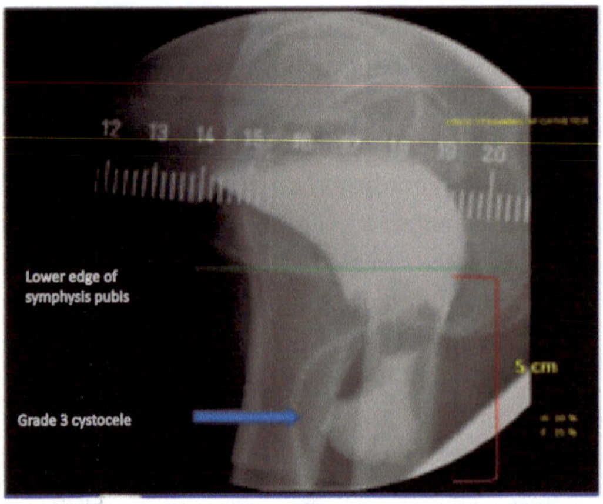

Fig. 16.6 Lateral VCUG showing bottleneck appearance of a Grade 3 cystocele on straining with poorly supported urethra represented by the axis of the urethral Foley catheter

Case 3

A 64-year-old presents with symptomatic uterine and bladder prolapse. She denies any urinary incontinence or bowel symptoms. Patient is still sexually active but denies dyspareunia. She gives a history of negative Pap smears. Previous surgical history includes a laparoscopic cholecystectomy but no other abdominal surgeries. Pelvic exam revealed a large cystocele and uterine prolapse with POP-Q: Ba +1, C −1, and D −3.

Given her symptoms and the presence of her reproductive organs, she was investigated with: (1) a pelvic ultrasound to evaluate for uterine size and to exclude a uterine or ovarian pathology, (2) standing cystogram to document the extent of her cystocele and degree of urethral hypermobility, and (3) a UDS with pack reduction of prolapse to unmask incontinence. Completed evaluation confirmed the following:

Pelvic ultrasound: small uterus and normal ovaries.

UDS: SUI with pack reduction.

VCUG: 600 mL bladder capacity with large cystocele Grade 3 and urethral hypermobility. No residual (Fig. 16.6).

This patient has significant dual compartment prolapses with occult SUI on UDS testing. The approach will depend on her decision regarding uterine preservation versus hysterectomy in addition to whether a concomitant anti-incontinence procedure should be undertaken (see discussion on controversies). If she desires uterine preservation, counseling with regard to an approach with laparoscopic or open abdominal mesh sacrohysteropexy with an anterior mesh segment to correct her cystocele and a Burch urethropexy or suburethral tape would be a reasonable option. If she decided on a hysterectomy, then a total vaginal approach could be a logical option including a vaginal hysterectomy with possible bilateral salpingo-oophorectomy (BSO), an enterocele repair with a Moschowitz-type purse-string closure of the peritoneal defect, a vault fixation procedure, and a cystocele repair with bladder neck suspension at the same setting. If she opted for an open repair, a supracervical hysterectomy would be considered to minimize the risks of mesh erosion at the vaginal cuff (see controversies).

Special Instruments

1. Da Vinci robotic-assisted mesh sacrocolpopexy has widened the minimally invasive options and seemingly requires fewer skills than needed for laparoscopy (Fig. 16.7). Single incision has been reported but is a very demanding procedure [13].
2. Covidien V-loc™ sutures—these unidirectional barbed absorbable sutures shorten suturing time and keep tissues on tension (Fig. 16.8).

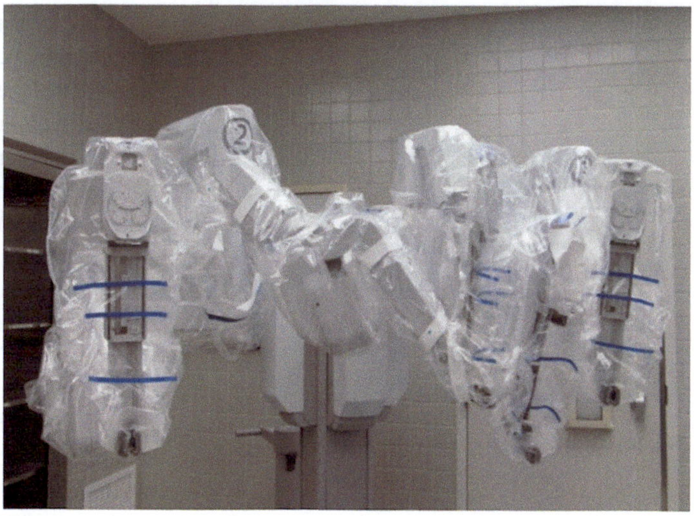

Fig. 16.7 Da Vinci robotic-assisted mesh sacrocolpopexy has widened the minimally invasive options and seemingly requires fewer skills than needed for laparoscopy

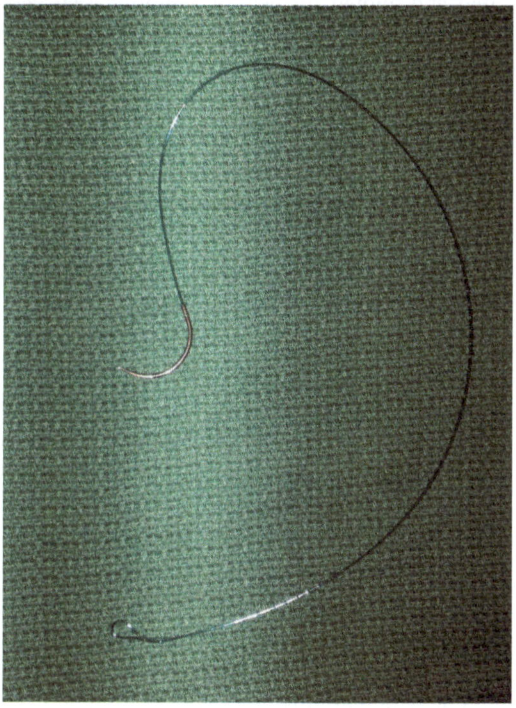

Fig. 16.8 Covidien V-loc™ sutures

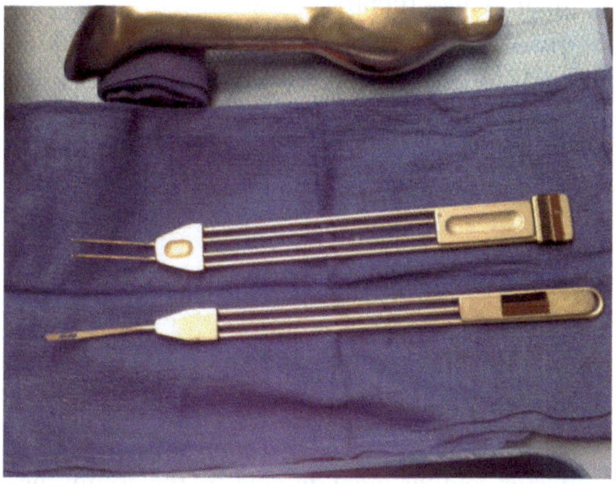

Fig. 16.9 Pereyra-Raz double prong or Pereyra or Stamey single prong needle passers

They are used primarily for peritoneal closure over the mesh.

3. Long blade-weighted vagina retractors—good vaginal access is imperative for cystocele repair and vaginal hysterectomy and depending on whether the patient is nulliparous or multiparous; the swan neck-contoured blades improve access and visibility.
4. Pereyra-Raz double prong or Pereyra or Stamey single prong needle passers are useful for suture transfers from the vaginal area to the suprapubic region during autologous pubovaginal sling and needle suspension procedures like the anterior vaginal wall suspension technique (Fig. 16.9).
5. Breisky-Navratil vaginal retractors and the Capio needle drivers are important to improve access to the ischial spine for a sacrospinous ligament fixation procedure (Fig. 16.10).

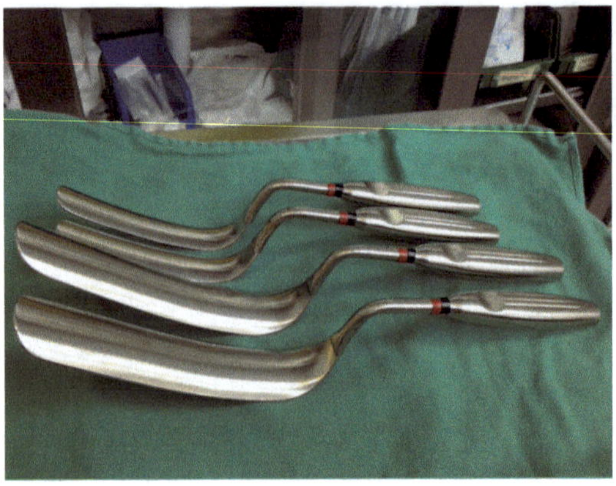

Fig. 16.10 Breisky-Navratil vaginal retractors

6. Betadine-soaked rectal packing can be used to mold the rectum during posterior compartment defect repairs.
7. EEA clamp or some form of vaginal molding tool (sponge stick) is needed to aid in the vaginal vault dissection during laparoscopic or robotic repairs.

Controversies

Mesh Versus No Mesh for Transvaginal Prolapse Repair

Anterior compartment defects are the commonest and also the most prone to recurrence following repair [14]. The definition of recurrence has changed over time further complicating the debate in this field. Data from a control group of women examined for non-prolapse symptomatology highlighted a natural tendency for anterior vaginal descent with ageing. Therefore, reconsideration of prior published studies with modified criteria for failure has led to a change in the rate of anatomic recurrence noted after native tissue cystocele repairs [15]. The assessment of postoperative outcomes following POP surgery lacks standardization leading to variable successes quoted in the literature for native tissue repairs. The initial emphasis on anatomical correction as the dominant outcome may have been too stringent as there may be less correlation with the patient's overall assessment of improvement. A study by Barber et al. using the colpopexy and urinary reduction efforts (CARE) trial data reevaluated their outcomes based on 18 definitions of surgical success. Treatment success varied widely depending on definitions used (19.2–97.2 %). Definition of surgical success correlated most with both treatment success and overall improvement when the following was utilized: (1) the absence of prolapse beyond the hymen (94 %), (2) the absence of bulge (92.1 %), and (3) the absence of re-treatment (97.2 %). Importantly, subjective cure was associated with significant improvements in the patient's assessment of both treatment success and overall improvement, more so than any other definition considered ($p<0.001$ and $p<0.001$, respectively) [16]. The original data of a landmark RCT by Weber et al., often cited and quoted for lack of anatomical success (30–46 %) with native repair, was reanalyzed using more clinically relevant definitions of success based on the NICHD Pelvic Floor Disorders Network's recommendation. Of the 114 subjects randomized to the three treatment arms, 88 % were successful based on the new definitions with no difference between the three groups. No reoperations were reported for complications or recurrence at 12 months [15].

Nonetheless, a legitimate approach to diminish these rates of anatomic failure included the interposition of a mesh material or net beneath the bladder base through a minimally invasive, transvaginal approach [17]. Fed by initial reports of anatomical success with short-term follow-up and byway of the US FDA 510 K-approval process, a plethora of mesh kits became rapidly available on the market [18]. However, a series of reports on "unique" mesh-related complications (mesh extrusion, erosion, and/or retraction, as well as pain and infection), some of which were found to be irreversible and crippling, prompted the US FDA to issue two consecutive notifications in 2008 and 2011. The second notification, based on a continued increase in complications reported on the MAUDE database, was directed to all involved, including patients for whom a list of 14 questions to ask their repair surgeon was recommended. Several other measures were activated including the process of reclassifying vaginal mesh products from a class II to class III device, which will mandate elaborate pre- and post-market investigations [9]. Just recently, Johnson and Johnson Ethicon Women's Health & Urology decided to remove the following meshes from the market: Prosima™, Prolift, and Prolift +M™ [19].

What Is the Current Evidence to Favor Transvaginal Mesh Use?

Most of the evidence base related to mesh use is at level 2–3 and there is only a handful of level 1 evidence to date. De Landsheere et al. reported on 3 % failure rate and 3.6 % mesh reoperation rate (2.7 % for mesh exposure) in their retrospective series of 524 patients with transvaginal Prolift™ mesh repair at a median follow-up of 38 months (range: 15–63). They concluded that the rate of prolapse recurrence and re-intervention for mesh-related complications was low in experienced hands [20]. In a large randomized trial by Altman et al. comparing anterior colporrhaphy versus trocar-guided mesh kit repairs in 389 women with stage ≥2 cystocele with composite (objective and subjective) outcomes, mesh kits performed better than native repair at 12 months: 60.8 % versus 34.1 %. The sexual function domains were not significantly different between the two groups ($p=0.99$) and the reoperation rate for mesh complications was 3.2 % [21]. Withagen et al. randomized 190 women with recurrent prolapse to trocar-guided mesh repair versus conventional repair and reported a lower anatomical failure rate for mesh repair compared to conventional repair; 9.6 % versus 45.2 % at 12 months follow-up [22].

What About Those Who Object to the Use of Transvaginal Mesh Placement?

Withagen et al., in the same study mentioned above, reported subjective improvement as equivocal between the two groups at 80 %, despite higher anatomical recurrence in the non-mesh group [22]. Similarly, Neiminen et al. at 3 years follow-up on their randomized trial of anterior colporrhaphy with mesh reinforcement versus traditional repair reported a lower recurrence rate in the mesh versus non-mesh arm: 13 % versus 41 % ($p<0.001$). Interestingly, no difference in symptomatic recurrence was noted between the two groups, and the mesh erosion rate was high at 19 % [23]. This debate can be summarized by reviewing the recent Cochrane publication issued in 2010 on 3,773 patients which reported that although mesh repairs showed superior anatomical outcomes, with a higher native repair failure risk (RR 3.55, 95 % CI 2.29–5.51), the current data sets were extracted from conference abstracts and should be interpreted with caution. Furthermore, it appears that there is insufficient evidence to support a clinically significant difference in subjective outcomes, QOL data, and reoperation rate for recurrent prolapse compared to traditional repairs [24]. Finally the FDA notification of 2011 emphasized the Cochrane review by stating that the anatomical outcome may be favorable for mesh, but there is no evidence that this finding changes functional outcomes or patient satisfaction, and can cause grief through mesh-related complications. "In particular, the literature review revealed that: while transvaginal surgical repair to correct weakened tissue between the bladder and vagina (anterior repair) with mesh augmentation may provide an anatomic benefit compared to traditional POP repair without mesh, this anatomic benefit may not result in better symptomatic results" [9].

How Safe Is Vaginal Mesh?

Data abstracted from a recent systematic review conducted by the Society of Obstetrics and Gynecology of Canada (SOGC) in 2010 reported that although mesh repairs had an anatomical success rate of 79–100 %, the mesh erosion rate was 5–19 % and the reoperation rate 3.2–22 % [25]. These numbers, derived from high volume and experienced centers, have implications for less well trained pelvic surgeons, although caseload and experience levels have not been officially quantitated to date. In recognition of the increased frequency and complexity of vaginal mesh-associated complications, the International Urogynecological Association (IUGA) and the International Continence Society (ICS) issued a joint terminology and classification system to

Table 16.1 Thirteen core discussion points with potential mesh patients as part of FDA 2011 notification

• Are you planning to use mesh in my surgery?
• Why do you think I am a good candidate for surgical mesh?
• Why is surgical mesh being chosen for my repair?
• What are the alternatives to transvaginal surgical mesh repair for POP, including nonsurgical options?
• What are the pros and cons of using surgical mesh in my particular case?
• How likely is it that my repair could be successfully performed without using surgical mesh?
• Will my partner be able to feel the surgical mesh during sexual intercourse?
• What if the surgical mesh erodes through my vaginal wall?
• If surgical mesh is to be used, how often have you implanted this particular product?
• What results have your other patients had with this product?
• What can I expect to feel after surgery and for how long?
• Which specific side effects should I report to you after the surgery?
• If I develop a complication, will you treat it or will I be referred to a specialist experienced with surgical mesh complications?
• What if the mesh surgery doesn't correct my problem?
• If I have a complication related to the surgical mesh, how likely is it that the surgical mesh could be removed and what could be the consequences?
• If a surgical mesh is to be used, is there patient information that comes with the product, and can I have a copy?

From http://www.fda.gov/MedicalDevices/ProductsandMedicalProcedures/ImplantsandProsthetics/UroGynSurgicalMesh/ucm345205.htm

standardize the reporting of mesh complications [26]. In addition, the FDA has proposed 13 points a mesh surgeon should discuss with suitable patients, which has become the core consensus requirement at present (Table 16.1) [9].

Falling short of a bipartisan divide between mesh supporters and mesh sceptics in "meshology," and leaving aside for a moment the patients' internet networks [27] and our volatile medicolegal environment regarding mesh use, we should debate the question of whether the time has come to reconsider the concept of vaginally placed mesh in the management of prolapse. First, a better understanding of mesh performance in tissues may be needed before human implantation. This could be obtained from animal studies allowing access to valuable information of in vivo mesh behaviors based on their properties (weight, porosity, fibrosis process, and composition) [28]. Second, once a mesh has been selected and tested in phase I studies [29], a process of gradual dissemination with surgeon mentors has to take place to try to reduce the effects of a learning curve. For now, transvaginal mesh may remain an option in well-selected cases, for example, a non-sexually active woman, with a symptomatic recurrent cystocele, in a high volume center and following thorough informed consent as recommended in the FDA notification of 2011. In this unique situation, the critical factor may well be the role of the surgeon experience as highlighted by Vaiyapuri et al. who reported on outcomes of Prolift™ mesh placement in Grade 4 POP by a single surgeon in 254 cases with 209 evaluated patients at 12 months. They noted improvements in both objective (Grade $\leq$ 1 POP: 92.4, 100, and 97 %) and subjective cure rates (absence of symptomatic bulge: 92.1, 92.1, and 97 %) for the consecutive 3 years of evaluation, respectively [30].

Mesh Placement, with or Without Hysterectomy

Mesh abdominal SCP is the current gold standard for the management of vault prolapse with well-established level 1 evidence in its favor [24]. The median mesh erosion rate from a large systemic review was reported at 3.4 % [31]. Most case series report an increased risk of mesh erosion when ASC was performed concurrent with total hysterectomy (TH) although RCTs are lacking. Culligan et al. reported an increase in mesh erosion in women who underwent a concurrent TH compared to those who did not: 27 % versus 1.3 % ($p < 0.001$) [32]. As part of the CARE trial, Cundiff et al. reported similar trends in 26 % of women who had concurrent TAH. The mesh erosion rate was 14 % in women with concomitant TAH compared to 4 % with SCP alone, which represented a fivefold increased risk. The increased risk was attributed to the direct contact between the mesh and the vaginal cuff suture line, in addition to possible mesh contamination from vaginal bacteria [33]. Bensinger et al. reported on a retrospective analysis of 121 women who were stratified into 3 groups: (1) SCH with SCP ($n=37$), (2) TH with SCP ($n=49$), and (3) SCP alone ($n=35$). The overall reported mesh erosion rate was 3.3 % and adjusted to 8.2 % ($p<0.039$) in Group 2 with all cases occurring exclusively within that group. Patients undergoing SCP at the time of TH had a sevenfold increase in erosion rate risk compared to SCH and ASC or SCP group alone [34]. A recent publication by Kim et al. explored the risk of mesh erosion with minimally invasive sacrocolpopexy (MISC), both robotic and laparoscopic-assisted SCP, in 188 women. They reported an overall 10 % mesh erosion rate, which is higher than most series. Women with concurrent transvaginal hysterectomy (TVH) had higher erosion rate (23 % versus 5 %, $p=0.109$) compared to SCH (5 %) or SCP alone (5 %). The odds of mesh erosion for concomitant TVH was 5.67 (95 % CI: 1.88–17.10) compared to SCP alone [35].

Over the last decade there has been a trend to perform uterine sparing surgery instead of the standard option of a total hysterectomy. Purported advantages of this approach include perioperative and psychosexual benefits in addition to preserving fertility in women who are still within child bearing age. Surgical treatment options for uterine prolapse include open, laparoscopic, or vaginal approaches. Uterine preservation techniques include the Manchester procedure and its variants, sacrospinous hysteropexy (SSH), laparoscopic sacral hysteropexy, and laparoscopic uterosacral vault suspension. Deciding on which operative approach is difficult as there is a paucity of head-to-head comparison trials.

SSH is the most studied vaginal technique with favorable outcomes. Most retrospective studies reported anatomical success rates between 74 and 93 % with short- to intermediate-term follow-up [36]. A recent multicenter randomized control trial by Dietz et al. compared TVH ($n=31$) with unilateral SSH ($n=35$) for stage 2–4 uterine prolapse with an intention to treat analysis. These authors reported a higher proportion of recurrent apical prolapse in the SSH group compared to TVH at 1 year: 27 % versus 3 %, which they attributed to a higher stage of POP. No statistical significance was detected for QOL or functional outcomes between the two groups although the time to return to work for SSH group was shorter [37].

Abdominal and laparoscopic sacrohysteropexy provide similar outcomes to TH and SCP with the advantage of shorter operative time, blood loss, and length of stay. Failure rates are estimated between 0 and 22 % and mesh erosion between 0 and 4.1 % [36]. However, most of the data for subjective and objective outcomes for these prolapse procedures are from uncontrolled retrospective case series. Costantini et al. reported on a prospective non-randomized series of 72 women comparing abdominal sacrohysteropexy ($n=34$) and SCP ($n=38$) alone. They reported shorter operating time in the uterine sparing group and although the rate of cystocele recurrence was higher in this group, 14.7 % versus 2.6 %, it did not reach statistical significance and no reoperations were performed for failures in either group [38].

The drawback with any uterine preservation technique is the requirement for lifelong surveillance for gynecological cancer. With a lack of definitive gold standard in uterine prolapse treatment, the operative approach will be dependent on multiple factors including compartments affected, patient's age, comorbidities and performance status, desire for future fertility, patient preference, family genetics, and the surgeon's skills set.

Global Versus Site-Specific Repair for Rectocele

Rectocele is a common clinical finding, often in association with other vaginal compartment defects with a prevalence of 50 % as reported by Olsen et al. Rectocele in isolation is less common with an estimated prevalence of 7 % [39]. Most rectoceles remain largely asymptomatic and conservative treatments with dietary modifications, stool softeners, vaginal pessaries, and/or pelvic floor therapy should be considered first. Symptoms related to a pronounced rectocele may include the presence of bulge, defecatory dysfunction requiring digital manipulation (vaginal splinting), and/or sexual dysfunction. The existence of a "rectovaginal septum" is controversial. Cadaveric studies by Richardson have demonstrated specific breaks within the "septum" resulting in site-specific defects [40]. On the contrary, histological studies by Farrell et al. on "fascia" biopsies at the time of colporrhaphy demonstrated a layer that consists of moderately dense connective tissue with smooth muscle similar to the deep aspects of the vaginal wall with a conclusion that the surgical "fascia" was an artifact of the surgical dissection [41]. Kleeman et al. reported similar findings on cadaveric studies with no evidence of a distinct septum identified [42].

Surgical management for rectocele is highly successful. Posterior colporrhaphy (PC) (with or without levator plication) is the most commonly used technique for repair with anatomical cure rates of 76–96 % [43, 44]. If surgical repair is to be considered, the impact on bowel and sexual dysfunction should be appropriately evaluated and the patient counseled accordingly, as rates of bowel dysfunction may not differ following surgery and postoperative dypareunia rates of 5–26 % have been reported [45, 46]. Levator plication should be reserved for nonsexually active women, as dyspareunia rates as high as 30 % have been reported [46]. For this reason, some pelvic floor surgeons have advocated for a more directed approach based on Richardson's "septum" theorem with site-specific repairs (SSR) on the premise of better functional outcomes. Anatomical cure rates for SSR have ranged between 56 and 100 %. Abramov et al. from a large retrospective series reported that SSR ($n=124$) is associated with higher anatomic recurrence rate and lower subjective outcome (symptomatic bulge) compared to traditional PC ($n=183$): (11 % versus 4 %, $p=0.02$) and (11 % versus 4 %, $p=0.02$), respectively. Rate of postoperative dyspareunia (16 % versus 17 %) was not significantly different between the two study groups [47]. Paraiso et al. reported on 106 women with stage $\geq$ II rectocele randomly assigned to PR ($n=37$), SSR ($n=37$), or SSR augmented with biologic graft. At 1 year, anatomical outcomes for PC (4/28; 14 %) and SSR (6/27; 22 %) were similar whereas those who received graft augmentation had a significantly greater anatomic failure rate (12/26; 46 %, $p=0.02$). There was no significant change in the rate of dyspareunia and overall sexual function improved significantly in all groups postoperatively at 1-year follow-up ($p<0.001$), with no differences between groups [48]. From the current literature, native tissue repair with PC remains the gold standard and SSR is an acceptable alternative [43].

Sling and POP Repair

To sling or not to sling? That is the question. But the answer is not so apparent. It is well known that a certain population of women will have postoperative stress urinary incontinence (POSUI) associated with prolapse repair. Multiple publications have attested to this problem but there is no easy solution. The estimated incidence of POSUI in women without preoperative SUI is estimated between 11 and 37 % [49, 50]. In patients with OSUI, especially in women with high-grade POP (stage $\geq$ 3), the risk may be as high as 80 % [51]. The intervention rate due to obstruction following mid-urethral sling in one study with POSUI was 8.5 % [52]. How does one justify an additional procedure that will offer benefit and yet not over-treat those that do not require the surgery to begin with and expose such individuals to material risks and complications? This frequent situation presents a particular conundrum to all treating clinicians. There are three proposed approaches: (1) concomitant prophylactic anti-incontinence procedure for all patients undergoing POP surgery, (2) staged approach, and (3) selective approach based on clinical and urodynamic parameters. For those who are in favor of prophylactic slings, we have level 1 evidence with the CARE trial. Women without significant symptoms of SUI on clinical evaluation who were randomized to receiving Burch urethropexy at the time of open abdominal SCP performed better than those without with respect to postoperative de novo SUI (6.1 % versus 24.5 %, $p<0.001$), without attracting additional risks at 3 months follow-up [53]. The same authors reported their 2-year data with a similar trend (32 % (Burch) versus 45.2 % (control), $p=0.026$) [54]. As cautioned by the authors, it is still a matter of debate as to whether these findings can be generalized to transvaginal route of prolapse repair and other associated anti-incontinence procedures. The OPUS trial aims to address this debate with a controlled study of planned accrual of 350 women, randomized to transvaginal prolapse repair with or without mid-urethra TVT sling [55]. Wei et al. reported on this recent data and concluded that prophylactic TVT during POP surgery resulted in superior continence rates at 3 and 12 months. Number needed to treat was six patients to prevent one urinary incontinence at 12 months, but benefits were tempered by higher rate of postoperative complications [56]. The counterpoint advocating for a staged approach favors the argument that there is scant high-level evidence evaluating clinical predictors that determine which women may require and ultimately benefit from a concomitant anti-incontinence procedure. A study by Borstad et al. gave further credence to this approach within a multicenter randomized trial between evident SUI women managed with concomitant prolapse repair and sling and delayed retropubic sling surgery at 3 months following repair. Of the women in the delayed group, 44 % did not proceed to sling surgery as they either were cured of their SUI (29 %) or improved (15 %) following POP repair alone at 3 months and at 1 year [57]. And finally the principles of first do no harm-"primum non nocere" needs to be factored into any surgical decision planning process. Anti-incontinence surgeries are not risk-free and a recent review by Daneshgari et al. reported on overall complication rates on synthetic mid-urethral slings (MUS) ranging from 4.3 % to 75.1 % for retropubic and 10.5 % to 31.3 % for transobturator MUS, respectively. De novo dyspareunia rate was 1.3–7.3 % and mesh extrusion rates were 0–10.9 % [58]. Furthermore, Deng et al. utilizing data from the MAUDE (manufacturer and user facility device experience) website concluded that MUS complications may be underreported [59].

On balance, most clinicians will prefer to exercise a balanced approach based on selective identification of women who may be at risk of POSUI and offer these women concomitant surgeries. Chaikin et al. reported from a small prospective study of 24 women that in 10 women with negative preoperative testing for SUI, none developed de novo SUI; and in the 14 women who tested positive for SUI on prolapse reduction and underwent sling surgery, 12 were cured and 2 were failures [60]. Ballert et al. in a prospective study evaluated 105 patients who were treated with a sling based on objective evidence of OSUI on UDS criteria. They reported an 8.3 % complication rate for obstruction in the sling group compared to an 8.5 % rate in those who required re-intervention for POSUI who had negative testing. Interestingly they also reported 30 % risk for POSUI in women with a history of SUI but negative urodynamics, suggesting that a remote history of SUI in the absence of clinical signs may also be a reason to consider an associated anti-incontinence procedure [52]. Liang et al. also reported similar trends when using OSUI on UDS with pessary reduction of high-grade prolapse as a predictor for POSUI. All women who tested negative did not develop POSUI and interestingly, of those that did and declined a TVT, 65 % developed POSUI [61]. From the various publications, performing anti-incontinence procedures with evident SUI is a reasonable approach. This is congruent with the recently published AUA adult urodynamics guidelines [62].

While there may be many facets on both sides of the argument, ultimately the overriding clinical principle is a thorough preoperative counseling that offers the patient a balanced perspective on risk to benefit ratio based on clinical and investigative predictors such as urodynamic findings.

Sexual Function and POP

Sexual dysfunction is common in women with POP but evidence on outcomes of sexual function following pelvic reconstructive surgery is limited. A prospective study by Dua et al. evaluated postoperative sexual function in 123 sexually active women undergoing prolapse repair stratified into four groups: posterior repair, anterior repair, anterior repair with vaginal hysterectomy, and combined anterior and posterior repair. The electronic personal assessment questionnaire-pelvic floor (ePAQ-PF) was used to assess symptoms and the authors reported that sexual function improved overall following pelvic reconstructive surgery, but greater improvement was seen following anterior repair either alone or in combination with a vaginal hysterectomy when compared with posterior repair [63].

Pain

Pain following pelvic floor reconstruction surgery is inherent to both native tissue and mesh prolapse repairs. Anterior colporrhaphy has a 5–9 % risk of dypareunia [24]. Posterior repair with levator plication is associated with dyspareunia rate as high as 30 % [46]. However, the advent of synthetic mesh and "mesh kits" with synthetic arm extensions into the ischiorectal fossa, transobturator foramen, and sacrospinous ligament for prolapse repair has given way to a new set of pain syndromes. De novo dyspareunia rate of up to 38 % has been reported following transvaginal mesh placement [64]. Withagen et al. attempted to identify risk factors for mesh complications and prospectively studied 294 women treated with tension-free trocar-guided mesh kits for POP. They reported a postoperative dypareunia and de novo dypareunia rate of 45 % and 26 %, respectively, and predictors for both were preexisting pain preoperatively [65]. The exact mechanism leading to pain is unknown. A combination of nerve damage/entrapment and tension on vaginal or perivaginal structures as a result of scarring seems probable. Feiner et al. defined the biomechanical characteristic of "mesh contraction" and reported on a case series of 17 women surgically managed with mesh excision. All subjects presented with intractable pelvic pain, global dyspareunia, and tenderness on pelvic examination associated with vaginal scarring. The reduction of pain postoperatively for pelvic pain and dypareunia was 88 % and 64 %, respectively, with 12 % reporting persistent pain symptoms [66]. Groin pain is a recognized complication of trocar-based mesh systems in up to 4 % with transobturator mesh placement. Most pain occurs transiently but can be intractable requiring extensive obturator dissection and mesh excision with variable success [67]. This is congruent with the FDA warnings that some complications are life altering and intervention "may or may not correct the complication."

References

1. Weber AM, Walters MD, Piedmonte MR, Ballard LA. Anterior colporrhaphy: a randomized trial of three surgical techniques. Am J Obstet Gynecol. 2001; 185(6):1299–304; discussion 1304–6.
2. DeLancey JO. Anatomic aspects of vaginal eversion after hysterectomy. Am J Obstet Gynecol. 1992;166(6 Pt 1):1717–24; discussion 1724–8.
3. Jackson SR, Avery NC, Tarlton JF, Eckford SD, Abrams P, Bailey AJ. Changes in metabolism of collagen in genitourinary prolapse. Lancet. 1996;347(9016): 1658–61.
4. Jia X, Glazener C, Mowatt G, MacLennan G, Bain C, Fraser C, Burr J. Efficacy and safety of using mesh or grafts in surgery for anterior and/or posterior vaginal wall prolapse: systematic review and meta-analysis. BJOG. 2008;115(11):1350–61.
5. Nguyen JN, Burchette RJ. Outcome after anterior vaginal prolapse repair: a randomized controlled trial. Obstet Gynecol. 2008;111(4):891–8.
6. Carey M, Higgs P, Goh J, Lim J, Leong A, Krause H, Cornish A. Vaginal repair with mesh versus colporrhaphy for prolapse: a randomised controlled trial. BJOG. 2009;116(10):1380–6.
7. Haylen BT, Freeman RM, Swift SE, Cosson M, Davila GW, Deprest J, Dwyer PL, et al. An International Urogynecological Association (IUGA)/ International Continence Society (ICS) joint terminology and classification of the complications related directly to the insertion of prostheses (meshes, implants, tapes) & grafts in female pelvic floor surgery. Int Urogynecol J. 2011;22(1):3–15.
8. FDA Public Health Notification: serious complications associated with transvaginal placement of surgical mesh in repair of pelvic organ prolapse and stress urinary incontinence. Issued: 2 Oct 2008.

9. FDA Public Health Notification: serious complications associated with transvaginal placement of surgical mesh in repair of pelvic organ prolapse and stress urinary incontinence. Issued: 13 July 2011.
10. Whiteside JL, Weber AM, Meyn LA, Walters MD. Risk factors for prolapse recurrence after vaginal repair. Am J Obstet Gynecol. 2004;191(5):1533–8.
11. Gilleran JP, Lemack GE, Zimmern PE. Reduction of moderate-to-large cystocele during urodynamic evaluation using a vaginal gauze pack: 8-year experience. BJU Int. 2006;97(2):292–5.
12. Takacs E, Zimmern PE. Chapter 32 role of needle suspensions. In: Raz S, Rodriguez L, editors. Female urology. 3rd ed. Philadelphia, PA: Saunders-Elsevier; 2008. p. 362–74.
13. Dillon BE, Cadeddu JA, Zimmern PE. Robotic laparoendoscopic single site (LESS) sacrocolpopexy. Journal of Endourology Part B, Videourology. 2012;26 DOI:10.1089/vid.2012.0005.
14. Swift SE. The distribution of pelvic organ support in a population of female subjects seen for routine gynecologic health care. Am J Obstet Gynecol. 2000; 183(2):277–85.
15. Chmielewski L, Walters MD, Weber AM, Barber MD. Re-analysis of a randomized trial of 3 techniques of anterior colporrhaphy using clinically relevant definitions of success. Am J Obstet Gynecol. 2011; 205(1):69.e1–8.
16. Barber MD, Brubaker L, Nygaard I, Wheeler TL II, Schaffer J, Chen Z, Spino C; Pelvic Floor Disorders Network. Defining success after surgery for pelvic organ prolapse. Obstet Gynecol. 2009;114(3):600–9.
17. Debodinance P, Berrocal J, Clavé H, Cosson M, Garbin O, Jacquetin B, Rosenthal C, Salet-Lizée D, Villet R. [Changing attitudes on the surgical treatment of urogenital prolapse: birth of the tension-free vaginal mesh]. J Gynecol Obstet Biol Reprod (Paris). 2004;33(7):577–88.
18. Washington JL. Commercial products for pelvic repair. Female Pelvic Med Reconstr Surg. 2011;17(5): 218–25.
19. http://www.nytimes.com/2012/06/06/business/johnson-johnson-unit-will-stop-selling-urinary-implants.html
20. de Landsheere L, Ismail S, Lucot JP, Deken V, Foidart JM, Cosson M. Surgical intervention after transvaginal prolift mesh repair: retrospective single-center study including 524 patients with 3 years' median follow-up. Am J Obstet Gynecol. 2012;206(1):83.e1–7.
21. Altman D, Väyrynen T, Engh ME, Axelsen S, Falconer C. Nordic transvaginal mesh group anterior colporrhaphy versus transvaginal mesh for pelvic-organ prolapse. N Engl J Med. 2011;364(19):1826–36.
22. Withagen MI, Milani AL, den Boon J, Vervest HA, Vierhout ME. Trocar-guided mesh compared with conventional vaginal repair in recurrent prolapse: a randomized controlled trial. Obstet Gynecol. 2011; 117(2 Pt 1):242–50.
23. Nieminen K, Hiltunen R, Takala T, Heiskanen E, Merikari M, Niemi K, Heinonen PK. Outcomes after anterior vaginal wall repair with mesh: a randomized, controlled trial with a 3 year follow-up. Am J Obstet Gynecol. 2010;203(3):235.e1–8.
24. Maher C, Feiner B, Baessler K, Adams EJ, Hagen S, Glazener CM. Surgical management of pelvic organ prolapse in women. Cochrane Database Syst Rev. 2010;(4):CD004014. Review.
25. Committee on Gynecologic Practice, Vaginal placement of synthetic mesh for pelvic organ prolapse. Female Pelvic Med Reconstr Surg. 2012;18(1):5–9.
26. Haylen BT, Freeman RM, Swift SE, Cosson M, Davila GW, Deprest J, et al. An International Urogynecological Association (IUGA)/International Continence Society (ICS) joint terminology and classification of the complications related directly to the insertion of prostheses (meshes, implants, tapes) and grafts in female pelvic floor surgery. Neurourol Urodyn. 2011;30(1):2–12.
27. Yanagisawa M, Rhodes M, Zimmern P. Mesh social networking: a patient-driven process. BJU Int. 2011;108(10):1539–41.
28. Shepherd JP, Feola AJ, Abramowitch SD, Moalli PA. Uniaxial biomechanical properties of seven different vaginally implanted meshes for pelvic organ prolapse. Int Urogynecol J. 2012;23(5):613–20.
29. Abrams P, Chapple CR, Drake M, El-Neil S, Ludgate S, Smith AR. Synthetic vaginal tapes for stress incontinence: proposals for improved regulation of new devices in Europe. Eur Urol. 2011;60(6):1207–11.
30. Vaiyapuri GR, Han HC, Lee LC, Tseng LA, Wong HF. Use of the gynecare prolift system in surgery for pelvic organ prolapse: 1-year outcome. Int Urogynecol J. 2011;22(7):869–77.
31. Nygaard IE, McCreery R, Brubaker L, Connolly A, Cundiff G, Weber AM, Zyczynski H; Pelvic Floor Disorders Network. Abdominal sacrocolpopexy: a comprehensive review. Obstet Gynecol. 2004; 104(4):805–23.
32. Culligan PJ, Murphy M, Blackwell L, Hammons G, Graham C, Heit MH. Long-term success of abdominal sacral colpopexy using synthetic mesh. Am J Obstet Gynecol. 2002;187(6):1473–80.
33. Cundiff GW, Varner E, Visco AG, Zyczynski HM, Nager CW, Norton PA, Schaffer J, Brown MB, Brubaker L; Pelvic Floor Disorders Network. Risk factors for mesh/suture erosion following sacral colpopexy. Am J Obstet Gynecol. 2008;199(6):688.e1–5.
34. Bensinger G, Lind L, Lesser M, Guess M, Winkler HA. Abdominal sacral suspensions: analysis of complications using permanent mesh. Am J Obstet Gynecol. 2005;193(6):2094–8.
35. Tan-Kim J, Menefee SA, Luber KM, Nager CW, Lukacz ES. Prevalence and risk factors for mesh erosion after laparoscopic-assisted sacrocolpopexy. Int Urogynecol J. 2011;22(2):205–12.
36. Zucchi A, Lazzeri M, Porena M, Mearini L, Costantini E. Uterus preservation in pelvic organ prolapse surgery. Nat Rev Urol. 2010;7(11):626–33.
37. Dietz V, van der Vaart CH, van der Graaf Y, Heintz P, Schraffordt Koops SE. One-year follow-up after

sacrospinous hysteropexy and vaginal hysterectomy for uterine descent: a randomized study. Int Urogynecol J. 2010;21(2):209–16.
38. Costantini E, Mearini L, Bini V, Zucchi A, Mearini E, Porena M. Uterus preservation in surgical correction of urogenital prolapse. Eur Urol. 2005;48(4):642–9.
39. Olsen AL, Smith VJ, Bergstrom JO, Colling JC, Clark AL. Epidemiology of surgically managed pelvic organ prolapse and urinary incontinence. Obstet Gynecol. 1997;89(4):501–6.
40. Richardson AC. The rectovaginal septum revisited: its relationship to rectocele and its importance in rectocele repair. Clin Obstet Gynecol. 1993;36(4):976–83.
41. Farrell SA, Dempsey T, Geldenhuys L. Histologic examination of "fascia" used in colporrhaphy. Obstet Gynecol. 2001;98(5 Pt 1):794–8.
42. Kleeman SD, Westermann C, Karram MM. Rectoceles and the anatomy of the posteriorvaginal wall: revisited. Am J Obstet Gynecol. 2005;193(6):2050–5.
43. Marks BK, Goldman HB. What is the gold standard for posterior vaginal wall prolapse repair: mesh or native tissue? Curr Urol Rep. 2012;13(3):216–21.
44. Maher CF, Qatawneh AM, Baessler K, Schluter PJ. Midline rectovaginal fascial plication for repair of rectocele and obstructed defecation. Obstet Gynecol. 2004;104(4):685–9.
45. Kenton K, Shott S, Brubaker L. Outcome after rectovaginal fascia reattachment for rectocele repair. Am J Obstet Gynecol. 1999;181(6):1360–3.
46. Cundiff GW, Fenner D. Evaluation and treatment of women with rectocele: focus on associated defecatory and sexual dysfunction. Obstet Gynecol. 2004;104(6):1403–21.
47. Abramov Y, Gandhi S, Goldberg RP, Botros SM, Kwon C, Sand PK. Site-specific rectocele repair compared with standard posterior colporrhaphy. Obstet Gynecol. 2005;105(2):314–8.
48. Paraiso MF, Barber MD, Muir TW, Walters MD. Rectocele repair: a randomized trial of three surgical techniques including graft augmentation. Am J Obstet Gynecol. 2006;195(6):1762–71.
49. Rosenzweig BA, Pushkin S, Blumenfeld D, Bhatia NN. Prevalence of abnormal urodynamic test results in continent women with severe genitourinary prolapse. Neurourol Urodyn. 1999;18(3):193–7.
50. Gordon D, Groutz A, Wolman I, Lessing JB, David MP. Development of postoperative urinary stress incontinence in clinically continent patients undergoing prophylactic Kelly plication during genitourinary prolapse repair. Obstet Gynecol. 1992;79(4):539–42.
51. Veronikis DK, Nichols DH, Wakamatsu MM. The incidence of low-pressure urethra as a function of prolapse-reducing technique in patients with massive pelvic organ prolapse (maximum descent at all vaginal sites). Am J Obstet Gynecol. 1997;177(6):1305–13.
52. Ballert KN, Biggs GY, Isenalumhe Jr A, Rosenblum N, Nitti VW. Managing the urethra at transvaginal pelvic organ prolapse repair: a urodynamic approach. J Urol. 2009;181(2):679–84.
53. Brubaker L, Cundiff GW, Fine P, Nygaard I, Richter HE, Visco AG, Zyczynski H, Brown MB, Weber AM; Pelvic Floor Disorders Network. Abdominal sacrocolpopexy with Burch colposuspension to reduce urinary stress incontinence. N Engl J Med. 2006;354(15):1557–66.
54. Brubaker L, Nygaard I, Richter HE, Visco A, Weber AM, Cundiff GW, Fine P, Ghetti C, Brown MB. Two-year outcomes after sacrocolpopexy with and without burch to prevent stress urinary incontinence. Obstet Gynecol. 2008;112(1):49–55.
55. Wei J, Nygaard I, Richter H, Brown M, Barber M, Xiao Xu, Kenton K, Nager C, Schaffer J, Visco A, Weber A; Pelvic Floor Disorders Network. Outcomes following vaginal prolapse repair and mid urethral sling (OPUS) trial—design and methods. Clin Trials. 2009;6(2):162–71.
56. Wei J, Nygaard I, Richter H, Brown M, Barber M, Xiao Xu, Kenton K, Nager C, Schaffer J, Visco A, Weber A; Pelvic Floor Disorders Network. A midurethral sling to reduce incontinence after vaginal prolapse repair. N Engl J Med. 2012;366(25):2358–67.
57. Borstad E, Abdelnoor M, Staff AC, Kulseng-Hanssen S. Surgical strategies for women with pelvic organ prolapse and urinary stress incontinence. Int Urogynecol J. 2010;21(2):179–86.
58. Daneshgari F, Kong W, Swartz M. Complications of mid urethral slings: important outcomes for future clinical trials. J Urol. 2008;180(5):1890–7. Review.
59. Deng DY, Rutman M, Raz S, Rodriguez LV. Presentation and management of major complications of midurethral slings: are complications under-reported? Neurourol Urodyn. 2007;26(1):46–52.
60. Chaikin DC, Groutz A, Blaivas JG. Predicting the need for anti-incontinence surgery in continent women undergoing repair of severe urogenital prolapse. J Urol. 2000;163(2):531–4.
61. Liang CC, Chang YL, Chang SD, Lo TS, Soong YK. Pessary test to predict postoperative urinary incontinence in women undergoing hysterectomy for prolapse. Obstet Gynecol. 2004;104(4):795–800.
62. AUA/SUFU Adult Urodynamics guidelines. 2012. http://www.auanet.org/content/media/adult_urodynamics_guideline.pdf
63. Dua A, Jha S, Farkas A, Radley S. The effect of prolapse repair on sexual function in women. J Sex Med. 2012;9:1459–65. doi:10.1111/j.1743-6109.2012.02660.x.
64. Bako A, Dhar R. Review of synthetic mesh-related complications in pelvic floor reconstructive surgery. Int Urogynecol J Pelvic Floor Dysfunct. 2009;20(1):103–11.
65. Withagen MI, Vierhout ME, Hendriks JC, Kluivers KB, Milani AL. Risk factors for exposure, pain, and dyspareunia after tension-free vaginal mesh procedure. Obstet Gynecol. 2011;118(3):629–36.
66. Feiner B, Maher C. Vaginal mesh contraction: definition, clinical presentation, and management. Obstet Gynecol. 2010;115(2 Pt 1):325–30.
67. Reynolds WS, Kit LC, Kaufman MR, Karram M, Bales GT, Dmochowski RR. Obturator foramen dissection for excision of symptomatic transobturator mesh. J Urol. 2012;187(5):1680–4.

Materials for Pelvic Repair

17

Tamer Aboushwareb

Pelvic organ prolapse (POP), with or without stress urinary incontinence (SUI), is a major healthcare problem. Nearly 200,000 women undergo prolapse surgery in the United States every year [1] and the annual cost of pelvic floor surgeries is estimated to be over $1 billion [2]. Olsen et al. reported that the lifetime risk for an American woman to undergo a single operation for prolapse or incontinence is 11.1 % and that a second operation is needed in 29.2 % of cases [3].

However, traditional surgery for POP seems to have limited effectiveness in preventing recurrences, and this disappointing result is due to the poor quality of tissues used. Recently, after the extended use of meshes in abdominal defects and hernias, application of meshed biomaterials for treatment of POP and SUI has been popularized with the hope of defining the most suitable biomaterial for this purpose.

Through the limited evidence available, it seems that the surgical repair of POP using vaginal meshes improves the outcome when compared to repair without the use of a mesh [4]. Maher et al. [5] suggested in their meta-analysis of the different repair methods that the concept of using a polyglactin mesh for anterior vaginal wall repair decreases the recurrence of cystocele.

In recent years, the use of grafts in gynecological surgery has proven to mandate special considerations when compared to materials used in other surgical procedures. Most relevant of those is the fact that these meshes are required to provide support not only for a herniated sac during rest, but also allow normal, strenuous, and painless sexual activity. Another important factor is the higher risk of infections in these procedures due to the nature of the surgical site in the vagina [4].

Consequently, surgery for POP aims at restoring physiologic anatomy as well as preserving lower urinary tract, intestinal, and sexual functions. These factors combined together have proven to be a true challenge for the modern urologist.

There are several points of debate within this problem, the most important of which are as follows:

1. Approach: vaginal, abdominal, or combined?
2. Is hysterectomy necessary or not?
3. Biomaterial: what's the most appropriate type [6]?

Due to the large number of points and counterpoints in all of those debates, we will focus only on the criteria, types, advantages, and disadvantages of the biomaterials used.

T. Aboushwareb, M.D., Ph.D. (✉)
RSS Urology, Mid Atlantic, Allergan Medical Affairs, P.O. Box 19534, Irvine, CA 92623, USA
e-mail: Aboushwareb_Tamer@allergan.com

G.H. Badlani (ed.), *Minimally Invasive Therapy for Urinary Incontinence and Pelvic Organ Prolapse*, Current Clinical Urology, DOI 10.1007/978-1-4939-0008-4_17,

Rationale for Biomaterial Use

In the past, large numbers of POP patients did not seek medical help; however, the number of patients seeking this help is increasing. This is mainly attributed to the improvement in available medical treatments and increased interest in the quality of life [7]. With the recent advances reported in the fields of tissue engineering and regenerative medicine, many technologies have emerged as possible treatment options for POP patients. Biomaterials have been central in those advances whether alone or in combination with cells. All approaches have focused on one of three goals:

1. Bulking biomaterials to support sphincteric continence.
2. Biomaterials that enhance local recruitment of autologous cells and maintain the tension needed for continence.
3. Pre-cell-seeded scaffolds that can integrate with tissue and serve as a permanent support.

There are four main outcomes for the evaluation of prolapse surgery illustrated by the following Venn diagram (Fig. 17.1):

1. Anatomy of the anterior and posterior vaginal walls, vaginal vault, and perineum.
2. Bladder, colon, and sexual function.
3. Patient satisfaction and impact on quality of life.
4. Avoidance of complications.

The successful treatment of POP patients must fulfill all or most of these outcomes to be considered as a viable alternative for management of those patients. The choice of the proper biomaterial is integral to achieving these goals and successful management of POP.

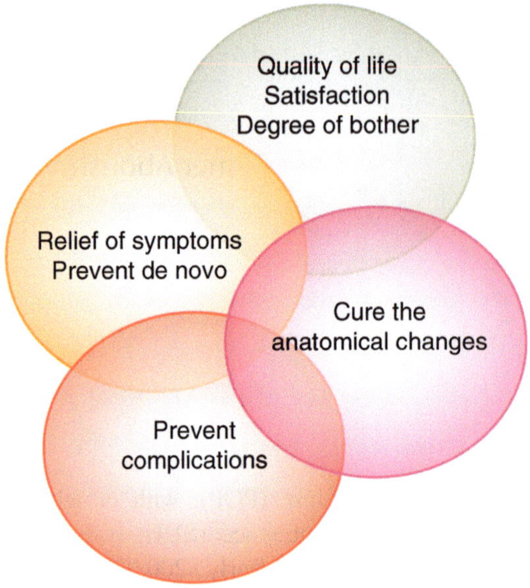

Fig. 17.1 Venn diagram. There are four main outcomes to evaluate prolapse surgery illustrated by the following Venn diagram. (1) Anatomy of the anterior and posterior vaginal walls, vaginal vault, and perineum. (2) Function of bladder and colon, and sexual function. (3) Patient satisfaction and impact on quality of life. (4) Avoidance of complications (From Lee, U. and S. Raz, *Emerging concepts for pelvic organ prolapse surgery*: *What is cure*? Curr Urol Rep, 2011. **12**(1): p. 62–7, with permission of Springer Science+Business Media)

Definition of a Biomaterial

A biomaterial is any natural or synthetic substance that incorporates or integrates into a patient's tissues during treatment. The ideal compound should be inert, sterile, noncarcinogenic, mechanically durable, noninflammatory, inexpensive, easy to use, and withstand modification by body tissues. The purpose of a biomaterial is to perform, supplement, or replace a natural function that is attenuated or lost [8].

Criteria of Biomaterials

Cumberland and Scales defined the criteria for an ideal implant material as [9, 10]:

(a) It should cause minimal or no foreign body reaction (biocompatible).
(b) It should mimic the original body strength and flexibility.
(c) It should be easily tailored to the appropriate size at an affordable price.
(d) It should allow native tissue integration with a permissible architecture.
(e) It should be well-tolerated even within a contaminated or infected environment.
(f) Local complication rates should be at a minimum.

To date, none of the biomaterials available meet all these criteria; however, many come close. The biochemical properties of biomaterials are determined by elasticity, viscosity, and plasticity. The biomaterial is said to be elastic when it regains its original shape after removal of a load without applying another load. When loading occurs for prolonged periods, some elongation of the material or tissue can occur depending on the viscosity of the material [11].

Difficulties Associated with Detecting the Best Material

In order to estimate the ideal graft characteristics for repair of POP, understanding the biomechanics of the normal patient's pelvic floor and its supports is useful; however, this is a difficult goal to achieve due to the size of tissue needed for testing. Usually only small biopsies can be obtained from normal women without prolapse and only strips of epithelium may be available from trimming of vaginal tissue as part of prolapse surgery. Also assessing cadaveric tissue has potential limitations such as age of donors, previous medical or surgical history that can affect biomechanical properties, postmortem changes, and potential tissue disintegration [11].

Additionally, when assessing biomechanical properties of the genital tract alone, other variables such as estrogen status, elastin, collagen, and genetic factors should be considered. Collagen and elastin content in tissue alter biomechanical outcomes. Collagen contributes to tensile strength and preliminary data indicated that collagenase activity was higher in women with SUI leading to increased urinary levels of collagen degradation products. This discovery revealed that the reduced collagen content represents a systemic process in tissues of women with SUI even in other tissues not involved in support of pelvic organs [12]. Elastin on the other hand is important in elasticity of pelvic floor connective tissue, and preliminary data have demonstrated elevated proteolytic activity in skin and endopelvic fascia in women with SUI compared to continent women [13]. Selecting a suitable biomaterial for prolapse or incontinence surgery should take these biochemical processes into consideration [14]. As an added level of complexity, the association of SUI with the onset of menopause suggests a role of estrogen [15]. There is also a threefold prevalence of SUI among first degree-related female patients suggesting the potential for predisposing genetic factors [12, 16]. It is also important to note that different studies offer different definitions about "cure" in prolapse surgery. This is mainly due to the variability of symptoms of prolapse and the lack of standardized definitions of "cure" other than depending on improvement of patient's own symptoms.

Types of Biomaterials

Biomaterials can be classified as either natural or synthetic. Natural biomaterials are typically acellular and may be *autologous* (harvested from the patient), *allogeneic* (harvested from cadaveric tissue), or *xenogeneic* (harvested from animal tissue). Synthetic biomaterials on the other hand differ in their degradation properties (absorbable or nonabsorbable), type of material (polyethylene, polypropylene, polypropylene terephthalate, Gore-Tex), structure (woven, knitted), fiber type (monofilament, multifilament, monofilament/multifilament), pore size, mechanical properties, shape, and surface characteristics [17].

Natural (Biological) Biomaterials

The potential advantages for biologic materials compared with synthetic meshes include in vivo tissue modeling, histological similarity, and reduced erosion rates. An important problem with some biologic grafts is their rapid degradation and lack of ability to provide long-term support to the grafted tissue [18, 19].

Rectus Fascia

Rectus fascia has remained the reference standard for fascial slings since its reintroduction as a treatment of SUI with reported cure rates of

82–83 % at 3.5–7 years [20]. It remains popular due to its autologous nature, ease of harvest, and durable characteristics. However, disadvantages of using this material include wound infection, increased operative time, patient morbidity associated with graft harvest, limitation of the material size, and susceptibility to degradation if the underlying host pathophysiology is not resolved [21]. One of the studies (Haab et al.) [20] found that urinary retention was found in 10 % of rectus fascia series slings used in women with SUI. This finding indicates that collagen degradation is systemic and implanted autologous tissue may lose durability over long time.

Fascia Lata

Fascia lata harvests can provide long specimens that are uniform in thickness while concurrently avoiding abdominal incision and subsequent risk of hernia. However, there is still long operative time, possibility of wound infection, susceptibility to degradation, as well as the possibility of peroneal nerve entrapment. This material also carries the risk of lack of experience of urologists with the harvest area [14].

Cadaveric Allografts

The goal of using this material is to decrease the morbidity, operative time, and complications seen with harvesting autologous fascia. Cadaveric fascia and dermis are the two most widely used materials from cadavers.

Strict criteria have to be met before donor harvesting. This usually includes a physical examination, screening for infectious pathogens (hepatitis B and C and human immunodeficiency virus), in addition to a brief medical and social review of the donor and family. The review usually targets previous bacterial sepsis, collagen vascular diseases, rabies, cancer, and intravenous drug abuse [14]. All tissue allografts must be harvested within 24 h of death, as regulated by the Food and Drug Administration (FDA). They must be retrieved under complete aseptic conditions and cultured to rule out bacterial infection before being placed in temporary ice storage [22].

Although good cure rates (65–98 %) with allograft slings have been reported [23], several other groups have reported high failure rates, with 20–38 % rate of dissolution of the cadaveric tissue [24, 25]. The reason for this discrepancy could possibly be due to variation in fascia integrity regarding tensile strength, collagen fiber orientation, region of harvest, donor's age, sex, and genetic background [14].

To remove the cellular content and sterilize the tissue while retaining structural integrity of the tissue is a multistep process involving irradiation, freeze-drying, or solvent dehydration, as reviewed by Gallentine and Cespedes [26]. However, controversy still exists as to whether irradiation and freeze-drying affect the strength of allograft collagen cross-linking. To date, no difference was noted between irradiated and nonirradiated fascia lata [27]; however, Lemer et al. [28] noted that freeze-dried fascia had 25 % less maximal load to failure than autografts or differently prepared allografts. These issues may still present a challenge for the wide use of these materials over larger populations of patients.

Xenograft

These grafts are harvested from animals (mostly porcine) and processed to remove all cellular components. Some examples of these grafts include small intestine submucosa (SIS) and dermis. Xenografts are strictly controlled by the FDA guidelines. These regulations include knowledge of the animal herd, vaccination status, feed source, and bovine spongiform encephalopathy clearance [19]. Surgisis (SIS, cook) and Pelvicol (Acellular Dermis, Bard) are common examples of xenogenic implants. Both products are extracted from porcine donors and undergo rigorous processes to ensure complete decellularization of the materials before human use. Both products claim retention of different growth factors like TGF-beta and FGR-2.

As these products are not cross-linked, they are easily remodeled and gradually replaced by host tissue. The rate of xenograft degradation usually ranges from 4 to 12 weeks and then it is fully replaced by normal regenerated tissue [29–31].

Because of the rapid tissue incorporation and minimal rate of infection, porcine SIS and dermis are promising biomaterials for pelvic floor reconstruction [14]. Collagen and other growth factors act as a signal for local epithelial cells to proliferate, causing a colonization of the SIS graft that promotes tissue healing without scarring. SIS produces the highest stimulus for the formation of collagen fibers around the graft [32].

Rutner et al. [33] demonstrated 93 % cure rate using SIS in 152 patients at 4 years, with no graft erosion or infection. A randomized comparison between porcine dermis sling and tension-free vaginal tape (TVT) found SUI cure rates of 85–89 % at 12 months, respectively [34]. However, a study by Ho et al. [35] indicates a less favorable outcome with SIS. In recent years, there has been more data emerging condemning the use of biomaterials in general (natural and synthetic) into higher rate of serious complications than previously reported. Recently, the FDA has issued a report warning patients against the use of meshes for SUI and POP repair unless highly indicated and with special risk criteria. However, many studies in the recent years have shown that the risks of use of such biomaterials are still acceptable and that when properly indicated, the use of meshes is still the most appropriate procedure for these patients [36–38]. A recently introduced approach makes use of regenerative medicine technologies along with naturally derived biomaterials to create a more biological method of repair for POP patients. The use of regenerative medicine has been popularized and is under investigation in many laboratories across the globe in hopes of creating an appropriately seeded biomaterial that not only repairs but also helps regenerate the area needed for long time success [12]. In the near future, it is expected that regenerative medicine technologies will provide the "perfect" seeded material for management of POP and SUI patients.

Synthetic Biomaterials

Surgical repair for POP patients usually involves repair of defects using native tissues. Due to this fact, failure rates are sometimes high due to the qualitative insufficiency of the tissues used. The native tissue usually shares the same decreased collagen content as the prolapsed tissue making it necessary for re-enforcement using synthetic materials.

These materials enforce the anatomical position, but they also induce an inflammatory reaction which can be chronic and potentially fibrotic [39]. This chronic inflammation results from the persistent remodeling of the connective tissue around the implant. This degree of reaction depends on the chemical and physical structure of the implant, as well as the amount of material and surface of the contact-area with the host; it can vary greatly according to the type of material used [40].

Thus, biomaterials have been classified into four groups according to pore size [41]:

1. Type I: macroporous with pores larger than 75 μm.
2. Type II: microporous with pores less than 10 μm in at least one of their three dimensions.
3. Type III: macroporous with multifilamentous or microporous components.
4. Type IV: submicronic pore size.

The pore size allows the host tissue to infiltrate and lay down a new collagen-based scaffold, which proves to be important for graft incorporation, erosion, and infection rates. Based on the previously mentioned classification, type I biomaterials are composed mainly of polypropylene monofilament with pore size more than 75 μm. These materials allow integration of fibroblasts and collagen to anchor the implant within the native tissue and for immune cells to scavenge for bacteria [42]. Type II biomaterials are multifilament with pores less than 10 μm. These materials allow passage of bacteria (usually 2 μm or less) but not leucocytes (9–15 μm) and macrophages (16–20 μm), which are both important for clearing an infection [43–45]. This property renders these materials less likely to be used in cases where infections are expected. Type III biomaterials are composed of polyester multifilaments with microporous components in at least one of the three dimensions, which don't allow macrophages or polymorph-nuclear cells to enter. Type IV biomaterials are coated with silicone and have pores smaller than 1 μm [14]. Iglesia et al. reported that multifilament polypropylene

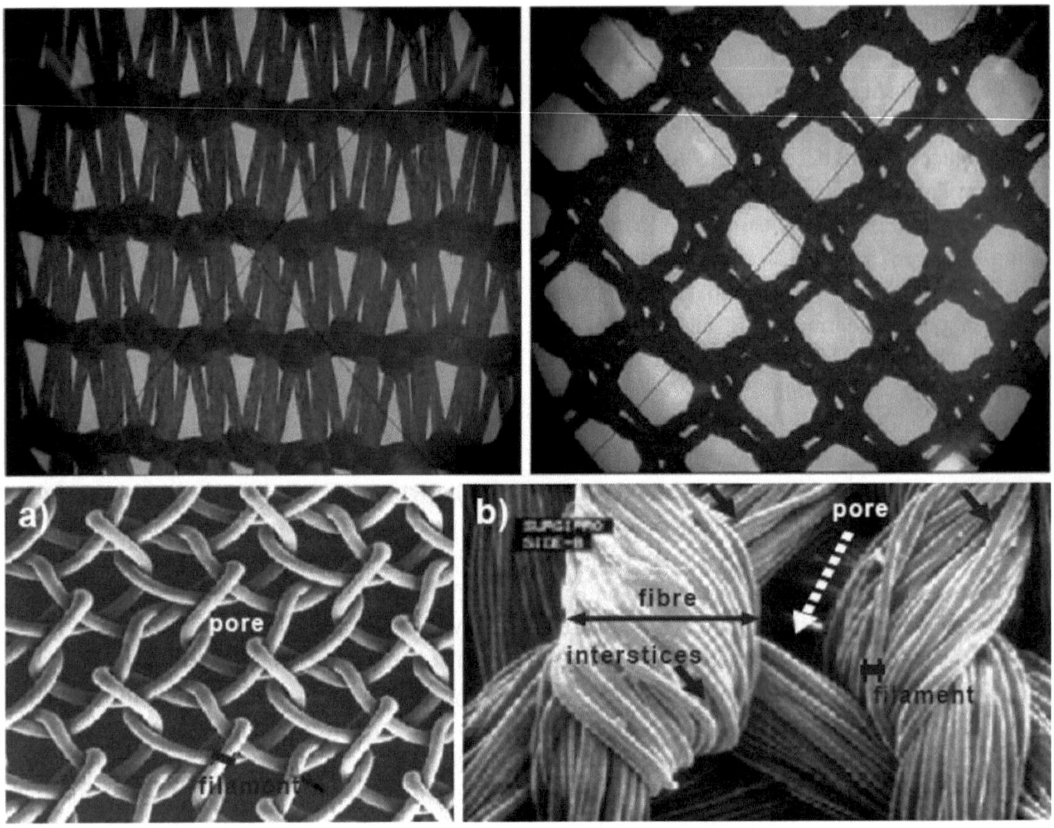

Fig. 17.2 Surgipro multifilament (*top left* and *right*) (×38; Auto Suture European Services Centre, Elancourt, France), and Marlex (**a**; Bard, Haasrode, Belgium) which is monofilament material; figure (**b**) shows at larger magnification the effect of multifilament weaving (From Deprest J., C.F., Zheng F., Konstantinovic M., Spelzini F., Guelinckx I., Pottier C., Verbeken E., De Ridder D., *Synthetic and biodegradable prostheses in pelvic floor surgery*. International Congress Series, 2005. **1279**: p. 387–397, with permission)

meshes (pore size < 10 μm) were at higher risk of infection than monofilament polypropylene meshes (pore size > 75 μm) due to difference in pore size of the mesh [46–48]. It has also identified that dead space between the mesh and host tissue, which contributes to seroma formation, is minimized by large pore type I synthetic biomaterials. Thus, type II and III meshes are usually removed in case of infection while with type I biomaterials, infection can be managed by local drainage and secondary healing [49]. One of the strategies implemented to reduce the possibility of infection is the use of a mesh embedded with antimicrobial agents. Such a mesh may prevent bacterial adhesion and colonization with reduction of intraoperative and postoperative infections [4].

Macroporous (type I) monofilament materials have been preferred in the clinical practice for decades. Polypropylene is the most commonly used fiber to construct strong, inert implants. The majority of clinically available materials are monofilament with limited local side effects such as infection and seroma formation. However, it can also be used to weave other types of fabrics as Surgipro (Tyco), which is a typical monofilament product but is also available as a multifilament mesh (Fig. 17.2).

Synthetic biomaterials can also be classified by their durability into (a) nonabsorbable materials [e.g., Prolene (Ethicon, Somerville, NJ, USA), Marlex (Bard, Cranston, RI, USA), Atrium (Atrium, Hudson, NH, USA), Gortex (Gore, Flagstaff, AZ, USA), Mersilene (Ethicon,

Somerville, NJ, USA), and Teflon (DuPont, Wilmington, DE, USA)] and (b) absorbable materials [e.g., Vypro, Vicryl (Ethicon, Somerville, NJ, USA)]. A prospective randomized controlled trial comparing fascia lata and synthetic mesh for sacral colpopexy showed level one evidence for increased durability of POP repair with nonabsorbable meshes [50].

Other physical properties required in a biomaterial are flexibility and strength. The flexibility of an implant depends on individual stiffness of its yarns, pore size, and knitting procedure of the implant. Implants with larger pores are more flexible than the ones with smaller pores; also multifilament meshes are usually more flexible than monofilament meshes. A stiff non-flexible implant may wrinkle and fold causing local pressure, erosion, and pain which would contradict the original requirement of being biocompatible with the native tissues [51, 52].

Use of Biomaterials in Different Approaches of Surgery for POP

Studies have reported use of prosthetic materials in different approaches (abdominal, vaginal, and laparoscopic) and in different vaginal compartments (anterior, posterior, and apical) for treatment of POP. They have been effectively used for abdominal sacrocolpopexy with minimal side effects. However, a strong debate still exists about their use for transvaginal repair of prolapse. The most recent FDA warning has sparked more active research into the efficacy and safety of using these meshes in patients with POP and SUI.

Abdominal Sacrocolpopexy

Abdominal sacrocolpopexy has undergone numerous modifications over the years. Those included the type of prosthesis used and placement onto the anterior and posterior walls of the vagina [48, 53, 54]. In a recent comprehensive review of 98 articles on abdominal sacrocolpopexy, the success rate (when defined as lack of apical prolapse postoperatively) was 78–100 %; however, when it was defined as *no* postoperative prolapse, success rate was 58–100 %. The follow-up duration in this study ranged from 6 months to 3 years and the median rate for a second operation was 4.4 % [54].

Culligan et al. [50] asserted that polypropylene mesh (91 % cure) was better than cadaveric fascia lata (68 % cure) for abdominal sacrocolpopexy ($p = 0.007$) at 1 year of follow-up.

FitzGerald et al. [53] also noted poor anatomic outcomes (a failure rate of 83 % at 17 months) when freeze-dried, irradiated donor fascia lata was used for abdominal sacrocolpopexy as compared to a near perfect success rate of polypropylene meshes.

Vaginal Repair of the Anterior and Posterior Compartments

Most studies reported on the use of synthetic biomaterials in vaginal repair of POP patients have reported good to excellent outcomes. However, most of these have been short-term studies and the rate of complications observed may not represent an accurate figure. A retrospective analysis by Flood et al. [55] of 142 women using Marlex revealed a success rate of 100 % with mean follow-up of 36 months, with no prosthetic-related complications. On the other hand Dwyer and O'Reilly [56] used a polypropylene prosthesis (Atrium) in the anterior and posterior compartments and showed a recurrence rate of 6 %.

De Tayrac et al. [57] reported a recurrence rate of 8 % and erosion rate of 8.3 % using polypropylene prosthesis on 87 women with a mean follow-up of 24 months. Milani et al. [58] reported a prospective observational cohort of 63 women who had anterior and posterior colporrhaphies using polypropylene mesh with excellent anatomic outcomes after 12 months of surgery but the rates of worsening dyspareunia reached 20 % for those who had anterior mesh repairs and 63 % for posterior mesh repairs.

Based on these results, the use of synthetic biomaterials for POP repair has excellent short-term outcomes; however, long-term studies are required to detect which is the best biomaterial with the least adverse effects and whether biological or synthetic materials are superior for use in treatment of POP.

Complications of Use of Prostheses in Pelvic Reconstructive Surgery

Multiple mesh complications have been reported in the literature that include vaginal wall exposure, vaginal pain, induration, bladder and urethral erosion, dyspareunia, vaginal mesh-related infections (bleeding, discharge, nonspecific pelvic pain, urinary and fecal incontinence), leg pain, neuropathy, and difficulty in walking. These complications have mostly been attributed to age-related changes of the vagina over time [59]. Various factors affect the development of mesh-related infections such as the kind of biomaterial used (pore size, filament structure), type of procedure (abdominal, vaginal, or laparoscopic), the preventive measures taken, age, and associated comorbidities of the patient [57]. Mesh erosion is one of the most important complications in the use of prostheses. The rate of such complication has been much higher in type II and type III (multifilament) synthetic materials reaching up to 20–30 % [60, 61]. On the other hand, the rate of erosion decreases to 0.5–5 % by using type I (monofilament) synthetic materials [62]. The erosion rate has been reported to vary in different materials: 0.5 % for polypropylene, 3.1 % for polyethylene terephthalate (Mersilene; Ethicon, NJ, USA), 3.4 % for Gore-Tex (Gore, Flagstaff, AZ, USA), 5.0 % for polyethylene (Marlex; Bard, Billerica, MA, USA), and 5.6 % for Teflon (DuPont, Wilmington, DE, USA) [54]. These results show that using the proper synthetic biomaterial may drastically decrease the risk of complications and result in very successful repair for the patient. Biological grafts on the other hand have a small risk of prion or viral infection that is estimated to be approximately 1 in 2 million [63].

Synthetic grafts have an overall higher success rates, but they also have higher erosion rates than biological materials. Current evidence based on available studies suggests that the use of monofilament macroporous polypropylene has the lowest incidence of infection and erosion when compared with other nonabsorbable meshes [64]. Other studies have shown that changing the surgical approach may also affect the rate of erosion even within the same material [65]. Visco et al. [65] analyzed Mersilene mesh erosion in 273 women who had undergone sacrocolpopexy or sacral colpoperineopexy and found that the risk was 3.2 % for abdominal sacrocolpopexy and 4.5 % for abdominal sacral colpoperineopexy. These results suggest that even though the risk of infection and erosion still exists with the use of synthetic biomaterials, the rate of complications can be drastically reduced by proper patient and biomaterial selections. Level one evidence for the exact rate of complications associated with these materials is still required to make a final decision on the appropriateness of their use [12, 38, 66].

Conclusion

Although several studies have demonstrated that both polypropylene and xenograft are promising materials for pelvic floor reconstruction and SUI treatment, level one evidence and long-term outcomes of prospective randomized trials for the use of biomaterials in pelvic floor prolapse are still needed. To date, no clear results have been reached in published studies about the best biomaterial suitable for any given pelvic floor defect [14].

Studies concerned with the biomechanical properties of each material have not proven to be sufficient to make this distinction. This is likely due to the fact that the behavior of the graft once implanted is usually different from the ex vivo test results. Another caveat is that studying the implanted material does not take into consideration the effect of regenerated or fibrotic surrounding tissues [11]. A final major issue is the fact that animal models for testing these materials do not test the flexibility needed to prevent vaginal complications once implanted.

The availability of different types of biomaterials, whether natural or synthetic, has expanded the options for management of SUI and POP. However, one has to take into consideration that the ultimate goal of treatment is to restore the physiological anatomy while incurring minimal side effects. The choice of the proper biomaterial is problematic due to the discrepancy of adverse events associated with different biomaterials, including cost, unexpected host response, risk of infection with xenografts [21], and increased morbidity and operative time for allografts. Other complications such as mesh erosion and dyspareunia are more common in synthetic grafts but can present in all cases on occasion [67].

The field of regenerative medicine may provide the correct path towards a combination (hybrid) biomaterial that could possess the benefits of both natural and synthetic materials [12]. Some studies have already shown that hybrid biomaterials consisting of type I collagen and PLGA can provide the correct properties of replacement tissues with the suitable biomechanical and biochemical characteristics as well as the feasibility of controlling the fiber diameter according to demand [68, 69].

There still exists a strong need for better and more appropriate biomaterials and identification of the optimal surgical approach. The quest for the ideal biomaterial is far from over and our only hope is to understand the needs of diseased tissue and pursue the right combination of materials to address these needs. Ideally, biomaterial would be developed that would provide the right tensile strength and flexibility while maintaining a natural tissue response that is not harmful to the patient. Longer-term studies are also needed to confirm the suitability of the currently used biomaterials for the management of SUI and POP patients. Until more appropriate level one evidence to the contrary, the use of the currently available biomaterials and meshes will continue to serve as an appropriate method of treatment for these patients [12, 70].

References

1. Boyles SH, Weber AM, Meyn L. Procedures for pelvic organ prolapse in the United States, 1979–1997. Am J Obstet Gynecol. 2003;188(1):108–15.
2. Subak LL, Waetjen LE, van den Eeden S, et al. Cost of pelvic organ prolapse surgery in the United States. Obstet Gynecol. 2001;98(4):646–51.
3. Olsen AL, Smith VJ, Bergstrom JO, et al. Epidemiology of surgically managed pelvic organ prolapse and urinary incontinence. Obstet Gynecol. 1997;89(4):501–6.
4. Falagas ME, Velakoulis S, Iavazzo C, et al. Mesh-related infections after pelvic organ prolapse repair surgery. Eur J Obstet Gynecol Reprod Biol. 2007;134(2):147–56.
5. Maher C, Baessler K, Glazener CM, et al. Surgical management of pelvic organ prolapse in women. Cochrane Database Syst Rev. 2004;4, CD004014.
6. Bartoletti R. Pelvic organ prolapse: a challenge for the urologist. Eur Urol. 2007;51(4):884–6.
7. Kim CM, Jeon MJ, Chung DJ, et al. Risk factors for pelvic organ prolapse. Int J Gynaecol Obstet. 2007;98(3):248–51.
8. Beiko DT, Knudsen BE, Watterson JD, et al. Biomaterials in urology. Curr Urol Rep. 2003;4(1): 51–5.
9. Cumberland VH. A preliminary report on the use of prefabricated nylon weave in the repair of ventral hernia. Med J Aust. 1952;1(5):143–4.
10. Scales JT. Materials for hernia repair. Proc R Soc Med. 1953;46:647–52.
11. Krause HG, Goh JT. Biomechanical properties of graft materials employed for pelvic floor reconstructive surgeries. Curr Opin Obstet Gynecol. 2009;21(5):419–23.
12. Aboushwareb T, McKenzie P, Wezel F, et al. Is tissue engineering and biomaterials the future for lower urinary tract dysfunction (LUTD)/pelvic organ prolapse (POP)? Neurourol Urodyn. 2011;30(5):775–82.
13. Kushner L, Mathrubutham M, Burney T, et al. Excretion of collagen derived peptides is increased in women with stress urinary incontinence. Neurourol Urodyn. 2004;23(3):198–203.
14. Karlovsky ME, Thakre AA, Rastinehad A, et al. Biomaterials for pelvic floor reconstruction. Urology. 2005;66(3):469–75.
15. McKenzie P, Rohozinski J, Badlani G. Genetic influences on stress urinary incontinence. Curr Opin Urol. 2010;20(4):291–5.
16. Mushkat Y, Bukovsky I, Langer R. Female urinary stress incontinence—does it have familial prevalence? Am J Obstet Gynecol. 1996;174(2):617–9.
17. Cosson M, Debodinance P, Boukerrou M, et al. Mechanical properties of synthetic implants used in the repair of prolapse and urinary incontinence in women: which is the ideal material? Int Urogynecol J Pelvic Floor Dysfunct. 2003;14(3):169–78; discussion 178.
18. Le TH, Kon L, Bhatia NN, et al. Update on the utilization of grafts in pelvic reconstruction surgeries. Curr Opin Obstet Gynecol. 2007;19(5):480–9.
19. Deprest J, Claerhout F, Zheng F, Konstantinovic M, Spelzini F, Guelinckx I, Pottier C, Verbeken E, De Ridder D. Synthetic and biodegradable prostheses in pelvic floor surgery. Int Congr Ser. 2005;1279: 387–97.
20. Haab F, Zimmern PE, Leach GE. Female stress urinary incontinence due to intrinsic sphincteric

deficiency: recognition and management. J Urol. 1996;156(1):3–17.
21. Rizk DE, El-Safty MM. Female pelvic floor dysfunction in the Middle East: a tale of three factors—culture, religion and socialization of health role stereotypes. Int Urogynecol J Pelvic Floor Dysfunct. 2006;17(5): 436–8.
22. Food and Drug Administration. The FDA intraagency guidelines for human tissue intended for transplantation. Fed Reg. 1993;58:65514–21.
23. Wright EJ, Iselin CE, Carr LK, et al. Pubovaginal sling using cadaveric allograft fascia for the treatment of intrinsic sphincter deficiency. J Urol. 1998;160(3 Pt 1):759–62.
24. Carbone JM, Kavaler E, Hu JC, et al. Pubovaginal sling using cadaveric fascia and bone anchors: disappointing early results. J Urol. 2001;165(5): 1605–11.
25. Fitzgerald MP, Mollenhauer J, Brubaker L. Failure of allograft suburethral slings. BJU Int. 1999;84(7): 785–8.
26. Gallentine ML, Cespedes RD. Review of cadaveric allografts in urology. Urology. 2002;59(3):318–24.
27. Bedrossian Jr EH. HIV and banked fascia lata. Ophthal Plast Reconstr Surg. 1991;7(4):284–8.
28. Lemer ML, Chaikin DC, Blaivas JG. Tissue strength analysis of autologous and cadaveric allografts for the pubovaginal sling. Neurourol Urodyn. 1999;18(5): 497–503.
29. Clarke KM, Lantz GC, Salisbury SK, et al. Intestine submucosa and polypropylene mesh for abdominal wall repair in dogs. J Surg Res. 1996;60(1):107–14.
30. Badylak S, Kokini K, Tullius B, et al. Strength over time of a resorbable bioscaffold for body wall repair in a dog model. J Surg Res. 2001;99(2):282–7.
31. Hiles MC, Badylak SF, Lantz GC, et al. Mechanical properties of xenogeneic small-intestinal submucosa when used as an aortic graft in the dog. J Biomed Mater Res. 1995;29(7):883–91.
32. Thiel M, Rodrigues Palma PC, Riccetto CL, et al. A stereological analysis of fibrosis and inflammatory reaction induced by four different synthetic slings. BJU Int. 2005;95(6):833–7.
33. Rutner AB, Levine SR, Schmaelzle JF. Processed porcine small intestine submucosa as a graft material for pubovaginal slings: durability and results. Urology. 2003;62(5):805–9.
34. Arunkalaivanan AS, Barrington JW. Randomized trial of porcine dermal sling (Pelvicol implant) vs. tension-free vaginal tape (TVT) in the surgical treatment of stress incontinence: a questionnaire-based study. Int Urogynecol J Pelvic Floor Dysfunct. 2003;14(1):17–23.
35. Ho KL, Witte MN, Bird ET. 8-ply small intestinal submucosa tension-free sling: spectrum of postoperative inflammation. J Urol. 2004;171(1):268–71.
36. Campeau L, Gorbachinsky I, Badlani GH, et al. Pelvic floor disorders: linking genetic risk factors to biochemical changes. BJU Int. 2011;108(8):1240–7.
37. Keys T, Campeau L, Badlani G. Synthetic mesh in the surgical repair of pelvic organ prolapse: current status and future directions. Urology. 2012;80(2):237–43.
38. Shah HN, Badlani GH. Mesh complications in female pelvic floor reconstructive surgery and their management: a systematic review. Indian J Urol. 2012; 28(2):129–53.
39. Postlethwait RW. Long-term comparative study of nonabsorbable sutures. Ann Surg. 1970;171(6): 892–8.
40. Klinge U, Conze J, Limberg W, et al. [Pathophysiology of the abdominal wall]. Chirurg. 1996;67(3):229–33.
41. Amid PK. Classification of biomaterials and their related complication in abdominal wall hernia surgery. Hernia. 1997;1:15–21.
42. Boublil V, Ciofu C, Traxer O, et al. Complications of urethral sling procedures. Curr Opin Obstet Gynecol. 2002;14(5):515–20.
43. Bobyn JD, Wilson GJ, MacGregor DC, et al. Effect of pore size on the peel strength of attachment of fibrous tissue to porous-surfaced implants. J Biomed Mater Res. 1982;16(5):571–84.
44. Law NW, Ellis H. A comparison of polypropylene mesh and expanded polytetrafluoroethylene patch for the repair of contaminated abdominal wall defects—an experimental study. Surgery. 1991;109(5):652–5.
45. Pourdeyhimi B. Porosity of surgical mesh fabrics: new technology. J Biomed Mater Res. 1989;23(A1 Suppl):145–52.
46. Iglesia CB. Synthetic vaginal mesh for pelvic organ prolapse. Curr Opin Obstet Gynecol. 2011;23(5):362–5.
47. Iglesia CB, Fenner DE, Brubaker L. The use of mesh in gynecologic surgery. Int Urogynecol J Pelvic Floor Dysfunct. 1997;8(2):105–15.
48. Iglesia CB, Hale DS, Lucente VR. Laparoscopic sacrocolpopexy versus transvaginal mesh for recurrent pelvic organ prolapse. Int Urogynecol J. 2012; 24(3):363–70.
49. Kobashi KC, Govier FE. Management of vaginal erosion of polypropylene mesh slings. J Urol. 2003;169(6): 2242–3.
50. Culligan PJ, Blackwell L, Goldsmith LJ, et al. A randomized controlled trial comparing fascia lata and synthetic mesh for sacral colpopexy. Obstet Gynecol. 2005;106(1):29–37.
51. Chu CC, Welch L. Characterization of morphologic and mechanical properties of surgical mesh fabrics. J Biomed Mater Res. 1985;19(8):903–16.
52. Beets GL, Go PM, van Mameren H. Foreign body reactions to monofilament and braided polypropylene mesh used as preperitoneal implants in pigs. Eur J Surg. 1996;162(10):823–5.
53. FitzGerald MP, Edwards SR, Fenner D. Medium-term follow-up on use of freeze-dried, irradiated donor fascia for sacrocolpopexy and sling procedures. Int Urogynecol J Pelvic Floor Dysfunct. 2004;15(4):238–42.
54. Nygaard IE, McCreery R, Brubaker L, et al. Abdominal sacrocolpopexy: a comprehensive review. Obstet Gynecol. 2004;104(4):805–23.

55. Flood CG, Drutz HP, Waja L. Anterior colporrhaphy reinforced with Marlex mesh for the treatment of cystoceles. Int Urogynecol J Pelvic Floor Dysfunct. 1998;9(4):200–4.
56. Dwyer PL, O'Reilly BA. Transvaginal repair of anterior and posterior compartment prolapse with Atrium polypropylene mesh. BJOG. 2004;111(8):831–6.
57. de Tayrac R, Gervaise A, Chauveaud A, et al. Tension-free polypropylene mesh for vaginal repair of anterior vaginal wall prolapse. J Reprod Med. 2005;50(2):75–80.
58. Milani R, Salvatore S, Soligo M, et al. Functional and anatomical outcome of anterior and posterior vaginal prolapse repair with prolene mesh. BJOG. 2005;112(1):107–11.
59. Lee U, Raz S. Emerging concepts for pelvic organ prolapse surgery: what is cure? Curr Urol Rep. 2011;12(1):62–7.
60. Winters JC, Fitzgerald MP, Barber MD. The use of synthetic mesh in female pelvic reconstructive surgery. BJU Int. 2006;98 Suppl 1:70–6; discussion 77.
61. Debodinance P, Cosson M, Burlet G. Tolerance of synthetic tissues in touch with vaginal scars: review to the point of 287 cases. Eur J Obstet Gynecol Reprod Biol. 1999;87(1):23–30.
62. Fatton B, Amblard J, Debodinance P, et al. Transvaginal repair of genital prolapse: preliminary results of a new tension-free vaginal mesh (Prolift technique)—a case series multicentric study. Int Urogynecol J Pelvic Floor Dysfunct. 2007;18(7):743–52.
63. Simonds RJ, Holmberg SD, Hurwitz RL, et al. Transmission of human immunodeficiency virus type 1 from a seronegative organ and tissue donor. N Engl J Med. 1992;326(11):726–32.
64. Birch C, Fynes MM. The role of synthetic and biological prostheses in reconstructive pelvic floor surgery. Curr Opin Obstet Gynecol. 2002;14(5):527–35.
65. Visco AG, Weidner AC, Barber MD, et al. Vaginal mesh erosion after abdominal sacral colpopexy. Am J Obstet Gynecol. 2001;184(3):297–302.
66. Badlani GH. Editorial comment. Urology. 2012;80(2):279; author reply 279.
67. Sonia Bishwajit CF, Badlani G. The biochemistry of wound healing in the pelvic floor: what have we learned? Curr Bladder Dysfunct Rep. 2009;4(1):13–9.
68. Lee SJ, Liu J, Oh SH, et al. Development of a composite vascular scaffolding system that withstands physiological vascular conditions. Biomaterials. 2008;29(19):2891–8.
69. Tillman BW, Yazdani SK, Lee SJ, et al. The in vivo stability of electrospun polycaprolactone-collagen scaffolds in vascular reconstruction. Biomaterials. 2009;30(4):583–8.
70. Badlani GH. Editorial comment. Urology. 2012;79(1):14; author reply 15.

Pelvic Organ Prolapse: Anterior Compartment—Kits and Customised Repairs

18

Ajay Rane and Jay Iyer

Introduction

Genital prolapse requiring surgery occurs roughly in one in ten women. The majority of these surgeries occur in the anterior compartment which is very vulnerable to recurrences. Primary surgery can itself prove problematic because the majority of cystoceles are treated with 'standard' midline fascial plication repairs in contrast to the anatomical defects which can be diverse in location (lateral paravaginal, midline fascial or apical). It is little surprise that in the 2001 study published by Weber et.al. comparing three different anterior repair procedures with a 23-month follow-up [1] reported up to a 70 % failure rate after a 'standard' anterior repair.

A robust anterior compartment repair should have the potential to support midline, paravaginal and apical portions of the anterior fascial hammock that support the urinary bladder. Cystocele repairs have traditionally been performed vaginally as these operations are inherently difficult to perform laparoscopically or transabdominally. Midline fascial plication repairs have never been reported via the abdominal route. It is important to appreciate that the results of both 'augmented' mesh repair (mesh overlay) and mesh 'replacement' (needle kit) grafts are typically encouraging in the short term and only studies with longer than a year's follow-up reveal the true picture [2].

In view of the high rates of post-operative recurrence with fascial and mesh overlay repairs, there was a genuine need felt to design an operation that could effectively address all 'parts' of the anterior hammock with or without the use of graft. This led to the invention of the needle-driven kits like PERIGEE™ (American Medical Systems, MN; Fig. 18.1). The idea was to use helical needles through the obturator foramen and place a new hammock that would effectively address multiple defects in the fascial hammock. Anterior PROLIFT™ (Johnson and Johnson, NJ) worked on a similar principle.

Indications: Symptomatic/Voiding Dysfunction

The main indication for an anterior repair should be a symptomatic prolapse POP-Q stage 2 or greater. We use mesh kits in our unit only for stage 3 and 4 cystoceles and mainly for recurrences. We tend to avoid use of grafts in smaller cystoceles principally because the defect is small and dissection to the sacrospinous ligament is technically difficult predisposing to cystotomy and bleeding complications. In addition the precut

A. Rane, M.B.B.S., M.Sc., M.D., F.R.C.S., F.R.C.O.G., F.R.A.N.Z.C.O.G., C.U., P.H.D., F.I.C.O.G. (Hon.), F.R.C.P.I. (Hon.) • J. Iyer, M.B.B.S., M.D., D.N.B., F.R.C.O.G., F.R.A.N.Z.C.O.G. (✉)
Department of Obstetrics and Gynaecology, James Cook University, Townsville, QLD, Australia

G.H. Badlani (ed.), *Minimally Invasive Therapy for Urinary Incontinence and Pelvic Organ Prolapse*, Current Clinical Urology, DOI 10.1007/978-1-4939-0008-4_18,

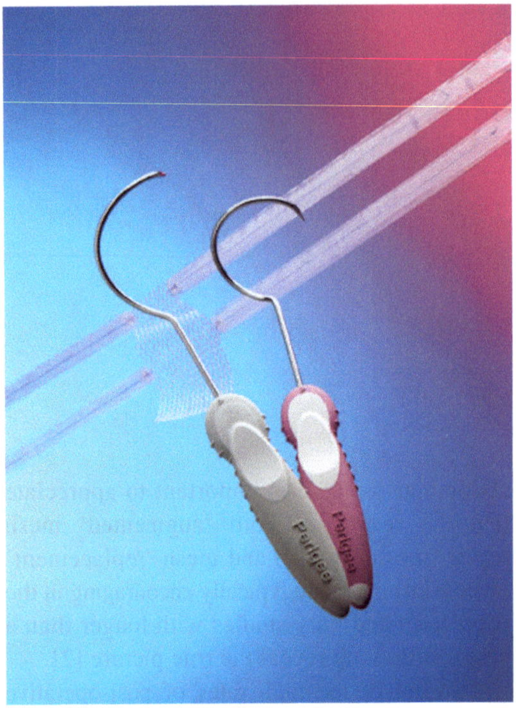

Fig. 18.1 Perigee system

mesh is typically large in surface area relative to the size of the prolapse, which may lead to bunching of mesh edges and symptomatic post-operative complications like mesh exposure and mesh-related pain. A smaller prolapse also indirect indicates partially intact fascial support and is typically best treated with a fascial repair.

Case Selection: Stage 3 and 4 Cystoceles and Recurrences

Cases for mesh repairs should be selected carefully. It is important that a conscious effort be made to ensure that the leading edge of the prolapse is beyond the level of the hymenal ring. We avoid the use of mesh in patients with previous irradiation, in poorly controlled diabetics and patients on high-dose immunosuppressants or corticosteroids. There is a small group of patients who do not want 'foreign material' used in their repairs—such patients should never be subjected to a mesh repair.

Special Instruments/Retractors/ Suture Materials

In our unit we tend not to use elaborate surgical equipment for either conventional surgery or for transvaginal mesh kit repairs. A Scott retractor is usually very handy. Although in recent times there has been a tendency to use the Lone Star™ Retractor System (Cooper Surgical, CT) for complicated vaginal repairs and mesh surgery, it is our practice to keep instrumentation simple and to a bare minimum. Apart from tissue holding forceps, sharp dissecting scissors and a good needle holder we do not insist upon any other special surgical tools. We also use standardised sutures and closure techniques. Our preference is to use 2/0 Vicryl for vaginal closure after all repairs, reserving 2/0 PDS for fascial repairs and mesh anchoring stitches.

Anaesthesia

The surgical time for most anterior compartment vaginal surgeries is around 30 min hence general anaesthesia is our preferred option. Surgeries under a spinal anaesthetic usually mandate the post-operative placement of an indwelling catheter, which delays our algorithmic 'trial of void' protocol and makes it problematic to ensure an ambulatory day surgery ethos [3, 4].

Positioning of Patient: Lithotomy

It is important that the surgeon either supervises or personally arranges the patient position. The use of hydraulic gas-aided stirrups makes adjusting patient position easier but also can lead to an asymmetric positioning of legs or excessive lithotomy.

Surface Anatomy

Following on from patient positioning, it is important to mark surface anatomy of the patient on each side so that asymmetric positioning of 'Yellow-fin' stirrups does not adversely affect (appropriate) siting of stab incisions during needle insertion and by corollary cause improper mesh placement.

We have abandoned a standardised approach to siting skin incisions and tend to individually vary them based on particular surgical requirements. The former ostensibly makes the operation appear simpler and more marketable, but the use of surface anatomy markings to individualise placement of incisions helps prevent complications. Using an indelible marker, the marking of the lower border of the adductor longus tendon and the genito-crural fold is outlined. The entry point (the 'first point') for the 'outside-in' transobturator needles or exit point for the inside-out transobturator tapes is at a point below the adductor longus tendon and medial to the genito-crural fold. This, in our opinion, measurably reduces tendon-related groin pain after surgery. On a related note, the aforementioned point on surface marking also serves as a guide to direct the trajectory of the needle when using 'minislings'.

The 'second point' that needs to be identified is the lowermost portion of the obturator foramen. This is marked by palpating the ischial tuberosity and using one's fingers to 'walk up' from this bony prominence till a distinct 'give' of the soft tissue over the obturator foramen is felt. This represents the lowermost portion of the obturator membrane. We tend to utilise this point to easily access the area around the ischial spine; this is useful for guiding transobturator needles mesh kits. By joining the first to the second points outlined above, one begins to appreciate the orientation and margin of the obturator foramen. This is particularly useful in defining the distance of the driving point of the helical needles from the obturator vessels (usually about 4.5 cm) constantly providing a visual feedback (point of reference) to the surgeon. This is especially important in difficult and obese patients when it is all too easy to 'lose' the needle when it traverses the obturator fossa. The movement of the needle tips is counter-intuitive; the needle tip moves away from the target location as the external handle is moved towards the surgeon. Needle vacillation is extremely dangerous and a documented cause of major pelvic vascular and visceral laceration. It is therefore imperative that the handle is kept 'flush' (in close contact) with the patient's obturator foramen and an attempt made to 'visualise' the three dimensional movement of the needle tip within the confined space between the obturator foramen, the sacrospinous ligament and the lateral pelvic wall.

Finally, prior to making an incision and in order to get a general idea of the topography of the pelvic structures, it is good practice to perform gynecologic pelvimetry, which helps assess the sub-pubic angle for adequacy of access, the accessibility of the ischial spines and the sacrospinous ligaments. These are the important landmarks that need to be identified prior any kind of pelvic floor reconstruction.

Instructions for Use

Stepwise Approach to Any Type of Vaginal Repair Surgery

We recommend the use of hydrodissection in all cases of vaginal repair surgery. This involves the use of Marcaine (0.5 %) with 1 in 200,000 Epinephrine; a volume of 20 millilitres (mL) diluted with 20 mL of normal saline per 'compartment'. Hydrodissection allows the surgeon to get in the right surgical plane in a bloodless manner (Fig. 18.2). Not only does it help in developing the natural, relatively avascular tissue planes in the pelvic floor, it also facilitates proper mesh placement, reducing the risk of visceral or neurovascular damage. In addition hydrodissection facilitates full thickness vaginal dissection and development of the paravesical space towards the ischial spines and sacrospinous ligaments [5]. We tend to follow the 'grey bubble' (Vincent Lucente, personal communication) which is the appearance created by the infiltrated fluid as it dissects the fascia off the viscus helping define the correct plane of dissection (Fig. 18.3). Sharp and blunt dissection is carried out in this plane that lies between the fascia and the serosa of the prolapsing viscus, NOT between the vagina and the fascia (Fig. 18.4). Dissection in the later plane leads to 'vaginal skinning' which regrettably, has for

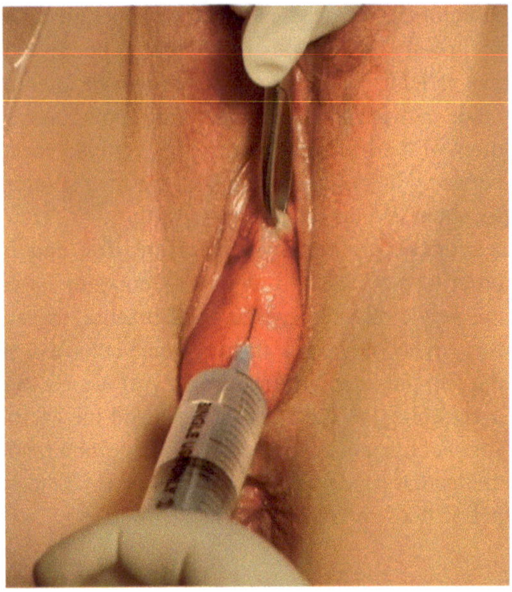

Fig. 18.2 Hydrodissection

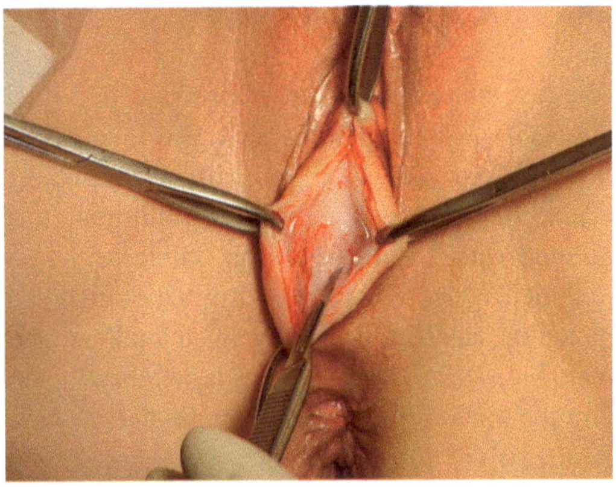

Fig. 18.3 Follow the 'grey bubble'

many years, been part of the standard technique for fascial repair. In some ways mesh surgery is counter-intuitive involving a degree of relearning, because it does mandate deeper dissection and placement of the mesh on the viscus–fascia interface rather than superficial fascia–vaginal skin plane.

Full thickness dissection not only permits adequate dissection of the bladder laterally to allow access to the obturator membrane and the sacrospinous ligament, it also allows sufficient dissection of the bladder from its attachment to

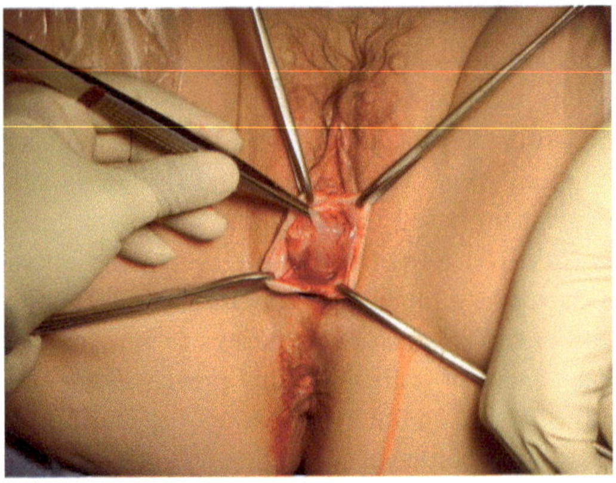

Fig. 18.4 'Four point hold'

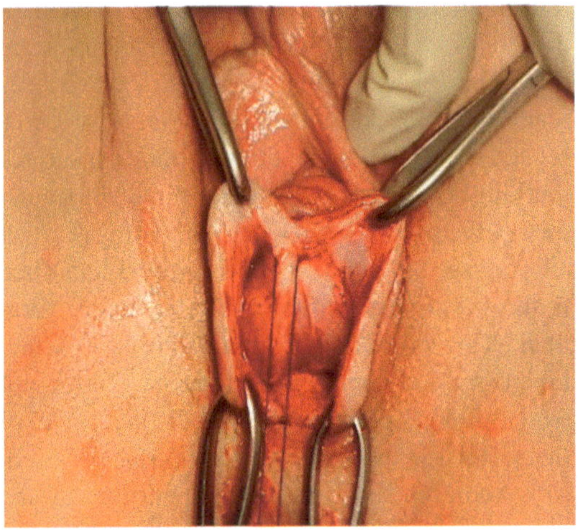

Fig. 18.5 Apical anchoring suture

the cervix or the vaginal vault (Figs. 18.4 and 18.5). This is a critical step for both mesh replacement and native tissue surgery. We employ sharp dissection at the base of the bladder with Metzenbaum scissors prior to the dissection of the tissues lateral to it, using gentle sweeping movements with the index finger from the lateral to medial aspect; keeping the pressure laterally prevents inadvertent bladder trauma. The tissue planes between the viscus and the lateral pelvic wall can usually be developed efficiently with a combination of blunt and sharp dissection. The foregoing techniques are usually sufficient to ensure that the mesh lies directly abutting the serosal surface of the prolapsing viscus, effectively reducing the incidence of

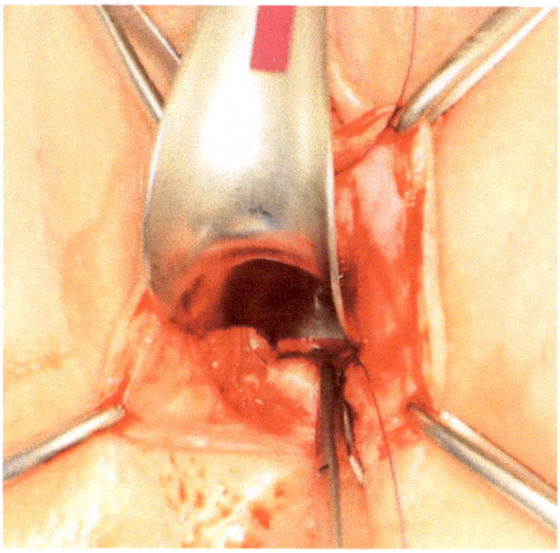

Fig. 18.6 Sacrospinous anchor loaded on to *Orange* needle and sheath

vaginal mesh exposure without increasing visceral mesh erosion. In addition this technique meets the core requirement of reducing the prolapse of the affected organ—not of its enveloping fascia/vaginal skin (M. Cosson, personal communication) [5]. A key element in all needle-driven mesh procedures is 'anchorage'; in the anterior compartment, this takes the form of a 'four-point anchor' inserted, respectively, into the obturator internus muscles and sacrospinous ligaments of either side, essentially mimicking the native fascial bladder hammock. This anatomical reproduction of Delancey's supports has been made possible with mesh surgery and is pivotal to its success (Figs. 18.6, 18.7, 18.8 and 18.9). The sacrospinous ligament forms the cornerstone for mesh surgery in both the anterior and posterior compartments–it is relatively avascular, has a fixed anatomic location with well-circumscribed boundaries, identifiable even in obese women or in the elderly, and acts as a sturdy anchor. The sacrospinous ligament is approached through the 'anterior approach', a technique that is essential for mesh surgery in the anterior compartment and which most pelvic floor surgeons can relearn [6, 7].

The mesh should be placed in situ in a 'tension-free' manner (Fig. 18.10) and there is no need to excise vaginal skin (minor trimming for

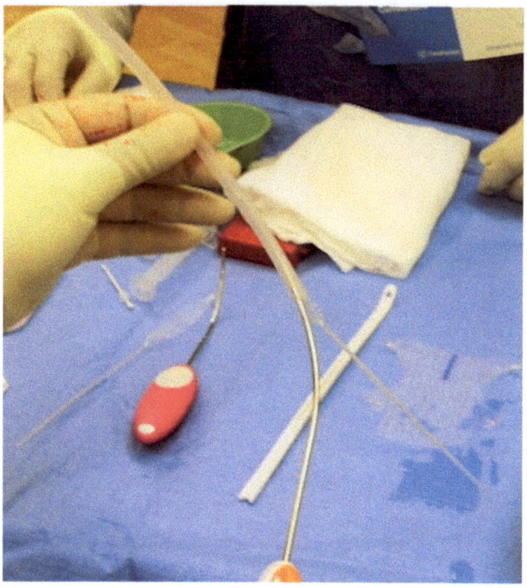

Fig. 18.7 Sacrospinous anchor being inserted (*Note*: Handle parallel to floor)

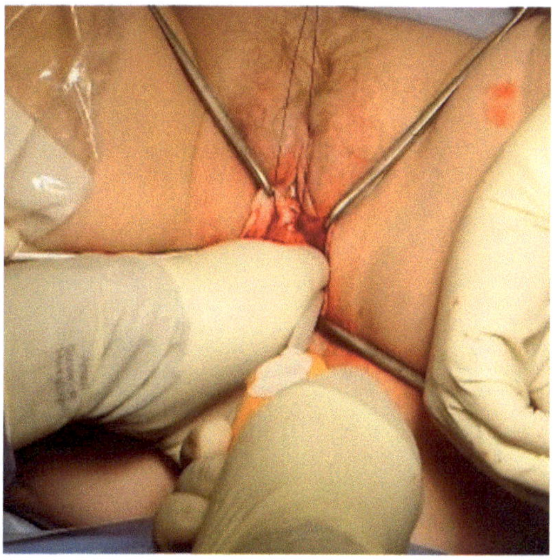

Fig. 18.8 Sacrospinous anchors in place

purposes of aligning the edges is acceptable). Oftentimes after vaginal closure, the operated area appears 'visually unpleasing' as if the prolapse has not been reduced at all—this in fact is an indirect indicator of appropriate mesh tensioning (Fig. 18.11) [5]. The beauty of mesh surgery lies in the fact that it factors in the concept of vaginal remodelling that allows surrounding

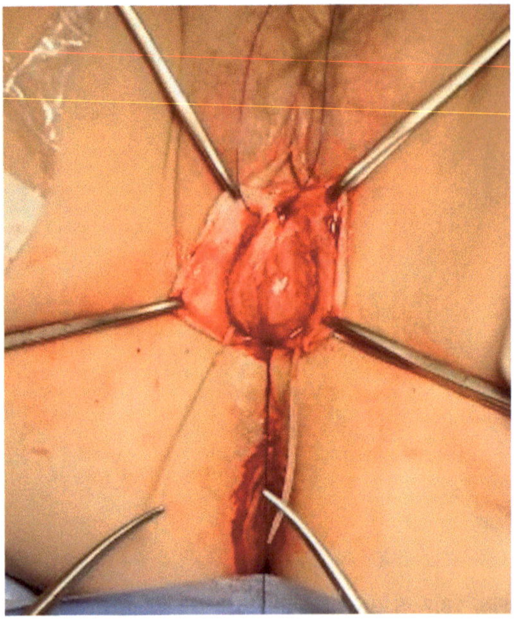

Fig. 18.9 Upper anchor in obturator internus muscle

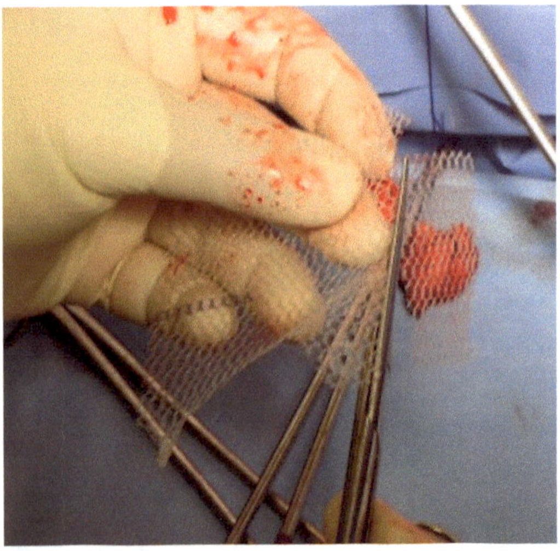

Fig. 18.10 Mesh locked in place

tissues to restructure in much the same way that the vagina involutes to its pre-pregnancy state following vaginal birth [8, 9].

It is important to appreciate that every 'needle' in every 'kit' is *different*; there is a variety to choose from—helical needles, open curve needles, self-retrieving needles, needles with inner and outer sheaths. It is imperative that surgeons

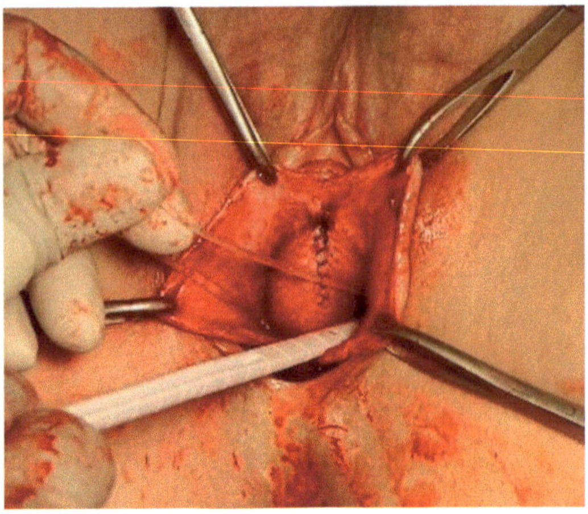

Fig. 18.11 Final result—'visually unpleasing'

have a detailed knowledge of anatomy to ensure surgical safety and therefore it is recommended that surgeons new to mesh surgery follow a 'three step training program' before using mesh. Step 1 usually involves cadaveric dissection and didactic teaching, which is then followed by preceptoring at the trainer's facility and finally proctoring at the nouveau surgeons operating rooms. Understanding the needle curvatures, the directional reversals of the needle tips with respect to the handles (this tends to be counter-intuitive) and last but perhaps most importantly, appreciating the spatial relationships within the three-dimensionality of female pelvic anatomy is paramount and effectively prevents major visceral and vascular injuries [5, 10]. This relatively new technology has not had the benefit of many robust randomised controlled trials or case-controlled studies done to address the pros and cons [11–14]. The proliferation of different types of synthetic and biologic meshes without comprehending their individual biodynamics could lead to delayed complications [13–23].

PERIGEE™ (American Medical Systems, MN)

The PERIGEE™ was the first needle-driven mesh replacement system introduced in 2003 to improve upon the results of anterior compartment fascial and mesh-augmented (mesh overlay) repairs. Mesh-augmented surgery was fundamentally inferior because these afforded little or no 'anchorage' and failed to provide 'arcus-to-arcus' support defined in John Delancey's seminal work on pelvic organ support [24].

The Superior or Pink Needles

At the commencement of the procedure, an important landmark to look out for is the bladder neck. Surface marking is carried out as discussed earlier. We perform all our anterior compartment repairs *below* the level of the bladder neck. This is marked by identifying the prominent sulcus at the point where the urethra meets the bladder or with the use of a Foley catheter balloon especially if anatomical landmarks are indistinct or have been obscured by previous surgery. In our opinion, avoiding dissection around the bladder neck potentially reduces the incidence of postoperative voiding dysfunction; therefore, a conscious effort needs to be made to stay above it for a sub-urethral sling and below it for an anterior compartment repair. A 'dry pass' is made outside the pelvis to get an idea of the position of the needle and its likely range of movement inside the pelvis. The needle is usually held at 45 ° to the vertical and the handle has to be pressed against the skin of the obturator foramen flush with the patient avoiding the tendency to draw the handle towards the operator. This technique ensures that the needle tip remains close to the inner aspect of the obturator internus/membrane rather than going deeper and vacillating in the pelvis around vital structures. The helix further prevents needle vacillation and protects the bladder and the obturator vessels. Tunnels of about 5 mm are created inferior to the ischiopubic rami; this allows palpation of the needles as they exit through the obturator fossa. These tunnels are dissected in a 'cone'-shape with the base towards the surgeon and the apex at the obturator membrane potentially reducing bleeding from vascular complications and forniceal punctures.

A skin stab incision is made on the external landmark and the needle is passed through the obturator membrane/internus; usually at least one 'pop' is felt, if not two. The first pop is through the obturator membrane and the second through the obturator internus. Once the 'pop' occurs the tip of the finger inside the tunnel should feel the needle tip and the needle should be brought out with the finger constantly guiding the tip to avoid puncturing the vaginal fornices. Once the tip exits the mesh arm can be attached to it with the connector and the needle is withdrawn in a 'reverse'-curved motion simultaneously pushing the connector in with the index finger from the vaginal end. This prevents unnecessary tissue distortion during needle withdrawal.

The Inferior or the Grey Needles

The design of these needles was crucial to the next part of the procedure; in order to allow optimal suspension in a 'hammock-like' fashion and ensure 'arcus-to-arcus support' the needles (and by extension the mesh arms) need to traverse the adductor brevis, adductor magnus, obturator externus, obturator membrane, obturator internus and finally the levator ani close to the ischial spine (about a centimetre medial and cranial). After numerous cadaver testings, two methods were derived for needle placement:

1. The direct placement method where the grey needles are held in a high-handed position like the handles of a 'Harley Davidson' or
2. The two-movement technique where the needle handle is initially held vertically in relation to the obturator foramen to ensure entry into the obturator membrane. In the second step the handle is swung by an angle of 90 ° with the handle perpendicular to its original position and then the needle is threaded through the obturator internus towards the levator muscle as close to the ischial spine as possible. The curvature of the needle usually achieves this without the surgeon needing to constantly feel the spine; the latter may lead to tearing/avulsion of the muscle secondary to unnecessary traction by the needle.

Tunnels of 5 mm are created at the lowermost lateral edge of the bladder dissection—these tunnels can be made bigger even allowing the

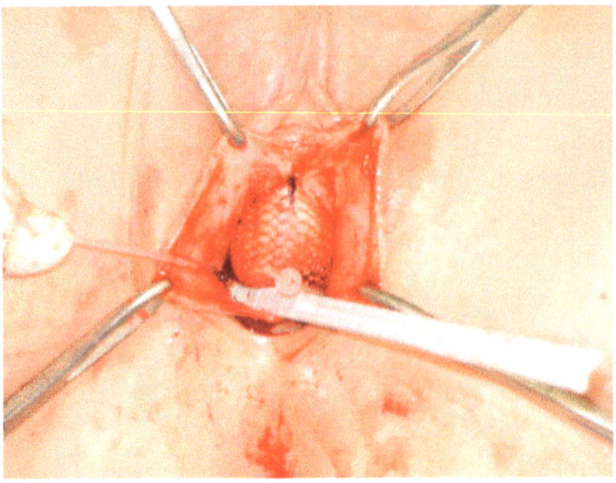

Fig. 18.12 Two-layered closure with 2/0 Vicryl

surgeon to 'sweep' the 'arcus' if necessary. We do not recommend this for the Perigee operation.

Stab incisions are made on the external surface and the needles are passed as indicated above preferably employing the second technique. The mesh is attached with the connectors and the needles are withdrawn with a reverse motion. The mesh is sited and covers the bladder in a 'tension-free' manner. The tail of the Perigee can be trimmed to suit the length of the vault. The mesh is then fixed with a 2-0 PDS suture both at its base and at its cranial portion in the midline below the bladder neck to ensure that the mesh is laid flat. A cystoscopy can be performed at this stage to ensure there has been no bladder trauma or perforation. We then recommend vaginal closure in two layers using 2-0 Vicryl without any vaginal trimming (Fig. 18.12).

Tensioning

Once the vagina is closed, we manually reposit the vagina as high as possible; we DO NOT recommend pulling on the mesh arms any further merely to make the operation 'look good'. A 'flat' non-sagging anterior vaginal wall invariably indicates that the mesh is too tight and virtually guarantees post-operative mesh pain in the fornices and predisposes to mesh exposure. Male dyspareunia ('His'pareunia) is invariably associated with vaginal exposure of mesh whilst female dyspareunia ('Her'pareunia) seems to be more associated with excessive graft tensioning or with shortening and narrowing of the vaginal canal secondary to skin excision [25–27]. We recommend pulling the slack off the mesh arms and then pulling the plastic off without further traction on the limbs. The limbs are then trimmed at skin level and a small dressing is placed on each stab wound.

We do not use an indwelling catheter post-operatively and a vaginal pack is placed only for 2 h. This has been our practice since 2005 and we have performed more than 600 operations (2011) with a readmission rate of 2.9 %.

Anterior Elevate (American Medical Systems, MN)

Following the warning by the FDA in 2008 and 2012, it became important to devise a mesh implantation system that avoided 'blind' needle passes in the obturator foramen, which at the same time maintained the success rates of the transobturator procedure. The Anterior Elevate™ transvaginal mesh replacement system was born out this concept (Fig. 2.13). It involves the passage of anchors into the sacrospinous ligament that provide surrogate anchorage for the mesh threaded through it. The system also provides for two additional anchors interwoven into the mesh that deploy into the obturator internus muscle.

Sacrospinous Needles (Orange), Plastic Sheath and Anchors

A full thickness vaginal incision is made below the bladder neck after ensuring adequate hydrodissection with local anaesthetic as described above (Fig. 18.2). A combination of blunt and sharp dissection allows the creation of adequate access laterally to the sacrospinous ligaments. It is very important to dissect the bladder away at the base free of the vaginal vault or cervix (as the case may be) in order to allow for the anchoring suture to be placed at the level of the vault or pericervical ring (Figs. 18.3, 18.4 and 18.13).

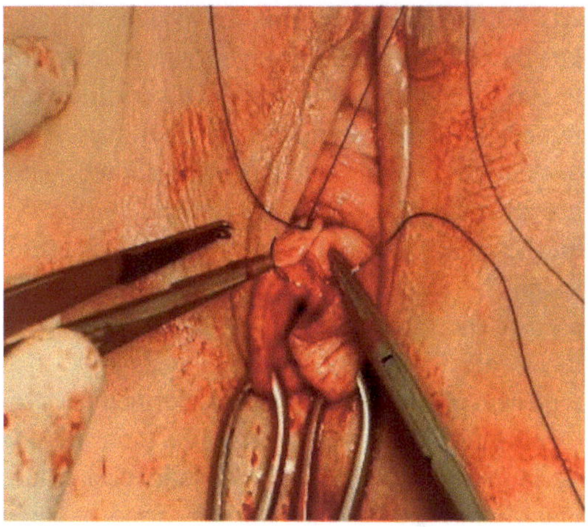

Fig. 18.13 Anchoring suture through peri-cervical ring

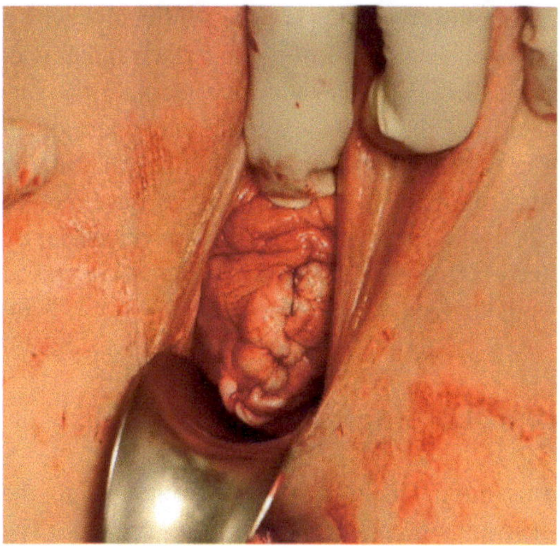

Fig. 18.14 Mesh trimmed to correct 'dose'

The anchors are loaded on to the Orange needles which are then sheathed by the plastic tube. Of note is the design of the tip of the needle that allows the anchor to slot in only one direction. The length of the tip of the needle is unique in that it limits the 'depth' to which the anchor treads into the sacrospinous ligament to 22 mm regardless of the driving force applied (Fig. 18.6). This is an important safety feature that protects against needle-induced neurovascular injury within the confines of the pelvis. Another tip to avoid complications is to gently grate the plastic sheath across the sacrospinous ligament about a finger's breadth medial to the ischial spine; this results in a characteristic 'grating' that is fed back to the surgeon's hand. This technique ensures that the needle driving system with the anchor is perpendicular to the sacrospinous ligament and this is also confirmed by the handle of the needle which lies parallel to the ground when placed correctly (Fig. 18.7). The perpendicular placement of the anchor affords excellent anchorage with pull-out forces of >8 psi and prevents 'splaying' of the sacrospinous ligament.

Pink Needle

Again staying clear of the bladder neck two small tunnels are made laterally carrying the dissection below and behind the ischiopubic ramus into belly of the obturator internus muscle. A second anchoring suture is placed just below the bladder neck which along with the other one at the vault helps in laying the mesh flat and prevents the edges from rolling up. These sutures do not in any way contribute to the strength of the repair (Figs. 18.5, 18.6 and 18.9). The 'tail' of the mesh is trimmed to size and threaded through the superior suture and tied into place (Fig. 18.14). The pink needles are inserted into the anchors fused with the mesh edges and passed into the obturator internus muscle via the tunnels described above taking care not to perforate the forniceal skin.

Further Steps

The vault/pericervical ring suture is then passed through the bottom edge of the mesh and tied in place. The vaginal end of the anchors that were placed in the sacrospinous ligament is then threaded through eyelets in the mesh and the mesh is sited in its appropriate position by means of a 'spoon' provided in the kit. This also allows for proper tensioning prior to locking the mesh in place with the 'buttons' included in the mesh kit (Figs. 18.13 and 18.10). The anchors are cut free and the vagina is closed in two layers using 2/0 Vicryl (Fig. 18.12). As described earlier, the end result of the operation is quite unattractive with a lot of residual laxity of the anterior vaginal wall (Fig. 18.11). This should help reassure the surgeon that the mesh is appropriately tensioned. The 6-week follow-up visit will reveal the true state of affairs as the vagina would have remodelled to a large extent and the perceived laxity that was seen in the immediate post-op period would have all but disappeared.

UPHOLD™ (Boston Scientific, MA)

This mesh kit utilises suture anchorage to the sacrospinous ligament instead of anchors. The Ethibond sutures attached to mesh arms are tacked in place by means of the Capio device which is a needle-driven system that delivers the suture to the appropriate location in the ligament and also retrieves the suture on its return journey. The mesh arms are then pulled through the sacrospinous ligament providing robust anchorage which provides level 1 support and some level 2 support. In cases where a large cystocele coexists with vault/cervical descent the PINNACLE™ device that has a larger mesh with two extra arms may be used. These arms are fixed via the Capio device into the arcus tendineus resulting in good arcus-to-arcus level 2 support like the PERIGEE™ device. Pinnacle has now been withdrawn from the market.

PROSIMA™ (Johnson and Johnson, NJ)

This mesh kit also involves the intravaginal introduction of mesh that is 'tucked' into the sacrospinous ligament using a metal carrier device and then held in place by means of inflatable balloon that remains in the vagina for 2 weeks. At the end of 2 weeks, it is expected that the mesh will 'stick in place'. This product has now been withdrawn from the market.

In our opinion, the Boston devices enshrine the philosophy of minimal mesh area in their kits; AMS kits have moderate mesh volume in their kits with the option of trimming to size whilst the kits by Johnson and Johnson have been relatively larger. So far studies have shown very little difference in clinical outcomes between these various devices. Having said that most studies do not use imaging like 3D/4D ultrasound to observe meshes over a period of time [28, 29]. It is useful to think of mesh as a medication that needs to be used in the 'correct dose'—so trim the mesh to meet individual requirements. It is vital that replacement mesh surgery be performed per protocol established by the manufacturer as any deviations from the accepted technique can cause untold damage to the woman besides being medico-legally indefensible.

The introduction of newer meshes that are lighter, softer and less dense has made a discernible change in patient outcomes in a few studies.

Tips and Pearls: Hydrodissection, Full Thickness and Remodelling

The most important lessons we have learnt in our unit over the last 9 years of mesh usage are:

- Proper patient selection—avoiding use of mesh in small prolapses, appropriate patient counselling before surgery
- Hydrodissection and full thickness dissection as mentioned before
- Gentle tissue handling
- Avoidance of excessive traction to the mesh
- Avoidance of vaginal trimming

Graft surgery at the end of the operation should not be 'visually pleasing' unlike fascial native tissue surgery. This does engender a 'leap of faith' and represents a shift in the surgical paradigm. In our experience tension-free placement does prevent mesh complications. The vagina is 'an innocent victim of prolapse' and once the proposing organ is supported with the mesh, vaginal remodelling takes over. Indeed a classic example of vaginal remodelling is the postpartum period where the vagina that is stretched to many times its normal size remodels back to its normal calibre (almost!) within 6 weeks.

Post-operative Orders and Management

In our patients the use of local anaesthetic for hydrodissection has reduced the need for post-operative narcotic analgesia to less than 3 %. We advise the use of intraoperative antibiotics like cephalosporins and metronidazole. We also routinely prescribe antibiotics for 5 days post-surgery. Pain relief is achieved by a diclofenac suppository post-surgery and oral ibuprofen, codeine and paracetamol. Patients using codeine are advised to use stool softeners like Lactulose.

All patients undergo a trial of void post-surgery and a post-void residual bladder volume (PVRBV) of <100 mL is our cut-off. We do not routinely use vaginal packing. Our patients are sent home the same day if they are pain-free, are not bleeding excessively and have passed their trial of void, with access to a 24-h hotline number. A nurse calls all patients the next day and performs a visual analogue score for pain, bleeding and bladder function with appropriate referral as necessary.

Table 18.1 Numbers sexually active

Status	Number	Percentage
Sexually active	111	64.91
Not sexually active	55	32.16
Not answered	5	2.93
Total	171	100

Table 18.2 Outcomes after operation

Dyspareunia	Number	Percentage
None	55	49.54
Same	15	13.51
Better	33	29.72
Worse	8	7.23
Total	111	100

Table 18.3 Mesh exposures in Perigee and Apogee

Year	Total number of perigee + apogee	Total number of mesh exposure	Percentage
2004	5	0	NA
2005	23	6	26.08
2006	43	18	41.8
2007	56	4	7.14
2008	44	1	2.27
2009	17	0	NA

Results: 5-Year Perigee Data with Data on Mesh Erosion and Sexual Function

Utilising the principles highlighted above, we followed up 350 data sets for a total of 5 years, the results of which were published in 2008 [2]. A total of 350 patients underwent surgery with the Perigee™ system between March 2004 and June 2008. There were no life-threatening complications with the procedure. Thirty-nine (11.1 %) patients were found to have small mesh extrusion through the vagina, and twenty (5.71 %) patients had recurrence of stage 2 cystocele. Of the subset of patients ($n = 171$) analysed 49.5 % reported no sexual dysfunction, 13.5 % reported no change in sexual function, 29.7 % reported improvement in sexual function whilst 7.2 % reported worsening of dyspareunia (Tables 18.1 and 18.2).

A recent audit of 188 of our patients over a 4-year period who had an Apogee and/or Perigee showed *29 (15.4 %) patients in total were diagnosed with mesh exposures*. Of the 29 patients, 20 (69 %) patients had Perigee and 9 (31 %) patients had Apogee procedures. Twenty-six patients required surgical management of mesh exposure under general anaesthesia and three patients were treated conservatively. On analysing the trend in occurrence of the mesh exposure, 80 % (16/20) among the Perigee exposure group and 88.9 % (8/9) among the Apogee exposure group had procedures performed at the introduction of the procedure during the years 2005 and 2006. The mesh was changed to InterProlite in 2008. In the following years 2007 and 2008, this significantly declined to 20 % (4/20) and 11.1 % (1/9) among the Perigee and Apogee exposure groups, respectively (Table 18.3).

Table 18.4 Analysis of mesh erosion data

Characteristics	Case group (total = 29) *n* (%)	Control group (total = 159) *n* (%)	*P* value (Chi squared test)
Age (29–90, mean age 63)			
<50	7 (24.1)	26 (16.5)	0.3108
50–70	21 (72.4)	120 (75.4)	0.7265
>80	1 (3.4)	13 (8.2)	0.3725
Diabetes mellitus	4 (13.8)	17 (10.7)	0.6258
Smoking	4 (13.8)	20 (12.6)	0.8570
Menopause	23 (79.3)	132 (83)	0.6292
Ovestin cream	1 (3.4)	8 (5)	0.71
Oral HRT	6 (20.7)	7 (4.4)	0.0015
Concomitant surgery	14 (48.3) (8/14 posterior repair, 6/14-sus)	97 (61)	0.1998

The time duration between the surgery and the mesh exposure revealed that 55 % had exposures within the first 6 months and 41.4 % had exposures from 6 months to 1 year. The exposure incidence reduced to 10.3 and 6.9 % at the end of second year and >2 years, respectively.

The risk factor parameters included for the analysis of characteristics of patients with mesh exposures included age, smoking, menopausal status, preoperative use of vaginal oestrogen cream, oral hormone replacement therapy, diabetes mellitus and concomitant surgery (Table 18.4). The phenomenon of mesh exposure into the vagina is not, in our opinion, a major worry, and can quite easily be managed either in clinic or in the operating theatre with few recurrences.

The study shows no significant risk factors identified to be associated with mesh exposure. The other significant finding is the dramatic reduction in the trend of incidence of mesh exposure over a period of 4 years since the introduction of the procedure. This can be well attributed to the skin closure technique or change in the type of the mesh used during the procedure.

Conclusion

Anterior compartment surgery is particularly fraught with increased recurrences. A robust surgical operation would be one that addresses all components of the anterior 'hammock'. The first generation of surgical kits like the PERIGEE™ and PROLIFT™ led the way to radical innovation in transvaginal mesh surgery. Our 5-year follow-up of 350 data sets of the Perigee suggests that careful patient selection is paramount when this modality of treatment is chosen.

Techniques of hydrodissection, full thickness vaginal dissection, anterior access to the sacrospinous ligament, tension-free mesh placement and a two-layered vaginal closure with no vaginal skin trimming have evolved over the years and have contributed significantly to our results. Longer term data continues to show these procedures to be safe, robust and durable particularly in the hands of sub-specialists who routinely perform them. Vaginal mesh exposure is on the decline and poses less of a problem owing to better ('softer') meshes, better closure techniques and perhaps a deeper placement of the mesh. Of paramount importance, however, is the change of 'mindset' of the surgeon performing mesh surgery.

References

1. Weber AM, Walters MD, Piedmonte MR, Ballard LA. Anterior colporrhaphy: a randomised trial of three surgical techniques. Am J Obstet Gynecol. 2001; 185(185):1299–306.
2. Rane A, Kannan K, Barry C, Balakrishnan S, Lim Y, Corstiaans A. A prospective study of the Perigee system for the management of cystocoeles—medium-term follow up. Aust N Z J Obstet Gynaecol. 2008;48(4):427–32.

3. Patwardhan S, Arunkalaivanan AS. Urogynaecology: an ambulatory approach. Br J Hosp Med. 2007;68(8): 414–7.
4. Penketh R, Griffiths A, Chawathe S. A prospective observational study of the safety and acceptability of vaginal hysterectomy performed in a 24-hour day case surgery setting. BJOG. 2007;114(4):430–6.
5. Muffly TM, Barber MD. Insertion and removal of vaginal mesh for pelvic organ prolapse. Clin Obstet Gynecol. 2010;53(1):99–114.
6. Cespedes RD. Anterior approach bilateral sacrospinous ligament fixation for vaginal vault prolapse. Urology. 2000;56(6 Suppl):70–5.
7. Rane A, Frazer M, Jain A, Kannan K, Iyer J. The sacrospinous ligament—conveniently effective or effectively convenient? J Obstet Gynaecol. 2011; 31(5):366–70.
8. Alperin M, Moalli PA. Remodeling of vaginal connective tissue in patients with prolapse. Curr Opin Obstet Gynecol. 2006;18(5):544–50.
9. Kannan K, McConnell A, McLeod M, Rane A. Microscopic alterations of vaginal tissue in women with pelvic organ prolapse. J Obstet Gynaecol. 2011;31(3):250–3.
10. Moore RD, Miklos JR. Vaginal mesh kits for pelvic organ prolapse, friend or foe: a comprehensive review. Scientific World Journal. 2009;9:163–89.
11. Davila GW, Drutz H, Deprest J. Clinical implications of the biology of grafts: conclusions of the 2005 IUGA grafts roundtable. Int Urogynecol J Pelvic Floor Dysfunct. 2006;17 Suppl 1:S51–5.
12. Galloway NT. Words of wisdom. Re: the perils of commercially driven surgical innovation. Eur Urol. 2010;58(1):179.
13. Ostergard DR. Lessons from the past: directions for the future. Do new marketed surgical procedures and grafts produce ethical, personal liability, and legal concerns for physicians? Int Urogynecol J Pelvic Floor Dysfunct. 2007;18(6):591–8.
14. Ostergard DR. Vaginal mesh grafts and the Food and Drug Administration. Int Urogynecol J Pelvic Floor Dysfunct. 2010;21:1181–3.
15. FDA public health notification. Serious complications associated with transvaginal placement of surgical mesh in repair of pelvic organ prolapse and stress urinary incontinence health; 2008.
16. FDA Safety Communication. UPDATE on serious complications associated with transvaginal placement of surgical mesh for pelvic organ prolapse; 2011.
17. National Institute of Clinical Excellence. Surgical repair of vaginal wall prolapse using mesh. UK; 2008.
18. Jacquetin B, Cosson M. Complications of vaginal mesh: our experience. Int Urogynecol J Pelvic Floor Dysfunct. 2009;20:893–6.
19. Rice NT, Hu Y, Slaughter JC, Ward RM. Pelvic mesh complications in women before and after the 2011 FDA public health notification. Female Pelvic Med Reconstr Surg. 2013;19(6):333–8.
20. Skoczylas LC, Turner LC, Wang L, Winger DG, Shepherd JP. Changes in prolapse surgery trends relative to FDA notifications regarding vaginal mesh. Int Urogynecol J. 2013.
21. Ellington DR, Richter HE. The role of vaginal mesh procedures in pelvic organ prolapse surgery in view of complication risk. Obstet Gynecol Int. 2013;2013: 356960. Epub 2013 Aug 28.
22. Nygaard I. Approval process for devices and mesh for surgical treatment of pelvic organ prolapse and urinary incontinence. Clin Obstet Gynecol. 2013;56(2): 229–31.
23. Rogers RG. To mesh or not to mesh: current debates in prolapse repair fueled by the U.S. Food and Drug Administration Safety Notification. Obstet Gynecol. 2011;118(4):771–3.
24. Wei JT, De Lancey J. Functional anatomy of the pelvic floor and lower urinary tract. Clin Obstet Gynecol. 2008;47(1):3–17.
25. Brubaker L. Editorial: partner dyspareunia (hispareunia). Int Urogynecol J Pelvic Floor Dysfunct. 2006;17(4):311.
26. Altman D, Elmér C, Kiilholma P, Kinne I, Tegerstedt G, Falconer C. Sexual dysfunction after trocar-guided transvaginal mesh repair of pelvic organ prolapse. Obstet Gynecol. 2009;113(1):127–33.
27. Feiner B, Maher C. Vaginal mesh contraction: definition, clinical presentation, and management. Obstet Gynecol. 2010;115(2):325–30.
28. Barry C, Dietz HP. The use of ultrasound in the evaluation of pelvic organ prolapse. Rev Gynaecol Perinat Med. 2005;5(3):182–95.
29. Dietz HP, Lekskulchai O. Ultrasound assessment of pelvic organ prolapse: the relationship between prolapse severity and symptoms. Ultrasound Obstet Gynecol. 2007;29:688–91.

Pelvic Organ Prolapse: Posterior Repairs

19

Bhavin N. Patel and Kathleen C. Kobashi

Rectoceles are defined as a herniation of the rectum through the posterior vaginal wall, resulting from weakness in the rectovaginal fascia that leads to compromised posterior compartment support. Although not life-threatening, rectoceles, like other forms of pelvic organ prolapse (POP), can have a negative effect on daily living and quality of life. Patients may complain of stool trapping/difficulty with passage of bowel movements, pain or difficulty with intercourse, pelvic pain/pressure, or lower back pain. The symptoms of a rectocele are most often the factor that drives patients to desire repair. The purpose of this chapter is to review the anatomy, pathophysiology, and surgical considerations or rectocele repairs.

Anatomy

Support of the posterior compartment is provided primarily by a thickened layer of tissue that lies beneath the posterior vaginal epithelium. This layer, often referred to as the rectovaginal fascia, is thought to be the female analog of Denonvillier's fascia in the male. This layer is a thick layer of subepithelial tissue of the posterior vagina composed mostly of smooth muscle, collagen, and elastin [1]. This tissue is anchored on all sides, apically by the cardinal-uterosacral complex, laterally by the posterior arcus tendineus fascia pelvis, and distally by the perineal body [2, 3].

Defects in the rectovaginal septum or its anchoring connections can result in a rectocele, with the location of the rectocele depending on the level of the defect. High rectoceles often result from an injury or defect of the upper third of the vagina and its attachment to the cardinal-uterosacral ligament complex. These rectoceles can be associated with uterine prolapse or enteroceles. Mid-level rectoceles are often associated with tears in the rectovaginal septum or in the attachment of the rectovaginal septum to the posterior arcus tendineus. Distal or low rectoceles are thought to be due to injury to or disruption of the perineal body and are often associated with widening of the posterior hiatus.

Etiology

The exact causes of compromised posterior vaginal support and rectoceles are not clear. Known risk factors include childbirth, defecation disorders, age/postmenopausal status, history of hysterectomy, and connective tissue disorders [4]. Although a rare patients with a rectocele may not have any of these risk factors, the majority of patients often have more than one risk factor.

Vaginal childbirth contributes to weakened posterior support as it is known to cause neural,

B.N. Patel, M.D. • K.C. Kobashi, M.D. (✉)
Department of Urology, Virginia Mason Medical Center, 1100 9th Avenue, Mailstop C7-URO, Seattle, WA 98101, USA
e-mail: Kathleen.Kobashi@vmmc.org

G.H. Badlani (ed.), *Minimally Invasive Therapy for Urinary Incontinence and Pelvic Organ Prolapse*, Current Clinical Urology, DOI 10.1007/978-1-4939-0008-4_19,

muscular, and connective tissue injury. Together these factors allow for vaginal laxities that can result in POP. Defecatory disorders, such as constipation, can damage support mechanisms through associated abdominal straining which may lead to nerve damage and stretch injury to the posterior vaginal support [4]. Prior hysterectomy may affect normal vaginal anatomy altering vaginal pressure vectors and causing pelvic denervation that can lead to weakened muscular support. Age is a risk factor for POP as aging females accrue increasing damage with time to their pelvic support. Finally, disorders of the connective tissues result in weakened or lax vaginal support that can lead to the development of POP.

Prevalence

Population-based studies on POP are difficult to accomplish as they require vaginal examinations on asymptomatic women. Furthermore, there is a difference in the prevalence of anatomic and functional rectoceles. For both of these reasons the true prevalence of rectoceles, symptomatic or not, is difficult to define as is the true prevalence of symptomatic rectoceles. In a study of primarily middle-aged and older women, Swift et al. found that 75 % of patients presenting to a gynecologist for their annual exam had some form of POP-Q gradable POP [5]. Furthermore, up to 76 % of women with POP had a documented rectocele [6]. Together these studies suggest a high prevalence of anatomic rectoceles in middle-aged and older women, which follows our clinical experience.

Clinical Aspects

Clinical Presentation and Evaluation

Many patients with anatomic POP are asymptomatic. Patients with rectoceles are no exception. However, symptomatic rectoceles can present with a variety of symptoms. General symptoms of POP include pelvic pressure or heaviness, visualization of a vaginal bulge, pelvic pain or discomfort, and difficulty with intercourse [7]. Other symptoms such as dyspareunia may also occur. Symptoms specific to rectoceles include a sensation of incomplete defecation and need to distally splint the vaginal wall or perineum to facilitate emptying [7].

Patients are seen and evaluated in the clinic. A thorough history is obtained with a focus on risk factors for POP, symptoms of POP, comorbidities, and previous pelvic surgeries. Patients are examined using the POP-Q system at rest and with strain. Levator ani muscle tone and strength are assessed. A rectal exam is done to evaluate for perineal body weakness and anal sphincter tone. The authors do not routinely order imaging, but in complex cases, dynamic MRI or endoanal ultrasonography may provide useful adjunctive information.

Indications/Patient Selection

The surgical indications for rectocele vary from provider to provider. Most pelvic floor surgeons will elect to proceed with repair of a rectocele if the patient has bothersome symptoms related to the posterior prolapse. These symptoms include those mentioned in the previous section. This repair is often performed in conjunction with other vaginal compartment repairs or anti-incontinence procedures.

The proper management of an asymptomatic rectocele present at the time of repair of anterior or apical compartment prolapse repair is controversial. Some clinicians feel that if a posterior compartment defect is left unrepaired while other compartments are repaired, then postoperatively the rectocele is exposed to higher abdominal force which may worsen the posterior defect [8]. Others believe that poor posterior vaginal wall support may provide improved resistance to urethral and bladder neck hypermobility, thereby increasing the success of anti-incontinence procedures [9]. Neither of these statements is supported by the literature. In the practice of the authors, rectoceles are generally only repaired if they are symptomatic or in asymptomatic cases if they have progressed beyond the hymen. In the latter scenario, it is our concern that in spite of being asymptomatic, a rectocele of this degree likely poses an increased risk of becoming symptomatic later in the patient's life.

Procedures

Vaginal Approaches

Vaginal approaches to rectocele repair include the traditional posterior colporrhaphy, plication of the prerectal and pararectal fascia with levator ani reconstruction, defect-specific repair, graft-augmented repair, and kit-based repairs. These approaches are all vaginal-based approaches that do not require abdominal access. As such, these procedures are reasonably well tolerated and suited for outpatient surgery.

Our preoperative and surgical preparations are the same for transvaginal rectocele repair techniques. All anticoagulant is stopped prior to surgery such that bleeding parameters have normalized prior to the day of surgery. The patient is asked to fast starting the night prior to surgery. Prior to beginning the procedure, the patient is given prophylactic antibiotics per the AUA best practice guidelines [10], which typically entails cefazolin intravenously administered 1 h prior to surgical incision.

Spinal anesthetic, laryngeal mask anesthetic, or general endotracheal anesthesia is used. Bilateral sequential compression devices are placed on the lower extremities for venous thromboembolism prophylaxis [11]. Once anesthesia is induced, the patient is placed in the dorsal lithotomy position. The lower extremities are padded and positioned appropriately to prevent nerve or muscle injury. The surgical field is then clipped with clippers, a betadine preparation is used to prepare the vagina, and a chlorahexadine-based preparation is used to prepare the surrounding perineal and lower abdominal skin. Once the patient is adequately draped, the Lone Star retractor (CooperSurgical™, Stafford, TX) is centered on the vaginal introitus and affixed to the perineum using penetrating towel clips. A Foley catheter is placed and the procedure is begun.

Once the vaginal procedure is completed, a vaginal packing is placed and the patients are transferred to the post-anesthesia care unit. One hour after arriving, the vaginal packing is removed and the patients are given a trial of void if they have had an associated anti-incontinence procedure or anterior compartment repair. Once they have recovered from the anesthetic and their pain is adequately controlled, they are discharged home with a prescription for pain medication, 24 h of oral antibiotic coverage, and an oral stool softener. They are given instructions to refrain from vaginal intercourse, avoid constipation, and avoid lifting greater than 10 lb or doing exercises that may put undue straining on the repair for 6 weeks.

Traditional Posterior Colporrhaphy

The standard or traditional posterior colporrhaphy is a method of rectocele repair that relies on reapproximation of the levator ani muscles and the rectovaginal fascia over the prolapsing rectum to provide posterior support. The patient is prepared and positioned as described above. Prior to rectocele repair all other concomitant pelvic floor surgeries, such as anti-incontinence procedures, cystocele repair, and hysterectomy, are done.

The posterior repair is begun by placing two Allis clamps on the posterior vaginal forchette at the 4 and 8 o'clock positions. The lateral positions of the Allis clamps are defined such that when the clamps are brought together in the midline, the introitus allows the passage of two fingers comfortably or three fingers snuggly. This avoids a stenotic introitus. An ellipse of tissue comprising the junction between the vaginal epithelium and the perineal skin is excised between the Allis clamps creating a diamond defect (Fig. 19.1). The previously described initial dissection is the same for all of the following vaginal approaches for rectocele repair.

Attention is then turned to the apical-most portion of the rectocele. From this point a V-shaped incision is made from the apical portion of the rectocele to the lateral aspects of the perineal incision. Working from the apex toward the introitus the vaginal epithelium is dissected off

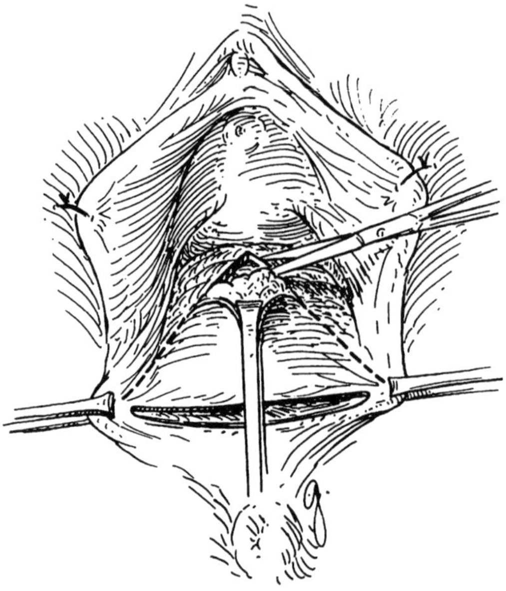

Fig. 19.1 An ellipse of tissue comprising the junction between the vaginal epithelium and the perineal skin between the Allis clamps is excised creating a defect at the posterior forchette. A V-shaped incision is made from the apical portion of the rectocele to the lateral aspects of the perineal incision. With counter-traction facilitated by placement of an Allis on the vaginal epithelium and working from the apex toward the perineum, the vaginal epithelium is dissected off of the rectovaginal septum in the white shiny layer (From Vaginal prolapse, in Raz S: Atlas of Transvaginal Surgery. Philadelphia, WB Saunders, 1992, with permission of Elsevier)

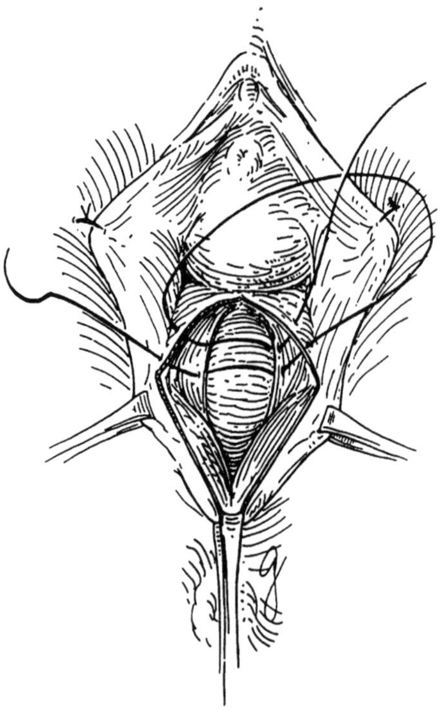

Fig. 19.2 Flaps are created by undermining the vaginal epithelium toward the levator ani muscles. Once the dissection laterally is completed hemostasis is achieved. Interrupted figure-of-eight sutures are placed in the levators and tied such that the levators meet in the midline along the entire rectocele defect (From Vaginal prolapse, in Raz S: Atlas of Transvaginal Surgery. Philadelphia, WB Saunders, 1992, with permission of Elsevier)

the rectovaginal septum. Dissection in the white shiny layer is aided by counter-traction with an appropriately placed Allis clamp (Fig. 19.1). Once the incision and dissection are completed, the excised vaginal epithelium is discarded. Flaps are created by undermining the vaginal epithelium toward the levator ani muscles. Once the dissection laterally is completed hemostasis is achieved. Interrupted figure-of-eight sutures are placed in the levators and tied such that the levators meet in the midline along the entire rectocele defect (Fig. 19.2). The prerectal fascia is closed with a running suture anterior to this layer. One should inspect the repair to ensure there are no ridges or acute drop-offs as these can be the source of postoperative pain or discomfort. The vaginal epithelium is then reapproximated in the midline and a vaginal packing is placed for 1 h and removed in the postoperative care unit prior to discharge.

In one of the largest published series on traditional posterior colporrhaphy, Abramov et al. reported on 183 women who underwent traditional posterior colporrhaphy [12]. These authors reported a 96 % cure rate at 1-year follow-up, with cure defined as no prolapse beyond the hymenal ring. In a more recent study using strict anatomic definitions and validated questionnaires, Paraiso et al. [13] reported on 37 patients randomized to traditional posterior colporrhaphy versus site-specific repair. With a strict definition of anatomic cure, POP-Q point Bp less than or equal to −2 at 1 year from surgery, they found that posterior colporrhaphy was associated with an 86 % anatomic cure rate. Seven percent of patients had posterior wall prolapse to the level of or beyond the hymen. Overall patients had statistically significant improvements in the prolapse and colorectal scales of PFDI-20 and PFIQ-7 after surgery indicating improvement in quality of life. There was no statistical difference in patients with dyspareunia pre- and postoperatively.

Although these 1-year follow-up studies show a high rate of anatomic success, longer term follow-up demonstrates lower rates of anatomic success and decreased functional bowel control after rectocele repair. With a mean follow-up of 3.5 years, Kahn and Stanton demonstrated a 76 % overall anatomic cure rate, with anatomic cure defined as grade 0 or I prolapse on the Baden-Walker scale, after traditional posterior colporrhaphy [14]. On interview, there was an improvement of bulge-related symptoms (64 % vs. 31 %), but despite this, most patients had worsening of bowel-related symptoms including constipation (22 % vs. 33 %), sensation of incomplete bowel emptying (27 % vs. 38 %), and incontinence of stool (4 % vs. 11 %). There was also an increased prevalence of sexual dysfunction postoperatively (18 % vs. 27 %).

Plication of Prerectal and Pararectal Fascia with Levator Reconstruction

In this repair a single layer of suture incorporates prerectal and pararectal fascia (rectal pillars) from the apex of the rectocele down to the lower third of the vagina. Distally, the same layers are incorporated, but the levator ani is included to reapproximate and support the levator hiatus. After the induction of anesthesia, the patient is placed in the dorsal lithotomy position. The patient is prepared in the dorsal lithotomy position as previously described. Prior to rectocele repair all other concomitant pelvic floor surgeries, such as anti-incontinence procedures, cystocele repair, and hysterectomy, are done.

The posterior repair is begun as previously described by excising an ellipse of tissue at the junction of the vaginal epithelium and perineal skin (Fig. 19.1). The subepithelial plane is developed with Metzenbaum scissors from the introitus to the apex of the rectocele and an incision in the midline overlying this dissected tissue is made. During this portion of the case, it is important to keep the tip of the scissors pointing anteriorly to avoid inadvertent damage to the rectal wall.

The reconstructive procedure is begun by using a 2-0 vicryl suture to reapproximate the vaginal epithelium, the pararectal fascia/rectal pillar, and the prerectal fascia from the level of the rectocele apex to the distal third of the vagina. The layers are incorporated with a running, interlocking suture. The running suture is tied down at the beginning of the distal third of the vagina. The remainder of the vaginal defect is closed with interrupted figure-of-eight sutures of 2-0 vicryl including the vaginal epithelium, the pararectal fascia, and the prerectal fascia as before, but the levator ani is also included to reduce and support the levator hiatus. Additionally, these distal vaginal sutures will help restore the vaginal axis. In performing this distal portion of the rectocele repair, one should ensure that the introitus is not too narrow and that there are no deformities or ridges created posteriorly as these can result in pain postoperatively. The remainder of the incision is closed to reapproximate the perineal skin and a vaginal packing is placed for 1 h and removed in the postoperative care unit prior to discharge.

There is limited published data on the outcomes of patients after plication of prerectal and pararectal fascia with levator reconstruction. Vasavada and colleagues reported that in 380 patients seen at a mean follow-up of 22 months after repair, there was a 96 % anatomic success rate with success being defined as a grade I or less posterior wall prolapse. There was a noted functional improvement as well with 67 % of those with preoperative constipation noting improvement in constipation postoperatively. It should be noted that in this study 69 % had asymptomatic rectoceles [4].

Defect-Specific Repair

In the defect-specific rectocele repair, the surgeon dissects the rectovaginal fascia and identifies deficiencies that are primarily repaired. The rectovaginal fascia, as previously mentioned, is a layer of collagen, elastin, and smooth muscle that separates the vagina and rectum. Injury to this layer of support from vaginal childbirth, constipation, abdominal straining, etc. can cause site-specific defects/damage that may result in rectocele. Damage to this posterior support may manifest as a tear in the body of the fascia, a lateral separation of the fascia from the iliococcygeus and pubococcygeus muscles, apical separation from its connection to the sacrum, or distal separation from the rectovaginal fascia's attachment to the perineal body [15].

The posterior repair is begun as previously described by excising an ellipse of tissue at the junction of the vaginal epithelium and perineal skin (Fig. 19.1). The subepithelial plane is developed with Metzenbaum scissors from the introitus to the apex of the rectocele and an incision in the midline overlying this dissected tissue is made. During this portion of the case, it is important to keep the tip of the scissors pointing anteriorly to avoid inadvertent damage to the rectal wall. Dissection is carried laterally allowing for appropriate exposure to the rectovaginal fascia. This exposure should allow for inspection of the rectovaginal fascia from the vaginal apex to the perineal body and out laterally to the tendinous arc of the levator ani.

A double glove is now placed on the non-dominant hand and the index finger of the non-dominant hand is placed transanally to elevate the anterior rectal wall. With lateral movement of the index finger, defects in the rectovaginal fascia are seen. Healthy, durable rectovaginal fascia is then plicated over the anterior rectal wall to address the defects resulting in correction of the rectocele. Once completed the vaginal epithelium is closed and if indicated a perineal body repair is undertaken.

A variation to the defect-specific repair adds another layer of support along the posterior vaginal wall. After the site-specific repair is completed, figure-of-eight sutures are placed to bring the lateral levator ani muscles together in the midline. The addition of the levator ani plication is thought to result in stronger posterior compartment support [16].

In one of the largest published series on site-specific defect repair, Abramov et al. reported on 124 women [12]. These authors reported an 89 % cure rate at 1-year follow-up, with cure defined as no prolapse beyond the hymenal ring. In a series of 89 women, with slightly longer follow-up, 1.5 years, Porter et al. had an anatomic success rate of 82 % [17]. Anatomic success was defined as no prolapse or a rectocele that did not descend beyond the hymenal ring on maximal straining. There were also functional improvements noted in stooling difficulties, pelvic pressure/pain, vaginal bulge/mass, and in need for splinting in the majority of patients. In the previously quoted series by Paraiso et al., 37 patients underwent defect-specific rectocele repair [13]. They described anatomic cure at 1 year as 78 %. Seven percent of patients had posterior wall prolapse to the level of or beyond the hymen. Overall patients had statistically significant improvements in the prolapse and colorectal scales of PFDI-20 and PFIQ-7 after surgery indicating improvement in quality of life. There was no statistical difference in patients with dyspareunia pre- and postoperatively.

Graft-Augmented Repairs

Grafts have been used to repair all compartments of vaginal prolapse and have been used as either a stand-alone support mechanism or an adjunctive to native-tissue repair. Grafts are classified as biologic or synthetic and are available either in a delivery kit or as stand-alone materials that are tailored by the surgeon at the time of surgery use. For rectocele repairs, the authors have used biological graft material as a stand-alone support mechanism. As previously mentioned, although surgeons have used a wide array of graft materials, it has been the authors' preference to use biologic graft over synthetic graft. The authors believe that the benefits of currently available synthetic (polypropylene) meshes do not outweigh the risks of vaginal exposure [18], rectal erosion [19], and mesh contraction [20] do not outweigh the benefits of currently available polypropylene mesh. On the other hand, biologic grafts provide adequate support [21] with little risk of graft contraction or vaginal narrowing. Additionally, vaginal epithelium more readily heals over exposed biologic graft when compared to exposed mesh, the latter of which often requires operative excision of exposed areas.

The posterior repair is begun as previously described by excising an ellipse of tissue at the junction of the vaginal epithelium and perineal skin (Fig. 19.1). Attention is then turned to the apical-most portion of the rectocele. From this point a V-shaped incision is made from the apical portion of the rectocele to the lateral aspect of the perineal incision. Working from the apex toward the introitus the vaginal epithelium is dissected off the rectovaginal septum. Dissection in the white shiny layer is aided by counter-traction with an appropriately placed Allis clamp (Fig. 19.1). Once the incision and dissection are completed, the excised vaginal epithelium is discarded. Flaps are created by undermining the vaginal epithelium in the white shiny layer toward the levator ani muscles.

A perineal repair is performed first, followed by placement of six 0 vicryl sutures prior to the graft being brought into the surgical field. Two sutures are placed proximally and distally in the levator ani/arcus complex bilaterally. One additional suture is placed at the apex of the rectocele and a final suture is placed at the perineal body. The pre-soaked cadaveric fascia (4 cm×7 cm, Tutoplast, Mentor Corporation, Santa Barbara, CA) is brought into the field and folded in half to maximize suture pull-out strength. It is then secured into place using the preplaced sutures thereby reducing the rectocele. The vagina is closed and a vaginal packing is left in place to be removed 1 h after the procedure. Using this technique with non-frozen cadaveric fascia lata, Kobashi et al. reported a 90 % rate of anatomic cure in 50 patients at a mean follow-up of 14 months [21]. Cure was defined as no gradable posterior wall prolapse. Of the 10 % of patients that failed, 40 % had a Baden-Walker grade I recurrence and 60 % had a Baden-Walker grade II recurrence. There were functional improvements in stool trapping, splinting, and dyspareunia.

Kit Repairs

There are many commercially available kits for POP repair. The kits combine graft material with needles passes in a package for treatment of prolapse or stress incontinence. These “all-inclusive” kits do not require tailoring of graft material or harvesting of tissues from patients. Furthermore, kits are designed to be minimally invasive, using passers to traverse anatomically “safe” spaces rather than requiring larger incisions and dissections. For these reasons, kits have been theorized to potentially reduce operative time and morbidity. The disadvantages of using kits to address prolapse or incontinence are the increased cost [22] and lack of long-term data on efficacy and complications related to each of the available kits. In the United States the following posterior repair kits are currently available: Prolift, Apogee, Posterior Elevate, and Pinnacle.

Gynecare Prolift™ Posterior, Ethicon® (Somerville, NJ). The Gynecare Prolift™ uses a pre-tailored piece of the Gynemesh PS™, Ethicon’s soft prolene mesh. The newer generation model, the Prolift+M™, uses a partially absorbable monocryl mesh. As in previous surgical procedures, the patient is positioned in the dorsal lithotomy position, a catheter is placed to drain the bladder, and Lone Star retractor (CooperSurgical™, Stafford, TX) is used for vaginal exposure. As previously described, the epithelium at the posterior forchette is excised and a midline incision is made in the posterior vagina. Vaginal flaps are created with lateral dissection toward the levator ani muscles. Care is taken to avoid rectal injury. The dissection is carried superiorly and posteriorly exposing the pararectal space to the level of the sacrospinous ligament bilaterally. At this point, plication of the rectovaginal fascia can be performed if desired, but this step is not mandatory.

Four-millimeter incisions are made at the skin 3 cm lateral and 3 cm posterior to the anus bilaterally. The cannula-equipped guide is placed into the incision and advanced to the posterior aspect of the sacrospinous ligament 3–4 cm medial to the ischial spine. The index finger of the non-dominant hand should ensure that as the guide is passed it stays posterior to the plane of the levator ani and lateral to the rectum. The guide is then passed through the ligament and the cannula is removed keeping the guide in place. The retrieval guide is passed down the cannula and brought through the vaginal dissection. The retrieval device is affixed to the arms of the mesh provided in the Prolift kit. The retrieval device is withdrawn, advancing the mesh arms from the posterior dissection, through the sacrospinous ligament and out toward the 4 mm skin incision. The mesh is tensioned at the level of the skin to eliminate redundancy or folding and the excess mesh is excised and the cannulas are removed. The lateral aspects of the mesh are sutured to the superior surface of the levator ani muscles to ensure proper positioning and the vaginal incision is closed.

In a large multicenter retrospective study, Abdel-Fattah and Ramsay reported on 70 women who underwent posterior compartment repair with the Prolift™ kit [23]. They reported 3-month outcomes and noted cure, Baden-Walker grade 1 or less, in 97 % of patients. There were five cases (7 %) of vaginal mesh exposures that all required mesh excision. In a study with 12-month follow-up, Lo noted that in combination prolapse cases repaired with anterior and posterior Prolift™ kits, there was a 95 % rate of success which was defined as POP-Q stage 1 or less recurrent prolapse [24]. Two patients developed recurrent rectoceles; they were both POP-Q grade II.

Apogee™, AMS® (Minnetonka, MN). The Apogee™ kit uses either a piece of IntePro® Lite™ prolene mesh or InteXen® LP™ cross-linked porcine dermis. Patient set up and exposure with the Lone Star (CooperSurgical™, Stafford, TX) retractor is the same as described with the other kits. As previously described, epithelium at the posterior forchette is excised and a midline incision is made in the posterior vagina to the apex of the rectocele. Vaginal flaps are created with lateral dissection toward the levator ani muscles. Care is taken to avoid rectal injury. The dissection is carried superiorly and posteriorly exposing the pararectal space to the level of the sacrospinous ligament bilaterally. At this point, plication of the rectovaginal fascia can be performed if desired, but this step is not mandatory.

Four-millimeter incisions are made at the skin 3 cm lateral and 3 cm posterior to the anus bilaterally. With the handle of the trocar pointed at the 12 o'clock position the trocar tip is advanced from the skin incision, below the levator ani muscles toward the ischial spine. One centimeter distal to the ischial spine the trocar handle is turned and the trocar tip is brought through the levator ani muscle. This procedure is repeated on the contralateral side. The mesh arms are connected to the trocar tip and the tip is then brought back to the level of the skin incision. Tension on the mesh arms is adjusted so the mesh or biologic used is free of redundancy and folding. The middle part of the superior portion of the graft is sutured to the vaginal apex. The excess mesh arms are trimmed at the skin and the vaginal epithelium is closed.

In a series of 195 patients who underwent Apogee™ kit for posterior compartment repair with IntePro® mesh, Lukban et al. reported that the success rate at a mean follow-up of 10.9 months was 96 % [25]. Success was defined as POP-Q grade I or less recurrent posterior wall prolapse. In a multicenter review, Abdel-Fattah and Ramsay [23] found a 94 % cure rate at 3 months in 30 patients treated with Apogee™. As mentioned previously, cure was defined as Baden-Walker grade 0 or I prolapse.

Posterior Elevate®, AMS® (Minnetonka, MN). Like the Apogee kit, the Posterior Elevate kit uses either a piece of IntePro® Lite™ prolene mesh or InteXen® LP™ cross-linked porcine dermis. Patient set up and exposure are the same as previous described. An elliptical portion of the posterior forchette epithelium is excised. Vaginal flaps are created toward the levator ani muscle. The dissection is carried superoposteriorly until the sacrospinous ligaments are palpable. At this point two apical sutures are placed with 3-0 vicryl suture. The tined arms are placed into the sacrospinous ligament and the graft is secured to the tined arms. The preplaced apical sutures are then passed through the superior portion of the graft to provide apical support. The graft is then advanced along the tined mesh arms toward the sacrospinous ligament and locked into place. The excess mesh arms are excised and lateral sutures are placed from the graft to the levator ani laterally to allow the graft to lay flat. The vaginal epithelium is then closed. At the time of this review, published outcomes on the Posterior Elevate® are lacking.

Pinnacle®, Boston Scientific (Natick, MA). The Pinnacle® kit provides a prolene mesh-based kit for posterior prolapse repair that uses the Capio® (Boston Scientific) needle driver for sacrospinous fixation. Once positioned and prepped, an ellipse of the posterior forchette is excised and this is carried into a midline vaginal dissection creating flaps laterally toward the levator ani muscles. Dissection is continued entering the pararectal space until the sacrospinous ligament is palpable bilaterally. A 3-0 vicryl suture is placed in the rectovaginal septum at the apex of the incision. The Capio® needle driver is used to deliver the mesh arms of the Pinnacle® kit through the sacrospinous ligament a finger breadth medial to the ischial spine. The preplaced apical suture is affixed to the mesh and the mesh arms are advanced until the graft is appropriately tensioned. 3-0 vicryl sutures are used to affix the lateral portions of the mesh to the levator ani muscles and excess mesh is trimmed. The vaginal incision is then closed. At the time of this review, published outcomes on the Pinnacle® kit are lacking.

Laparoscopic or Robotic-Assisted-Laparoscopic Rectocele Repairs

With the widespread use of the vaginal approach, laparoscopic rectocele repairs are relatively uncommon procedures. Although classified as a minimally invasive approach, laparoscopic repair does involve entering the peritoneal cavity and may be considered difficult to perform as it involves laparoscopic suturing and a potentially difficult exposure. The advent of the da Vinci robot (Intuitive Surgical®, Sunnyvale, CA) has allowed for improved visualization and easier suturing; however, as a stand-alone procedure, laparoscopic rectocele repair is rarely done.

For laparoscopic or robotic cases the patient is positioned in the low lithotomy position so that vaginal access is maintained once general endotracheal anesthesia is induced. Once prepared, access to the peritoneal cavity is gained and ports are placed. The cuff of the vagina is identified with the aid of a vaginal dilator. The dilator is then used to displace the cuff of the vagina anteriorly toward the umbilicus and an incision is made in the peritoneum overlying the vaginal cuff. With a combination of sharp and blunt dissection the posterior vaginal wall is dissected off of the rectovaginal septum and the rectum. In certain cases identification of the rectum is facilitated by placement of a betadine-soaked kerlex into the rectum at the start of the case. The dissection is carried down to the perineal body.

If placed, the rectal kerlex is removed and a vicryl suture is used to reapproximate the perineal body to the rectovaginal fascia. At this point, specific defects in the rectovaginal fascia or its lateral connections are repaired. Another approach involves a running plication of the rectovaginal fascia. Next, figure-of-eight sutures are placed in the levator ani muscles and they are bought together in the midline reinforcing the repair. Care should be taken to avoid painful ridges that can develop with aggressive repair. Introital width should also be assessed during the case to ensure that the posterior forchette of the vagina is not overly narrowed; the introitus should allow the passage of two fingers comfortably or three fingers snuggly.

Modifications to this procedure have been made to include mesh. Lee and colleagues report a method of laparoscopic prolene-augmented mesh repair. In this procedure, mesh is placed in the dissected bed between the vagina and the rectovaginal septum. It is placed flat and sutured laterally with permanent suture to the levator ani muscles. The superior-most portion is fixed to the uterosacral ligaments in the same fashion. The mesh is then retroperitonealized [26].

Transanal Repairs: Stapled Transanal Rectal Resection

In an attempt to minimize the risks of dyspareunia, wound complications, and rectocele recurrence, Longo described the stapled transanal rectal resection (STARR) as a means of rectocele repair in 2004 [27]. Rather than augmenting support of the rectovaginal fascia, the STARR procedure focuses on reducing the bulging rectocele.

Prior to the procedure the patients undergo a mechanical colon preparation with an enema and are given preoperative antibiotics covering colonic bacterial flora. After the induction of spinal or general anesthetic the patient is positioned in the Lloyd-Davis position (Trendelenburg position with the legs apart). A transparent anuscope is inserted into the anus and secured to the skin. Purse-string sutures are placed in the redundant, prolapsing rectum. A circular hemorrhoidectomy stapler (Ethicon®, Somerville, NJ) is fired along the anterior rectum, incorporating the mucosa, submucosa, and rectal wall, while excluding the posterior rectum. The procedure is repeated on the posterior rectal wall, but only incorporating the mucosa and submucosa.

At a mean follow-up of 24 months 95 % of patients treated for rectocele or intussusception were clinically and radiographically free of recurrence [8]. In a retrospective review, comparing STARR to traditional transvaginal rectocele repair, the STARR procedure had less blood loss and a faster operating time when compared to transvaginal rectocele repair, but a significantly higher complication rate (61 % vs. 19 %) [9]. Recurrence rates, failure rates, and postoperative dyspareunia rates were not statistically different [9]. Complications in the STARR group include rectal bleeding, rectal pressure/tenesmus, fecal incontinence, diarrhea, pruritus ani, rectal pain, and Clostridium difficile infection [9]. This and other methods of transanal repairs are not indicated in high rectoceles or rectoceles associated with enteroceles. When compared to the traditional vaginal approach, transanal repairs are associated with less pain [28].

Conclusion

Rectoceles are the result of defects in posterior vaginal wall support. The exact mechanisms that lead to posterior vaginal weakness are not clear, although advancing age, defecation disorders, connective tissue disorders, and childbirth injury may play a role. Although many patients with rectoceles are asymptomatic, symptomatic patients with rectoceles may present with pelvic pressure, pelvic bulge, pelvic pain, dyspareunia, and/or difficulty with defecation.

The indications for surgery vary from surgeon to surgeon. Common surgical procedures for rectocele repairs include traditional posterior colporrhaphy, plication of rectal fascia with levator reconstruction, site-specific defect repair, graft-augmented repairs, and kit-based repairs. Transanal approaches and endoscopic approaches to rectocele repair are described, but are less commonly done. Although data exists on the effectiveness of these procedures, true long-term data with report of functional and anatomic outcomes is lacking. Prospective, randomized trials with long-term follow-up are needed to compare these surgical procedures with regard to patient outcome and complication.

References

1. Kleeman SD, Westermann C, Karram MM. Rectoceles and the anatomy of the posterior vaginal wall: revisited. Am J Obstet Gynecol. 2005;193(6):2050–5.
2. Hsu Y, Lewicky-Gaupp C, De Lancy JQ. Posterior compartment anatomy as seen in MI and 3-D reconstruction from asymptomatic nulliparas. Am J Obstet Gynecol. 2008;198(6):651.e1–7.
3. Leffler KS, Thompson JR, Cundiff GW, Buller JL, Burrows LJ, Schon Ybarra MA. Attachment of the rectovaginal septum to the pelvic sidewall. Am J Obstet Gynecol. 2001;185(1):41–3.
4. Segal JL, Kirram MM. Evaluation and management of rectoceles. In: Vasavada A, Sand R, editors. Female urology, urogynecology and voiding dysfunction. New York: Marcel Dekker, Chapter 52. 2005, p. 735–59.
5. Swift S, Woodman P, O'Boyle A, Kahn M, Valley M, Bland D, Wang W, Schaffer J. Pelvic organ support study (POSST): the distribution, clinical definition, and epidemiologic condition of pelvic organ support defects. Am J Obstet Gynecol. 2005;192(3):795–806.
6. Olsen AL, Smith VJ, Berkstrom JO, et al. Epidemiology of surgically managed pelvic organ prolapse and urinary incontinence. Obstet Gynecol. 1997;89(4):501–6.
7. Ellerkmann RM, Cundiff GW, Melick CF, Nihira MA, Leffler K, Bent AE. Correlation of symptoms with location and severity of pelvic organ prolapse. Am J Obstet Gynecol. 2001;185(6):1332–7.
8. Arroyo A, Vicente F, Serrano P, Sanchez A, Miranda E, Navarro JM, Candela F, Calpena R. Evaluation of the stapled transanal rectal resection technique with tow staplers in the treatment of obstructive defecation syndrome. J Am Coll Surg. 2007;204(1):56–63.

9. Harris MA, Ferrara A, Gallagher J, DeJesus S, Williamson P, Larach S. Stapled transanal rectal resection versus transvaginal rectocele repair for treatment of obstructive defecation syndrome. Dis Colon Rectum. 2009;52(4):592–7.
10. Wolf JS, Bennet CJ, Dmochowski RR, et al. Best practice statement on urologic surgery antimicrobial prophylaxis. J Urol. 2008;179(4):1379–90.
11. Turner GM, Cole SE, Brook JH. The efficacy of graduated compression stocking in the prevention of deep vein thrombosis after major gynecologic surgery. Br J Obstet Gynecol. 1984;91(6):588–91.
12. Abramov Y, Gandhi S, Goldberg RP, et al. Site-specific rectocele repair compared with standard posterior colporrhaphy. Obstet Gynecol. 2005;105: 314–8.
13. Paraiso MF, Barber MD, Muir TW, Walters MD. Rectocele repair: a randomized trial of three surgical techniques including graft augmentation. Am J Obstet Gynecol. 2006;195(6):1762–71.
14. Kahn MA, Stanton SL. Posterior colporrhaphy: its effects on bowel and sexual function. Br J Obstet Gynaecol. 1997;104:82–6.
15. Richarson AC. The rectovaginal septum revisited: its relationship to rectocele and its importance in rectocele repair. Clin Obstet Gynecol. 1993;36(4):976–83.
16. Mellgren A, Anzén B, Nilsson BY, Johansson C, Dolk A, Gillgren P, Bremmer S, Holmström B. Results of rectocele repair: a prospective study. Dis Colon Rectum. 1995;38(1):7–13.
17. Porter WE, Steele A, Walsh P, Kohli N, Karram MM. The anatomic and functional outcomes of defect specific rectocele repairs. Am J Obstet Gynecol. 1999; 181(6):1353–8.
18. Garcia SL, Ramirez DL, Rey JR, Calvo JF, Iglesias BR, Calvo AO. Complications of polypropylene mesh for the treatment of female pelvic disorders. Arch Esp Urol. 2011;64(7):620–8.
19. Hurtado EA, Bailey HR, Reeves KO. Rectal erosion of synthetic mesh used in posterior colporrhaphy requiring surgical removal. Int Urogynecol J Pelvic Floor Dysfunct. 2007;18(12):1499–501.
20. Feiner B, Maher C. Vaginal mesh contraction: definition, clinical presentation, and management. Obstet Gynecol. 2010;115(2 Pt 1):325–30.
21. Kobashi KC, Leach GE, Frederick R, et al. Initial experience with rectocele repair using nonfrozen cadaveric fascia lata interposition. Urology. 2005;66:1203–7; discussion 1207–8.
22. Patel BN, Smith JJ, Badlani GH. Minimizing the cost of surgical correction of stress urinary incontinence and prolapse. Urology. 2009;74(4):762–4.
23. Abdel-Fattah M, Ramsay I. Retrospective multicenter study of the new minimally invasive mesh repair devices for pelvic organ prolapse. BJOG. 2008; 115(1):22–30.
24. Lo TS. One year outcome of concurrent anterior and posterior transvaginal mesh surgery for treatment of advanced urogenital prolapse: case series. J Minim Invasive Gynecol. 2010;17(4):473–9.
25. Lukban JC, Beyer RD, Moore RD. Incidence of extrusion following type 1 polypropylene mesh 'kit' repairs in correction of pelvic organ prolapse. Obstet Gynecol Int. 2012;2012:354897.
26. Lee HK, Lee YS, Koo TB, Cho YL, Park IS. Laparoscopic management of uterine prolapse with cystocele and rectocele using 'Gynemesh PS'. J Laparoendosc Adv Surg Tech A. 2008;18(1):93–8.
27. Longo A. Obstructed defecation because of rectal pathologies. Novel surgical treatment: stapled transanal rectal resection (STARR). Presented at the international colorectal disease symposium, Fort Lauderdale, FL, June 7Y11, 2008.
28. Arnold MW, Stewart WR, Aguitar PS. Rectocele repair: four years' experience. Dis Colon Rectum. 1990;33:684–7.

Apical Repairs

20

Leon N. Plowright and G. Willy Davila

Presentation and Symptoms

Pelvic organ prolapse (POP) is a common condition affecting adult women. Epidemiologic studies suggest the lifetime risk of prolapse or incontinence surgery is between 7 and 19 % [1]. The most common complaint reported by women with genital prolapse is a sensation of a vaginal bulge. Women may also report pelvic discomfort or pressure and may have associated voiding or defecatory dysfunction. Well established risk factors for POP development include pregnancy, vaginal delivery, increased parity, age, increased body mass index, race, chronic diseases associated with increased intra-abdominal pressure, postmenopausal status, and previous hysterectomy.

POP can be categorized as an anterior or posterior vaginal wall defect, an enterocele, or a vaginal vault support defect. While listed separately, these sites of vaginal laxity are often found in combination. There is growing evidence in the literature that apical support is the key element in maintaining normal vaginal anatomy [2–4]. Given such evidence, it is of the utmost importance that patients being evaluated for POP undergo a proper inspection of the vaginal apex as identifying the sites of apical support can be challenging. In particular, any woman with an exteriorized, large cystocele should be assumed to also have some degree of apical support weakness, until proven otherwise on careful pelvic exam. Any degree of support weakness of the vaginal vault should be addressed at the time of anterior or posterior POP surgery.

Anatomy

Our current working understanding of pelvic organ support is that it requires a complex interplay of adequately functioning pelvic floor muscles, and intact ligamentous support and endopelvic fascia. In the early 1990s DeLancey popularized the concept of levels of pelvic support. Level I support encompasses the vaginal apex and cervix which are held in place by the surrounding endopelvic connective tissue which includes the cardinal and uterosacral ligaments. Level II support refers to the mid-vagina which is supported by the lateral connective-tissue attachments to the levator muscles while Level III support involves the distal connective-tissue attachments of the urethra to the pubic bone and levator muscle support to the distal hymen [5].

L.N. Plowright, M.D.
Department of Gynecology, Cleveland Clinic Florida, Weston, FL 33331, USA

G.W. Davila, M.D. (✉)
Department of Gynecology, Cleveland Clinic Florida, 2950 Cleveland Clinic Boulevard, Weston, FL 33331, USA
e-mail: DAVILAG@ccf.org

G.H. Badlani (ed.), *Minimally Invasive Therapy for Urinary Incontinence and Pelvic Organ Prolapse*, Current Clinical Urology, DOI 10.1007/978-1-4939-0008-4_20,

When we take a closer look at the supportive structures of the apex it becomes evident as to why it is such an integral component of vaginal support. The principal ligaments involved in cervical/vault support are the uterosacral and cardinal ligaments. The uterosacral ligaments are fibromuscular tissue bands extending from the apex to the sacrum while the cardinal ligaments extend laterally from the apex to the pelvic sidewall adjacent to the ischial spines. The coalescence of both ligaments is often referred to as the uterosacral–cardinal ligament complex. The cervix, if present, also acts as an attachment site for connective tissue and ligamentous fibers from the uterosacral-ligament complex. Women who have undergone a complete hysterectomy lose this pivotal supportive structure, which often leads to vaginal laxity and eventual prolapse [6]. It is thus crucial to methodically reattach the apical supports to the vaginal cuff during closure once the uterus is removed at the time of hysterectomy—regardless of the route utilized.

Another important supportive component to consider is endopelvic fascia. This supportive structure is the fibromuscular tissue layer that underlies the vaginal epithelium as an integral component of the vaginal wall. Endopelvic fascia can be found supporting the entire vaginal canal, extending from the apex to the perineum. A tear in this layer, whether anterior or posterior, typically presents as a detachment of endopelvic fascia from the apex resulting in subsequent herniation and subsequent downward displacement of the affected vaginal segment. This displacement can place undue strain on the vaginal apex and weaken apical support.

Proper understanding of the anatomy of normal vault support is therefore important in surgical planning. The complexity of vaginal support is being better understood today using a variety of tools including ultrasound and other imaging modalities. Current research is being focused on using modeling techniques, physics, and basic sciences to explain how the coalescence of ligaments, fascia, and neuromuscular tissue interact to maintain pelvic support.

Physical Examination and Diagnosis

In order to achieve successful restoration of pelvic anatomy, proper identification of vault support defects is as important as understanding normal vault support anatomy. Even for the experienced surgeon, this can represent a challenging endeavour. The key is a systematic and careful pelvic examination. Tools that may be used in evaluating apical support include a bivalve speculum and a right angle or Sims retractor.

The approach to vaginal vault assessment is dependent on the presence or absence of the uterus. When the uterus is present it is important to make the distinction between vault prolapse and cervical hypertrophy, as the cervix may be exteriorized while vault support is intact. First, the posterior blade of a speculum may be inserted into the posterior fornix, elevating the vault to its fullest extent. The patient is then asked to Valsalva while the speculum is slowly being removed. If a defect of vaginal vault support is present, descent of the uterus will be noted. Reinsertion of the speculum will re-suspend the uterus. If the vault is well supported the uterus and cervix will remain in place. The degree of apical prolapse can be measured using the POP-Q system (the difference between TVL and point D).

In a previously hysterectomized woman, the apical portion of the vagina is represented by a dense band of scar tissue horizontally across the top of the vagina. This represents the vaginal cuff. The previous apical attachments of the uterosacral–cardinal ligament complex are noted by "dimples" located at the lateral edges of vaginal cuff. These landmarks can be challenging to identify at times. Placing the posterior blade of the right-angle speculum to support the anterior vaginal wall, while using the index and middle finger of the right hand to support the posterior vaginal wall, the dimples can usually be identified. The patient is then asked to Valsalva and the degree of apical prolapse quantified. In some instances, complete evaluation of the vaginal vault requires an exam in the standing position.

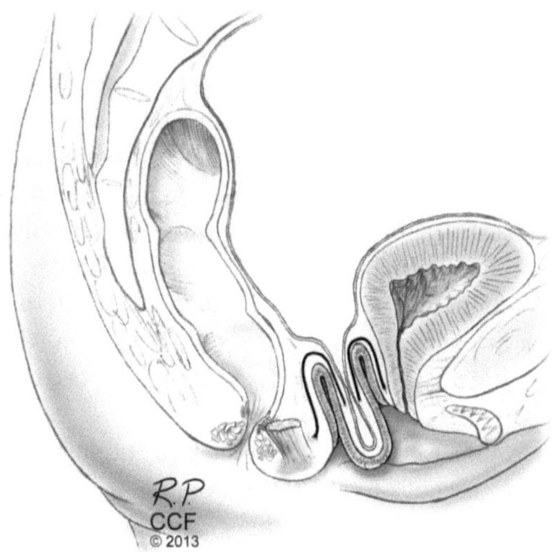

Fig. 20.1 Vaginal vault prolapse with associated anterior and posterior fascial tears off the apex (*dark lines*). (Courtesy of the Cleveland Clinic Foundation)

In addition, a bimanual and/or rectal examination may also be helpful in identifying the presence of an enterocele. An adequate evaluation of the vaginal vault cannot be overemphasized as this dictates surgical planning [6].

Assessing anterior and posterior vaginal wall support is then performed, with a focus on identifying fascial tears which require repair (Fig. 20.1). These are usually seen as areas where normal vaginal rugation is absent—representing separation of the endopelvic fascia from the vaginal cuff, lateral attachments, or perineal body.

There are many effective approaches to restoring apical vaginal support. These include vaginal as well as laparoscopic/robotic approaches. Choice of the best approach for an individual patient should be based on a variety of individual factors as well as surgeon expertise (Table 20.1). Patient age may dictate anesthetic approach preference and as a consequence a choice for a vaginal approach under regional anesthesia for an elderly patient in order to avoid postoperative cognitive problems. A vaginal depth greater than 9 cm is unlikely to be maintained with a vaginal approach to apical prolapse—and may lead to a preference for an abdominal approach if sexual function is of key importance. Recurrent POP, especially when associated with a large cystocele, may dictate the need for mesh or biologic graft augmentation in order to optimize success.

Table 20.1 Factors in deciding the approach to vault suspension surgery

1. Presence of the uterus
2. Cervical hypertrophy
3. Vaginal length
4. Sexual activity
5. Previous POP surgeries
6. Previous abdominal surgeries
7. Presence of vaginal atrophy
8. Needed concomitant prolapse/incontinence procedures
9. Patient age
10. Patient-associated morbidities
11. Patient's degree of physical activity

Traditional surgical options for vault prolapse include vaginal and abdominal approaches. Minimally invasive options have been developed in an effort to improve surgical outcomes while reducing hospitalization and recovery times. Vaginal surgery—the ultimate natural orifice surgery—is appropriate for most postmenopausal women, but requires special training and expertise. Endoscopic approaches require prolonged general anesthesia and steep Trendelenburg positioning, and thus may be more appropriate for the younger patient. Since most techniques for apical support restoration are proven to be effective, individualization of the approach based on a patient's specific functional and anatomic characteristics is the key consideration [7]. Of the many apical suspension procedures described, the following have acceptable published outcomes and are the most commonly used.

Minimal Invasive Surgery for Apical Prolapse

Laparoscopy

Laparoscopic techniques are typically an adaptation of the open abdominal surgical approaches used for vault prolapse. In order to attain equivalent outcomes, the surgeon must be proficient and experienced.

Open abdominal sacral colpopexy is considered to be gold standard for vault prolapse repair. Multiple publications have demonstrated its high efficacy and durability. Success rate is reported as ranging from 78 to 100 % [8]. The laparoscopic adaptation does not differ significantly from the open technique. In fact, laparoscopic sacral colpopexy is said to have comparable clinical outcomes [9].

One landmark study demonstrating this was a comparative cohort study done by Paraiso et al. [9]. This study investigated the efficacy and safety of laparoscopic versus open sacral colpopexy. While they concluded that the operative time was greater in the laparoscopic group the estimated blood loss and the hospital stay were significantly less in the laparoscopic group. In addition, complications and need for re-operation were the same between groups. Paraiso's findings were upheld by a similar study in 2007 comparing laparoscopic and abdominal sacrocolpopexy for vault prolapse. In this study, Hsiao et al. compared 25 patients who underwent laparoscopic sacrocolpopexy to 22 patients who underwent open abdominal sacrocolpopexy. Again, the operative time was longer for the laparoscopic group but the mean estimated blood loss and length of hospital stay were significantly more for the open abdominal approach. The anatomical success rate at 5.9 months was 100 % for the laparoscopic approach and 95 % success at 11 months for the open approach [10]. With the recent decline in vaginal mesh use, there has been a resurgence of interest in the performance of laparoscopic sacrocolpopexy. Tools to facilitate performance of this technique will certainly become available in the near future, further increasing its popularity.

Does sacrocolpopexy require the use of synthetic mesh? This question has been asked by many patients who prefer to not have any synthetic mesh implanted, whether vaginally or abdominally. This question has been at least partially answered by studies performed by Culligan et al., looking at two biologic materials in an RCT study format. Processed fascia lata was found to be equivalent to polypropylene in terms of apical support with the only differences in POP staging being in the lower anterior points, which may have been affected by the performance of more anti-incontinence procedures [11]. Evaluating cross-linked porcine dermis in an RCT against polypropylene mesh, objective anatomic and clinical cure rates were similar at 12-month follow-up [12]. Thus, there are alternative available biologic materials for women who require a sacrocolpopexy and are opposed to receiving synthetic mesh.

Another laparoscopic procedure employed by some surgeons to elevate the vault is uterosacral ligament suspension. In this procedure the uterosacral ligaments are essentially sutured to the apex of the vagina thereby elevating the apex. A permanent suture is used for this purpose. In the literature there are several case series, retrospective trials, and some prospective studies. One study done in 2005 by Lin et al. reported on 133 laparoscopic uterosacral ligament vault suspensions. In their study, they found an 87 % anatomic success rate with a mean follow-up of 3.2 years [13]. Comparing laparoscopic uterosacral colpopexy at the time of vaginal hysterectomy to vaginal colpopexy, Rardin et al. found a higher recurrent symptomatic prolapse rate and increased risk of ureteral injury in the vaginal colpopexy group [14]. Though review of the literature revealed a variety of techniques used to suspend the uterus, taken together these studies make a strong case for laparoscopic uterosacral ligament suspension as a feasible safe and effective approach to treatment of vault prolapse.

Women requesting uterine sparing prolapse surgery may be candidates for sacrohysterocolpopexy or uterosacral ligament suspension. For this purpose, surgeons have employed a variety of laparoscopic techniques to re-suspend the vaginal vault [15]. The uterosacral ligaments can be plicated bilaterally from the level of the ischial spines to their insertion on the uterus. Diwan et al. reported on 25 patients who underwent the above procedure and were compared to 25 patients who underwent a total vaginal hysterectomy with vaginal vault suspension. There were a superior anatomic and clinical outcomes associated with laparoscopic uterosacral ligament uterine suspension compared to vaginal hysterectomy and vault suspension as demonstrated by a significant difference in points C and D, and the fact that three patients in the vaginal hysterectomy group required re-operation for recurrent prolapse [16]. These findings have been confirmed by several other articles in the literature making it a safe and effective option for women desiring uterine preservation [17, 18]. The use of permanent sutures is recommended, and the recent availability of barbed, self-fixating sutures has facilitated the performance of laparoscopic vault suspension surgery.

Robotics

Robotic surgery has rapidly emerged as a popular minimally invasive tool for prolapse repair. Robotic assistance adds yet another option to the minimally invasive armamentarium for apical POP. The use of robotics started to gain popularity in the early 2000s and today is a very popular component of the residency training curriculum. Due to its durability, robotic sacrocolpopexy is the most commonly performed robotic pelvic reconstructive procedure [19].

The first case series to evaluate the use of robotic-assisted laparoscopic sacrocolpopexy was published by DiMarco et al. [20]. They reported on 5 women who underwent the procedure, three with concomitant pubovaginal sling placement. The only complication encountered was associated with the sling placement. There was no recurrent, anterior, posterior, or vault prolapse at 4 months of follow-up. Since this study there have been several other case series and retrospective studies looking at anatomic and clinical outcomes. Robotic and laparoscopic surgery has demonstrated equivalent anatomic outcomes with shorter hospital stay and decreased blood loss when compared to open sacrocolpopexy [9, 21]. To date the only prospective randomized trial comparing conventional laparoscopy to robotic-assisted laparoscopic colpopexy was published in 2011 by Paraiso et al. The study was a single-center randomized controlled trial of women with stage 2–4 posthysterectomy vault prolapse. There were 38 women in the laparoscopic group and 40 women in the robotic group. Though both groups demonstrated equivalent surgical and functional outcomes 1 year after surgery, robotic-assisted sacrocolpopexy resulted in longer operating time, increased pain, and increased cost when compared to traditional laparoscopy [22]. Cost being an increasingly important consideration, cost-minimization analysis has demonstrated that open ASC is less expensive then laparoscopic, and the robotic approach exceeded the cost of both [23]. While more long-term surgical follow-up is needed to clarify the role of robotic surgery, preliminary data seems to endorse its use for certain indications, POP management being one of them. Surgeon experience is a key factor in optimizing outcomes and reducing morbidity. Recently, the safety and cost-effectiveness of robotic surgery have been brought into question by professional associations and the FDA. The dust is yet to settle on this novel MIS approach.

Vaginal Mesh

Over the last several years vaginal mesh kits have also grown in popularity as a minimally invasive alternative to traditional native tissue POP repairs. The purpose of the kits was to provide a durable, standardized, reproducible, and effective product that can be easily placed after adequate training. Through the use of pelvic landmarks and employing principles of tradition repairs these mesh kits are used to augment or replace conventional vaginal repairs.

The Apogee system (American Medical Systems, Minnetonka, MN) was the initial kit to be widely marketed. It requires a transperineal trocar passage to suspend the apex via a mesh bridge from ischial spine to ischial spine. As with traditional sacrospinous fixation, a posterior dissection is first performed to the level of the apex. The para-rectal space is entered and the ischial spine identified. An incision is made on each buttock, 3 cm lateral and 3 cm posterior to the anus. A trocar is passed through this incision just lateral to the rectum and exits anterior to the ischial spine and into the arcus tendineus fascia pelvis. This is done bilaterally. Next, each of the mesh arms is fastened to the tips of the trocars and pulled through the para-anal incisions. The graft is then attached to the apex and the vault elevated accordingly. Concomitant anterior and posterior colporrhaphy can be performed. The remainder of the graft is trimmed to size and sutured distally, just before the hymen. This kit comes as a composite with polypropylene mesh arms attached to a biologic graft or simply polypropylene material is used throughout [6]. Review of the literature reveals an objective success rate ranging from 81 to 100 % [24].

The Prolift kit (Gynecare), also a trocar-based kit for anterior, posterior, and apical prolapse management, went on to become the most popular kit based on sales volumes. Multiple studies demonstrated its success in anterior compartment prolapse when compared to native tissue repairs. It was also studied in the population of patients in whom a synthetic mesh may be most clearly indicated, those with recurrent prolapse. In this population, this mesh kit was associated with a significantly better anatomic result relative to native tissue repair, but subjective outcome was no different at 12 months. Mesh exposure rates in the synthetic group were 16.9 % [25]. This kit was removed from the market by the manufacturer in 2012. Multiple other trocar-based kits were available and continue to be marketed.

Novel mesh kits utilize direct internal fixation techniques, and are thus trocar-free. They include the Elevate (AMS), Uphold, and Pinnacle (Boston Scientific). The Elevate kit system (American Medical Systems, Minnetonka, MN) which comes in a composite biologic graft/polypropylene mesh or total polypropylene mesh requires dissection down to the level of the ischial spine and identification of the sacrospinous ligaments. Once identified, a trocar is used to deploy a fixation soft tissue anchor into the ligament to which the graft is attached. After attaching the graft to the apex, it is then elevated using a pusher and locking eyelets. In a similar fashion the Uphold (Boston Scientific, Natick, MA) kit suspends the apex by using the sacrospinous ligaments.

The recent public health announcement released in 2011 by the Food and Drug Administration again called into question the use of transvaginal mesh. This was a follow-up to a 2008 notification. The associated risk of erosion, pelvic pain, and other morbidities as well as the lack of data demonstrating superiority to native tissue repairs led to the requirement that manufacturers perform a prospective surveillance program in order to be able to continue to market their products. This process is projected to last 3 years and requires methodical data collection. Due to this scrutiny, multiple other kits have been taken off the market over the past year, and are therefore not mentioned in this discussion. Moving forward there will be more studies focused on not only the efficacy but also the complication profile of transvaginal mesh. It is unlikely that mesh kits will regain a significant market share once the FDA's 522 process is completed. It is very unclear what role mesh implanted via the vaginal route will have in future of POP surgery.

Native Tissue POP Repairs

Using a patient's endogenous support structures via the vaginal approach has been the leading principle followed by traditional surgical practice for POP. Due to the lack of tools to accurately report outcomes, most of the older surgical reports were subjective, short term, and in small case series. As a consequence, the true success rates were unclear. Due to the recent controversies surrounding vaginal mesh, there has been a large degree of interest in performing native tissue repairs, but with improved techniques relative to older reports.

For apical support, various structures are available to anchor the vaginal apex. Reaching the sacral promontory—as for a sacrocolpopexy—via a vaginal approach has not been achievable until the present time. Thus, all vaginal vault suspension procedures are performed with either unilateral or bilateral attachment to a firm pelvic structure. In general, the available structures are connected to the ischial spines—landmark body structures located along the

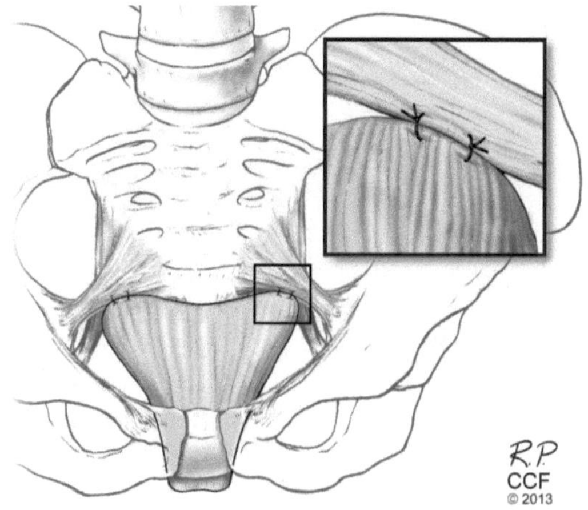

Fig. 20.2 Bilateral sacrospinous fixation maintains bilateral vaginal symmetry. (Courtesy of the Cleveland Clinic Foundation)

posterior lateral pelvis. The spines are located lateral to the site of cardinal ligament attachment to the cervix and thus are located along a physiological level in the pelvis. Successfully utilized support structures emanating from the ischial spine include the sacrospinous ligaments (thick bands extending to the sacrum), arcus tendineus fascia pelvis (extending laterally towards the pubic symphysis), and the ileococcygeus fascia (overlying the ileococcygeus muscle along the lateral pelvic sidewall, inferior to the arcus tendineus). These structures are readily accessible via a posterior or anterior pelvic dissection, and have been reported to allow effective apical support restoration by various fixation mechanisms. Among the accepted native tissue repair techniques for apical POP, the most commonly used ones are as follows:

Sacrospinous Ligament Fixation

Because these ligaments are predictably strong and easy to identify along the posterior margin of the para-rectal space, sacrospinous fixation is likely the most commonly performed minimally invasive native tissue apical suspension technique. The procedure was initially performed unilaterally on the patient's right side. It has now been reported in a bilateral configuration in order to maintain vaginal symmetry (Fig. 20.2). There is, however, no objective data to demonstrate superiority for either approach. One or two sutures, preferably permanent monofilament, are placed thru the ligament approximately 1–2 cm from the ischial spine, using one of a variety of available suture passers. The suture is then passed through the apical cuff scar tissue (or posterior cervix if a hysteropexy is being performed) and then tied, elevating the apex to the ligament. If a bilateral approach is performed, the procedure is repeated on the opposite side. Correction of anterior and/or posterior vaginal prolapse is usually required and can then be performed.

Complications of sacrospinous fixation include buttock pain and sciatic nerve pain if the fixation sutures are placed too deeply into the ligament, or distal to the ligament's inferior edge. Since the procedure deviates the vaginal axis somewhat horizontally relative to the physiologic axis, cystocele formation is a recognized consequence of this procedure. The resultant cystocele rate is >20 %, but typically asymptomatic, not requiring re-operation. Sacrospinous fixation has been compared to mesh kit repair in a randomized, controlled format, with better success rate for the mesh kit (POP recurrence 39.4 % vs. 16.9 %), but a 20.8 % erosion rate was identified with the mesh kit [26].

Uterosacral Ligament Suspension

Perhaps the most physiologic approach to vault suspension is to suspend the vault to the ligaments which originally gave support to the uterus and vaginal apex, the uterosacral ligaments. Attaching the vault to a more proximal site along these ligaments can maintain a normal vaginal axis. When this procedure is performed at the time of a vaginal hysterectomy it is commonly termed a McCall culdoplasty. When performed for posthysterectomy vault prolapse, it is termed a high uterosacral vault suspension. Neither term is exclusive for that application. In either case, the ligaments can be plicated in the midline and attached to the midpoint of the apex or each ligament can be attached to the ipsilateral apex (Fig. 20.3). There is no data to specify which is more effective. The success rate of this technique is very high, and both anterior and posterior vaginal fascial defects should be corrected at the same time [27]. The technique can be accomplished via an intraperitoneal or retroperitoneal approach, the former recently being more commonly used. When performed in a

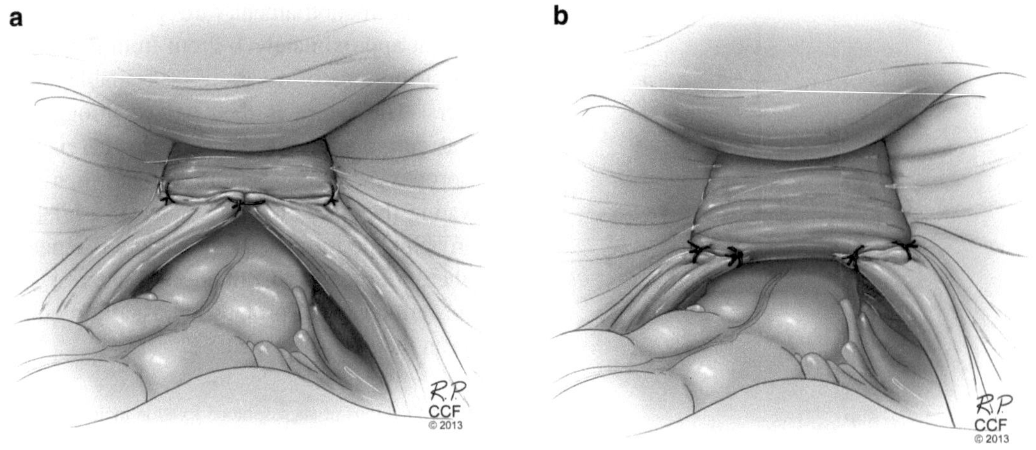

Fig. 20.3 Uterosacral ligament suspension can be performed with midline (**a**) or bilateral (**b**) fixation. (Courtesy of the Cleveland Clinic Foundation)

posthysterectomy scenario, it may be challenging to identify the ligaments, especially if the prolapse is large and the apex wide. Care must be taken to avoid ureteral kinking or ligation, as rates of 2–12 % have been reported. The sutures should never be placed anterior to the ischial spines, and intraoperative cystoscopy is mandatory to confirm ureteral patency. A more recently recognized risk is sacral root nerve entrapment during this procedure. Although the risk is only 1.6 %, this complication requires suture removal and thus jeopardizes the success of the surgery [28, 29].

Ileococcygeus Suspension

Utilizing the ileococcygeus fascia may be the safest means to achieve vault suspension. This support structure can be reached via a posterior vaginal dissection into the para-rectal space, identification of the ischial spine, and palpation of the fascia immediately below the arcus tendineus fascia pelvis. Permanent sutures can be placed through this fascia and attached to the ipsilateral vaginal apex. Acceptable success rates have been reported [30]. Vaginal depth may be difficult to maintain if the vagina has an original depth of >8 cm. Reported complication rates are very low as no major structures are located deep to the ileococcygeus fascia. This technique can be used as primary therapy, or as salvage therapy for a patient who underwent a unilateral sacrospinous fixation and weakness of the opposite apex is noted. In this scenario, a transmucosal ileococcygeus "hitch" can be performed with a monofilament suture.

Colpocleisis

Another minimally invasive surgery to address vault prolapse is a LeFort colpocleisis. This obliterative procedure was first described in 1877 by Leon LeFort. It is a minimal risk procedure requiring short operative time and can be performed under spinal or local anesthesia thereby decreasing anesthetic morbidity. Candidates for this type of surgery are elderly women who do not plan on having intercourse, and/or who may have significant medical comorbidities.

The surgical technique entails denuding rectangular segments of the anterior and posterior vaginal epithelium. The rectangles are sutured together in the midline from front to back, such that the middle portion of the vaginal canal is obliterated. A high perineoplasty is performed allowing the passage of only one finger into the vagina, exposing only the urethra. This procedure can be performed using the same technique regardless of the presence or absence of a uterus.

The largest published series confirmed the high success rate and satisfaction with this procedure [31]. We reported on 355 patients who underwent a LeFort colpocleisis. The mean age was 81.3 ± 5.3 years, and a mean follow-up of 45 weeks. Anatomic success rate and patient satisfaction were 98.1 % and 92.9 %, respectively. Using a protocol focused on regional anesthesia, careful preoperative clearance, and early ambulation, associated morbidity is minimal, despite the advanced age of these patients.

Summary

There are many safe and effective minimally invasive means for re-suspending a prolapsed vaginal apex. Individual patient characteristics should be considered primarily when selecting a surgical approach. Surgeon experience and comfort should also be realistically taken into account. As such, very active young woman for whom maintaining optimal sexual activity is important may best be served with a laparoscopic or robotic sacrocolpopexy, a postmenopausal woman may be optimally treated via a vaginal approach vault suspension, and an elderly woman who has not been, and will not be, sexually active with a colpocleisis.

Regardless of the approach, assessment of bladder function preoperatively, tissue preparation with local estrogen cream as indicated, and allowing unstressed healing during the early postoperative healing phase are all keys to optimizing surgical outcomes.

References

1. Cvach K, Dwyer P. Surgical management of pelvic organ prolapse: abdominal and vaginal approaches. World J Urol. 2012;30(4):471–7.
2. Rooney K, Kenton K, Mueller ER, et al. Advanced anterior vaginal wall prolapse is highly correlated with apical prolapse. Am J Obstet Gynecol. 2006; 195:1837–40.
3. Lowder JL, Park AJ, Ellison R, et al. The role of apical vaginal support in the appearance of anterior and posterior vaginal prolapse. Obstet Gynecol. 2008; 111:152–7.
4. Summers A, Winkle LA, Hussain HK, et al. The relationship between anterior and apical compartment support. Am J Obstet Gynecol. 2006;194:1438–43.
5. DeLancey JO. The anatomy of the pelvic floor. Curr Opin Obstet Gynecol. 1994;6:313–6.
6. Biller DH, Davila GW. Vaginal vault prolapse: identification and surgical options. Cleve Clin J Med. 2005;72 Suppl 4:S12–9.
7. Walters MD, Ridgeway B. Surgical treatment of vaginal apex prolapse. Obstet Gynecol. 2013;121: 354–74.
8. Nygaard I, McCreery R, Brubaker L, Connoly AM, et al. Abdominal sacrocolpopexy: a comprehensive review. Obstet Gynecol. 2004;104(4):805–23.
9. Paraiso MF, Walters MD, Rackley RR, Melek S, Hugney C. Laparoscopic and abdominal sacral colpopexies: a comparative cohort study. Am J Obstet Gynecol. 2005;192(5):1752–8.
10. Hsiao KC, Latchamsetty K, Grovier FE, et al. Comparison of laparoscopic and abdominal sacrocolpopexy for the treatment of vaginal vault prolapse. J Endourol. 2007;21(8):926–30.
11. Culligan PJ, Blackwell L, Goldsmith LJ, Graham CA, Rogers A, Heit MH. A randomized controlled trial comparing fascia lata and synthetic mesh for sacral colpopexy. Obstet Gynecol. 2005;106:29–37.
12. Culligan PJ, Salamon C, Priestly JL, Shariati A. Porcine dermis compared with polypropylene mesh for laparoscopic sacrocolpopexy. Obstet Gynecol. 2013;121:143–51.
13. Lin L, Phelps JY, Liu CY. Laparoscopic vaginal vault suspension using uterosacral ligaments: a review of 133 cases. J Minim Invasive Gynecol. 2005;12: 216–20.
14. Rardin C, Ereckson E, Sung V, Ward R, Myers D. Uterosacral colpopexy at the time of vaginal hysterectomy: comparison of laparoscopic and vaginal approaches. J Reprod Med. 2009;54:273–80.
15. Diwan A, Rardin CR, Kohli N. Uterine preservation during surgery for uterovaginal prolapse: a review. Int Urogynecol J. 2004;15:286–92.
16. Diwan A, Rardin C, Strohsnitter W, Weld A, Rosenblatt P, Kohli N. Laparoscopic uterosacral ligament uterine suspension compared with vaginal hysterectomy with vaginal vault suspension for uterovaginal prolapse. Int Urogynecol J. 2005;17:79–83.
17. Medina C, Tukacs P. Laparoscopic uterosacral uterine suspension: a minimally invasive technique for treating pelvic organ prolapse. J Minim Invasive Gynecol. 2006;13:472–5.
18. Uccella S, Ghezzi F, Bergamini V. Laparoscopic uterosacral ligaments plication for the treatment of uterine prolapse. Arch Gynecol Obstet. 2007;276: 225–9.
19. Visco AG, Advincula AP. Robotic gynecology surgery. Obstet Gynecol. 2008;112(6):1369–84.
20. DiMarco DS, Chow GK, Gettman MT, Elliot DS. Robotic-assisted laparoscopic sacrocolpopexy for the treatment of vaginal vault prolapse. Urology. 2004; 63(2):373–6.
21. Geller EJ, Siddique S, Wu J, Visco A. Comparison of short-term outcomes of robotic sacrocolpopexy. J Pelvic Med Surg. 2008;14(4):233–4.

22. Paraiso MF, Jelovsek JE, Frick A, Chen C, Barber M. Laparoscopic compared with robotic sacrocolpopexy for vaginal prolapse. Obstet Gynecol. 2011;118: 1005–13.
23. Judd JP, Siddiqui NY, Barnett JC, Visco AG, Havrilesky LJ, Wu JM. Cost-minimization analysis of robotic-assisted, laparoscopic, and abdominal sacrocolpopexy. J Minim Invasive Gynecol. 2010;17:493–9.
24. Fiener B, Jelovsek JE, Maher C. Efficacy and safety of transvaginal mesh kits in the treatment of prolapse of the vaginal apex: a systematic review. BJOG. 2009;116(1):15–24.
25. Withagen MI, Milani AL, den Boon J, Vervest HA, Vierhout ME. Trocar-guided mesh compared with conventional vaginal repair in recurrent prolapse. A randomized controlled trial. Obstet Gynecol. 2011; 117:242–50.
26. Halaska M, Maxova K, Sottner O, et al. A multicenter, randomized, prospective, controlled study comparing sacrospinous fixation and transvaginal mesh in the treatment of posthysterectomy vaginal vault prolapse. Am J Obstet Gynecol. 2012;207:301.e1–7.
27. Shull BL, Bachofen C, Coates KW, Kuehl TJ. A transvaginal approach to repair apical and other associated sites of pelvic organ prolapse with uterosacral ligaments. Am J Obstet Gynecol. 2000;183: 1365–73.
28. Chung CP, Kuehk TJ, Larsen WI, Yandell PM, Shull BL. Recognition and management of nerve entrapment pain after uterosacral ligament suspension. Obstet Gynecol. 2012;120:292–5.
29. Siddiqui NY, Mitchell TRT, Bentley RC, Weidner AC. Neural entrapment during uterosacral ligament suspension: an anatomic study of female cadavers. Obstet Gynecol. 2010;116:708–13.
30. Shull BT, Capen CV, Riggs MW, Kuehl TJ. Bilateral attachment of the vagina cuff to ileococcygeus fascia: an effective method for cuff suspension. Am J Obstet Gynecol. 1993;168: 1669–74.
31. Zebede S, Smith AL, Plowright L, Hegde A, Aguilar VC, Davila GW. Obliterative LeFort colpocleisis in a large group of elderly women. Obstet Gynecol. 2013;121:1–7.

21 POP Complications and Their Management

Denise Chow, Shlomo Raz, and Forrest Jellison

Pelvic organ prolapse (POP) is a condition affecting approximately 30 % of the population. Eleven to 19 % of the population will undergo surgery for symptomatic cure [1, 2]. Nearly 166,000 patients per year undergo surgical procedures for the treatment of POP [3]. With an expected increase in life expectancy, there will be an increasing number of patients who present with POP. It is forecasted that the total number of women who will undergo surgery for POP will increase from 166,000 in 2010 to 245,970 in 2050 based on rates of inpatient and outpatient surgeries and the growing US census data [3]. Predisposing factors contributing to the development of POP include age, parity, obesity, menopause, number of vaginal deliveries, chronic strain, genetics, and connective tissue disorders [4, 5]. There has been a higher reported predominance of POP amongst Caucasian women than in African American and Hispanic women [6]. Despite its prevalence, POP is a condition that many women are not aware of until they become symptomatic and seek medical attention. One population-based observational study revealed that 68–73 % of women greater than age 60 had stage 2 or greater prolapse [7]. Of those, 30 % had stage 3 POP. In women between the ages of 60 and 69, 68 % of women had POP-Q stage 2 or greater. In women greater than 70 years old, over 73 % had POP-Q stage 2 or greater. There are many women who have stage 2 or greater prolapse that are asymptomatic and do not seek surgical treatment. Therefore, a small number of those patients who become symptomatic will eventually seek treatment. Despite over half of patients having had POP, a significantly smaller number, approximately 11 %, will eventually undergo surgery for symptomatic prolapse. Adequate counseling regarding the expectations and inherent risks for POP surgery is necessary, as reoperation carries a high risk of up to 30 % [3].

D. Chow, M.D. • F. Jellison, M.D.
Division of Pelvic Medicine and Reconstructive Surgery, Department of Urology, University of California, Los Angeles, CA, USA

S. Raz, M.D. (✉)
Division of Pelvic Medicine and Reconstructive Surgery, UCLA School of Medicine, Los Angeles, CA, USA

Department of Urology, UCLA School of Medicine, 200 UCLA Medical Plaza, Suite 140, Los Angeles, CA, USA
e-mail: sraz@mednet.ucla.edu

General Complications

Patients must be informed of the potential risks associated with undergoing an elective procedure. All patients undergo informed consent prior to POP surgery. General risks including bleeding; pain; infection; injury to proximate organs such as the bladder, bowels, rectum, ureter, and urethra; injury to blood vessels; and injury to

G.H. Badlani (ed.), *Minimally Invasive Therapy for Urinary Incontinence and Pelvic Organ Prolapse*, Current Clinical Urology, DOI 10.1007/978-1-4939-0008-4_21,

nearby nerves are discussed with the patient. In addition, further counseling including risks for prolapse recurrence and for urinary incontinence are discussed with the patient. It is important to address the potential risks beforehand to ensure that patient's expectations are met postoperatively. A patient who experiences deviation from what she expects may perceive the surgery as a failure even though her prolapse is repaired. Therefore, it is important to set expectations early.

Evaluation of Patient After Complication

Patients who present with complications after a prolapse procedure require a comprehensive history and physical examination. If the patient is able to obtain operative notes, it is extremely helpful in the patient's management, as key components of the procedure, which may have been technically complex, can help with understanding the patient's condition. After a complication from prolapse surgery, the patient's primary complaint should be first and foremost addressed. There may be multiple presenting complaints (Table 21.1). The surgeon should focus the examination and diagnostic evaluation based on the patient's primary complaint. A complete history should be obtained including the specific onset and timing of symptoms relative to the surgery. Aggravating and alleviating factors should be elicited. A complete physical examination and focused genitourinary exam should be performed. If the patient complains of pain, the specific area needs to be completely evaluated. If it is pain or weakness in the leg, assessment of the leg and basic neurologic evaluation should be performed. Each vaginal compartment needs to be closely examined. Evaluation of tissue quality and evidence of mesh-related issues should be noted.

In addition to a physical and genital examination, additional diagnostic evaluation may be available. Some centers have employed the use of the translabial ultrasound (TLUS) for the evaluation of mesh-related complications. As mesh is not visible on CT scan or MRI, utilization of TLUS allows the characteristics of the mesh to be visualized in 2D and 3D. Characteristics such as residual segments, fragmentation, folding, proximity to the bladder neck, and depth of placement can be visualized. We have found this modality especially useful for patients who have undergone prior excisional attempts and who have residual fragments of mesh in place; this modality can also be useful where we suspect the proximity of the mesh may penetrate into bladder or urethra and consequently require reconstruction. TLUS is particularly helpful in visualizing remnant pieces of mesh and helps preoperative surgical planning and patient counseling regarding the potential risks and outcome. It can also be used to rule out any evidence of mesh if the patient does not have an operative note or does not recall if mesh was placed. Other anatomic findings visible on TLUS are urethral mobility and anterior compartment prolapse.

In this chapter, we will discuss transvaginal, transabdominal, and mesh-augmented POP-related complications. We will seek to (1) define the complications of prolapse surgery in general and by compartment, (2) define complications by mesh, and (3) offer ways to treat complication from POP surgery.

General Complications

Lower Urinary Tract Complications

Lower urinary tract (LUT) injuries during benign gynecologic surgeries are rare. During prolapse surgery for the anterior and apical compartments, the LUT is in close proximity and thus at risk for injury. If these injuries are not recognized intraoperatively, patients may develop symptoms of unexplained postoperative pain, fever, malaise, peritonitis, or ileus. They may be associated with loss of renal function, prolonged catheter drainage, urinary tract infections (UTIs),

Table 21.1 Classifying complications

Vagina	Lower urinary tract	Bowel or rectal	Skin/musculoskeletal/neurological
Vaginal bleeding	Urinary obstruction (a) Urethral (b) Ureteric	Fistula (a) Rectovaginal (b) Enterovaginal	Skin infection (a) Cutaneous sinus tract (b) Abscess (c) Labial or suprapubic cellulitis
Vaginal discharge	Urethral incontinence (a) Stress (b) Positional	Mesh erosion (a) Rectum (b) Small bowel	Pain (a) Suprapubic (b) Hip/pelvic/sacrum (c) Lower extremity
Vaginal infection	Bladder incontinence (a) De novo OAB (b) Worsening OAB (c) Overflow	Defecatory dysfunction (a) Diarrhea (b) Obstructive (c) Defecation (d) Constipation (e) Stool urgency (f) Stool incontinence	Subcutaneous (a) Hematoma (b) Seroma
Recurrent prolapse	Fistula (a) Urethral (b) Vesicovaginal (c) Ureteral	Bowel obstruction	Neurological: with or without neurological deficit (a) Sciatic pain (b) Pudendal (c) Ilioinguinal (d) Femoro-cutaneous
Dyspareunia/vaginal pain	Urethral mesh erosion Bladder mesh erosion	Perineal abscess	
Vaginal stenosis/shortening	Recurrent urinary tract infections		
Mesh exposure/extrusion/ intraepithelial infiltration	Stones		

ureterovaginal or vesicovaginal fistulas, and a consequent return to the operating room may be warranted. A systematic review was performed [8] from 1966 to 1998 to examine the frequency of LUT injuries after major benign gynecologic surgery. The overall frequency of bladder injury was 2.6–10.4 per 1,000; overall frequency of ureteral injury was 1.6–6.2 per 1,000. In cases where routine cystoscopy was performed, there was a higher rate of recognition, and 90 % of unsuspected ureteral injuries and 85 % of unsuspected bladder injuries were identified and managed successfully intraoperatively. About 70 % of recognized ureteral injuries were repaired by the release of a suture. However, when injuries are not recognized intraoperatively, patients may return with findings of a urinary fistula and need for operation.

Bladder Injury

Bladder perforations are rare during benign gynecologic procedures. One study [9] reported a 0.5 % rate of bladder perforation in patients with anterior colporrhaphy versus 3.5 % in mesh-augmented repairs. In benign gynecology evaluating hysterectomies, another study [10] reported that the incidence of bladder injury was highest in patients undergoing laparoscopic-assisted hysterectomy (LAH) and vaginal hysterectomy (VH), 13.8 per 1,000 and 13.1 per 1,000, respectively. Total abdominal hysterectomy, subtotal hysterectomy, and radical hysterectomy had a lower risk of bladder injury. An unrecognized intraoperative bladder injury may lead to a vesicovaginal fistula. In mesh-augmented repairs, bladder erosion due to unrecognized penetration may be present and will be further discussed later in this chapter. Performing intraoperative cystoscopy is essential during cystocele repair. Recognized bladder injuries may be closed in two layers with absorbable suture. Injection of indigo carmine or methylene blue may be used to test for leakage and to ensure water-tight closure. A Martius flap is not required unless there is a concern for a high risk of vesicovaginal fistula, for instance in a patient who has had radiation to the pelvis. We do not advocate the use of mesh in the anterior compartment after recognition of a bladder injury. The Foley catheter should be left in place for 7–10 days and some may consider performing a cystogram prior to removal of the Foley catheter.

Ureteral Injury

Patients who undergo anterior and apical repairs should undergo evaluation for ureteral patency, as there is a risk for ureteral injury. Ureteral injury during hysterectomy was higher during LAH [11] and less likely recognized [10] versus open hysterectomy. The incidence of ureteral injury was much lower during VH at 0.7 per 1,000, and routine cystoscopy is not recommended unless there is a high index of suspicion. Cystoscopy with the use of indigo carmine may be administered, and the ureteral orifices may be examined for efflux to ensure ureteral patency, ruling out ureteral obstruction. If injury is suspected a guide wire or 5-French open-ended ureteral catheter may be passed. If it passes smoothly and subsequent efflux is visualized, no injury is present. If fluoroscopy is available, retrograde instillation of contrast may be placed up the ureteral orifice to assess the ureter. If live fluoroscopy is not available, a one-shot intravenous pyelogram can be performed by injecting intravenous contrast at 1 mL per pound of body weight up to a maximum of 150 mL and performing an X-ray 10 min after administration.

If ureteral obstruction is found from an anterior or apical repair, sutures will need to be released in order to alleviate the obstruction. Intraoperatively, the cystocele or apical sutures may be released, and patency of the ureter can be evaluated. A retrograde pyelogram may be performed, and the ureter may be evaluated if unable to pass a catheter or stent. If there is no extravasation but the ureteral appears deviated, a suture can be released and a stent inserted. If extravasation is noted, a ureteroureterostomy may be attempted. A ureteral reimplant may be done if necessary and all other measures have been exhausted. Postoperatively, however, if a patient presents with flank pain and/or diminished renal function, evaluation to rule out hydronephrosis is required. A renal ultrasound or CT urogram (with delay of the collecting system imperative) may be performed to evaluate the upper tract. The passage of a ureteral stent can be attempted if signs of obstruction are observed postoperatively. If this fails, then a percutaneous nephrostomy tube may be placed, and an antegrade stent may also be attempted. Depending on the location and length of ureteric injury, a ureteral reimplant with or without a psoas hitch may be needed, and in rare instances a Boari flap may be necessary.

Ureteral transection is a possible, albeit rare, occurrence during POP surgery. There is a higher risk of ureteral transection during any transabdominal surgery for prolapse. During abdominal sacral colpopexy, for instance, the ureter is in close proximity to the fixation point of sacral promontory. If concern exists intraoperatively for a ureteral transection, the evaluation is similar to that discussed previously. In addition, the ureter may be directly examined intraoperatively. If injury is observed, depending on the location of injury, a ureteral reimplantation, psoas hitch, or Boari flap may be necessary.

Urinary Incontinence

A good history is key to the discussion of new onset postoperative urinary incontinence. Patients need to be queried regarding the specific onset of symptoms and their duration. Discussion with the patient regarding the timing of events is essential. Was the patient dry prior to surgery? Had she ever had episodes of urinary incontinence prior to surgery? When does the incontinence occur—is it constant, or does it occur with stress or urgency? A careful history is essential in identifying the factors contributing to the patient's complaint. It is imperative that the physician rule out a urinary fistula. If suspicion is high for a fistula, investigation for a urethrovaginal, vesicovaginal, or ureterovaginal fistula must be performed. This can be done with a pyridium-indigo carmine dye test, retrograde pyelogram, or CT cystogram. When asking a patient to perform the pyridium test, a tampon should be placed in the vagina. At the time of removal of the tampon, the patient should note the location of the site of orange discoloration, if any. The patient may save the stained tampon or may take a photo to show the region of stain. This will help facilitate localizing the fistula. If obtaining a VCUG, it is essential to obtain static lateral films, voiding phase images at 30° lateral, and a post-void film to rule out the presence of a urethrovaginal or vesicovaginal fistula. Patients who present with incontinence after prolapse surgery need to be evaluated with urodynamics. The addition of fluoroscopy may also be helpful.

De Novo Stress Urinary Incontinence

Preoperative counseling in high grade anterior wall and apical prolapse should include the discussion of de novo stress urinary incontinence (SUI). Management of the urethra at the time of POP surgery has been largely dependent on surgeon preference and patient counseling. During high grade anterior vaginal wall prolapse, urethral kinking may mask occult SUI. Preoperatively, patients may have their prolapse reduced via vaginal pack, half speculum, pessary, or rectal swabs during physical examination or urodynamics study to check for occult SUI. However, methods of prolapse reduction measures in unmasking SUI have been inconsistent, ranging from 6 to 30 % [12]. There are advocates of performing an anti-incontinence procedure at the time of high grade prolapse repair versus selective management of the urethra. Advocates of performing a prophylactic sling at the time of prolapse repair believe that creating the anatomic support is essential in high grade prolapse repair. The recent OPUS trial has also reinforced that performing a prophylactic transvaginal tape (TVT) during vaginal POP surgery demonstrated superior continence rates at 12 months [13].

In contrast, those in favor of selective management believe that there may be risks in performing a prophylactic sling that may outweigh the benefits. One study reported that the risk of intervention with a second surgery due to postoperative urinary obstruction from a sling versus the risk of having to place a sling in the future in patients without demonstrable preoperative SUI was 8.5 % and 8.3 %, respectively [14]. Thus, the risk of placing a sling that causes obstruction is nearly equivalent to the risk of intervention due to SUI. Therefore, patients may require a second surgery for a procedure that may not have been necessary. If, however, the patients reported clinical SUI, which was unable to be demonstrated by urodynamics or prolapse reduction, those patients had a 30 % risk of postoperative SUI. One can expect that risk would be higher for those with clinical SUI. Therefore, an informed discussion with the patient is of utmost importance when undergoing POP surgery involving the choice of whether an anti-incontinence procedure should be performed at that time.

Urge Incontinence

Patients may have symptoms of overactive bladder (OAB) and urge urinary incontinence preoperatively or may develop it de novo postoperatively. When evaluating a postoperative patient, urinary obstruction must be ruled out as a cause of her presenting symptoms of OAB. Preoperatively, patients must be counseled that their symptoms of OAB may not resolve after POP surgery and that they may need to continue taking medication or seek other therapies for OAB. de Boer et al. reported that patients who did not have OAB preoperatively would likely not experience it postoperatively. Furthermore, in symptomatic patients with OAB, 69 % of women had improvement after POP surgery [15]. Thus, 30 % of symptomatic OAB patients may continue to have symptoms. A retrospective review of women who underwent primary POP surgery and who did not have OAB preoperatively developed de novo OAB in ~20 % of patients. Of those patients, 75 % of them had a TVT procedure. The study showed that older age, BMI, and history of a TVT procedure were risk factors for de novo OAB [16]. It is important to counsel patients that there is a risk of developing symptoms of OAB postoperatively.

Fistula

Vesicovaginal, urethrovaginal, and ureterovaginal fistula may occur during hysterectomy or any pelvic reconstructive surgery. Predisposing factors include unrecognized intraoperative perforation of the ureter, urethra or bladder, pelvic radiation, prior uterine surgery [17], fibroids or pelvic mass, endometriosis, or steroid use. Urethrovaginal fistulas may occur after sling placement. Rectovaginal fistula can form rarely after rectocele repair however, factors that may increase risk are inflammatory bowel conditions, malignancy, and pelvic radiation. Evaluation for vesicovaginal fistula may include the indigo carmine dye test or other diagnostic imaging as discussed earlier in this chapter. A urethrovaginal fistula may be diagnosed with a VCUG with lateral static and voiding images. A rectovaginal fistula may be diagnosed on physical examination or diagnostically by obtaining a rectogram or gastrograffin enema. Once diagnosis is confirmed, discussion with the patient for surgical intervention will need to be undertaken.

Nerve Injury

Nerve injury may result from the surgical procedure or from patient positioning prior to surgery. Positioning in the dorsal lithotomy position for vaginal surgery may result in injury of the common peroneal nerve from direct compression against the stirrup, which results in foot drop. A retractor placed around the inguinal area during open surgery may compress the femoral or femoro-cutaneous nerves resulting in pain in the inguinal region, difficulty with hip flexion, knee extension, or numbness in the anteromedial thigh. Over-flexion of the hip may cause stretching of the sciatic or femoral nerves and can be prevented by limiting abduction and outward rotation of the hip. As a result of over-flexion, patients may perceive weakness in hip flexion or decreased sensation of the ipsilateral thigh. Most of these positional cases of nerve injury will resolve over time. Physical therapy consultation may be helpful. Direct nerve injury to the ilioinginual, anterior, lateral, and posterior cutaneous, pudendal, and sciatic nerve all may occur during surgery.

Recurrence and Definition of Failure

Due to a high failure rate of POP surgery there have been efforts to develop new technologies to improve outcomes. Not only does the technology need to have equivalent or better anatomical outcomes, but important factors include patient satisfaction and low rates of complications. The definition of failure no longer is restricted to the anatomic outcome, as quality of life and symptoms are also factored. If the patient has a stage 2 POP-Q, but is asymptomatic, that should not be considered a failure. Previously, mesh- and graft-augmented repairs were noted to give an anatomic success defined as POP-Q stage 1 or 0. However, with the proliferation of mesh and the ensuing complications associated with it, many have further probed the definition of success after prolapse repair. Is it the anatomy or the symptomatic improvement that defines a successful repair? Native tissue repair has had variable success rates with high failure rate leading to the use of mesh-augmented repairs. Anatomic improvement with mesh-augmented repairs has demonstrated to be superior to that of native tissue repairs. However, mesh-induced complications, including mesh extrusion, erosion, vaginal pain, dyspareunia, leg and groin pain, difficulty ambulating, and neuropathy, have led pelvic floor surgeons to reexamine the pros and cons of mesh-augmented repairs.

Transvaginal Pelvic Organ Prolapse Repairs and Their Complications

POP complications resulting from a transvaginal approach will be addressed according to compartments. Intraoperative risks during transvaginal POP surgery include hemorrhage requiring transfusion; however, they are rare. Postoperative complications for transvaginal POP surgery include urinary or bowel fistula, urinary incontinence or obstruction, and recurrent prolapse. Each compartment will be discussed individually for its respective, unique complications.

The Anterior Compartment

Cystoceles are the most prevalent prolapsed compartment [18]. The determining factor to intervention for prolapse is the symptomatic bother to the patient. Traditional anterior colporrhaphy is described as reapproximation/plication of the pubocervical fascia [19]. Failure rates have been wide ranging dependent on the measurement of failure being symptomatic versus anatomic success with reports of failures in the range from 40 [20] to 70 % [21].

Recurrence

After anterior colporrhaphy, anatomic success has been noted as low as 30 % [21]. In order to repair a recurrent cystocele, one has to assess tissue quality and other compartmental defects. If there is apical descent, a vault suspension procedure will need to be performed, as failure to correct the vault results in a high incidence of recurrent prolapse. Not surprisingly though, the recurrence rate after recurrent cystocele repair is less than primary repair. One study [22] reported a success rate at 2 years of 42 % versus 71 % for recurrent and primary anterior colporrhaphy, respectively. Because of high recurrence rates, augmented procedures were introduced. These procedures have shown improvement in anatomic outcomes but not necessarily functional outcomes with higher complication rates. Mesh-augmented repairs will be discussed later in this chapter.

Urinary Obstruction

A patient may present with urinary retention and obstructive voiding symptoms after a cystocele repair and/or sling procedure. A recurrent or de novo cystocele may lead to urethral kinking and obstruction. However, if a sling procedure was performed, the patient may require urethrolysis and/or sling excision in additional to anatomic correction of the cystocele. If a patient presents with new onset urinary obstruction after a cystocele repair, a complete workup including urodynamics and cystoscopy is needed to determine the etiology. Obstruction after a sling may be due to excessive tensioning, position of the sling (too distal or too proximal), deep insertion (penetration of periurethral fascia reaching the submucosa), urethral fibrosis due to scarring, or the effect of a primary or secondary cystocele (primary was present at the time of surgery and not corrected or secondary due to later development). Some patients may present with a history of recurrent UTIs due to urinary obstruction and incomplete voiding. In patients that fail sling incision or excision, primary urethrolysis may be required. In recurrent obstruction, urethrolysis with placement of a retropubic Martius fat pad may be performed to prevent scarring and fixation of the urethra. If a bladder neck suspension was performed initially, some advocate for a suprameatal urethrolysis. These techniques are dependent on surgeon experience and comfort level in performing these procedures. In very selective cases with failed urethrolysis, where bladder neck obstruction is found secondary to urethral fibrosis or fixation, an incision of the bladder neck may be performed.

The Vaginal Apex

Vaginal apical support plays a significant role in POP surgery. The ideal procedure provides a durable suspension that does not affect sexual or visceral function and is associated with minimal complications. Transvaginal procedures that provide restoration to vaginal apical support include uterosacral ligament suspension (USLS), SSL fixation (SSLF), and iliococcygeus fascial fixation (ICFF). The abdominal sacrocolpopexy (ASC), which is a transabdominal procedure, is also effective for vaginal vault suspension and considered by some experts as one of the most durable repairs for apical prolapse. Indications for ASC over a vaginal approach would be a young patient, preoperative vaginal shortening, and failed prior repairs. The vaginal approaches, however, provide patients with a faster recovery, shorter hospital stay, and avoidance of an intra-abdominal procedure. In addition, all compartments may be addressed transvaginally. The approach to POP surgery greatly depends on surgeon's experience, as the best operation is the one that works best in that particular surgeon hands.

Transvaginal Vault Suspensions

Transvaginal vault suspensions include USLS, SSLF, and iliococcygeus suspension. These suspension and fixation procedures involve suturing of the apex to each respective ligament or muscle and fascia.

Uterosacral Ligament Suspension Procedure

USLS has been described as suturing the apex of the vagina to the origin of the uterosacral ligament. This procedure may be performed transvaginally or abdominally. Delayed absorbable or permanent suture may be used for the suspension. Transvaginal USLS has had reported successful apical outcomes in 98 % of patients with a median follow-up of 25 months [23].

Intraoperative complications from USLS most commonly occur at the urinary tract where ureteral injury and kinking have been reported as low as 1.8 % [24] and as high as 11 % in patients where cystoscopy was utilized [25]. If the injury is recognized immediately, the suture may be removed and resolution of the occlusion may be noted. However, if recognition of the injury is delayed, a ureteral reimplantation may be required. Ureteral injury may be avoided by placing the suspension sutures at the level of the ischial spine, which has been shown to be the furthest position, approximately 4.9 cm from the ureter and vascular structures [26]. Avoiding ureteric injury depends on the direction or axis of the sutures placement. Our method involves a posterior insertion in the groove between the rectum and levator, which will avoid the ureter.

Most common postoperative complications from a USLS include nerve or musculoskeletal complications. The pain in the buttock or posterior thigh may be due to the incorporation of sutures into the levator and obturator muscles without definitive nerve injury. A retrospective review of 278 women who underwent transvaginal USLS was performed, identifying 19 (6.8 %) women who had sensory neuropathy. Most commonly, buttock pain (73.7 %) and posterior thigh pain (57.9 %) were present. Some women underwent suture removal approximately 2 months after surgery and most of the women had full symptomatic improvement, while partial improvement was noted in the remaining patients [27]. Neural complications have been studied in cadaver specimens, the sacral nerve roots being the most vulnerable neural structures involved during USLS [28]. Bowel complications are rare with 0.5 % injury and only 3 reported cases of bowel obstruction [29, 30]. Hemorrhage requiring transfusion for apical vault suspension procedures is rare.

Sacrospinous Ligament (SSL) Fixation Procedure

The SSLF has been shown to be effective in correcting apical prolapse. Long-term success rates have been reported as high as 84–99 % [31]. The ligament may be palpated and a suture is placed one to two fingerbreadths medial from the spine to avoid damage to the pudendal nerve and vessels. Sutures may be placed unilaterally or bilaterally directly or with a suture carrying device. In recent years, vaginal vault procedures have been substituted by the use of mesh in different anchoring system to the SSL. With the recent FDA warnings, a decline of mesh use is expected.

Intraoperative complications of SSLF include injury to the bladder, rectum, or ureter, which are rare. Intraoperative bleeding requiring blood transfusion has been reported as 0.5–2.5 % [31]. The inferior gluteal artery has been cited as the most common vessel injured during SSLF [32]. Nearby vessels including superior gluteal, internal pudendal, vertebral, middle sacral, lateral sacral and external iliac, and other anastomosing vessels posterior to the SSL can also be injured and hemorrhage during SSLF. Intraoperatively, diffuse venous bleeding may be controlled using pressure and packing. Prohemostatic agents such as surgical Nuknit or Surgicel may also be used if necessary. During suture placement, sutures are placed 1–2 cm medial to the ischial spine to prevent vascular and nerve injuries.

Some postoperative complications include reports of fever, abscess, and hemorrhage requiring transfusion [24]. Pain symptoms include gluteal pain, buttock pain, or posterior thigh pain, which has been cited to resolve in as little as weeks to 6 months. De novo dyspareunia has been reported in approximately 1–7 % of cases [33–36]. One factor which may contribute to dyspareunia is narrowing of the introitus during perineorraphy. Release of the SSLF sutures may lead to resolution of dyspareunia [33].

The development of anterior compartment prolapse after SSLF has been described as the most common site of failure [37]. This failure has been cited due to retroversion of the vagina, displacing the vaginal apex posteriorly and allowing anterior descensus. Patients need to be thoroughly counseled prior to procedures of the risks of recurrence and potential risks of other compartmental defects.

Iliococcygeus Suspension Procedure

Iliococcygeus suspension entails attachment of the vaginal vault to the fascia of the iliococcygeus muscle and has been reported to have long-term anatomic success [38]. Iliococcygeus suspension involves bilateral fixation of the vaginal apex. The point of fixation is located 1–2 cm caudad and posterior to the ischial spine. This is an alternative choice to the SSLF, as the proposed advantage is the decreased risk of neurovascular injury and decreased risk of future cystocele.

Intraoperative complications are similar to those of SSLF including risks of bladder and rectal injury and hemorrhage requiring transfusion; however, they are rare. Postoperative complications include vaginal cuff abscess, fever, transient neuropathy, and buttock pain; however, these complications are uncommon. In a study comparing SSLF and iliococcygeus fixation, the most frequent postoperative complaint in both groups was buttock pain and sciatica and all cases resolved in 2–3 months [39]. In addition, there was no statistically significant difference between patients who underwent SSLF or iliococcygeus fixation in regard to postoperative cystocele formation or dyspareunia.

Transabdominal Open Versus Lap/Robotic

Transabdominal procedures share risks of complications including vascular, bowel, and urinary tract injuries. Other complications include ileus, venous thrombosis, and urinary and wound infections. Paraiso et al. reported on laparoscopic and open ASC and did not find significant differences in cystotomy, enterotomy, rate of blood transfusions, deep venous thrombosis, wound infection, or ventral hernia [40]. Patients presenting with either febrile illness, bowel distension, and abdominal pain, or any signs of peritonitis require work up for bowel and urinary injuries. A CT scan with oral and IV contrast with delayed ureteral images should be obtained to adequately assess the patient. Overall, there is a low rate of less than 1% in gynecologic laparoscopic related surgeries [41].

Presence of the Uterus

If the uterus is present, discussion with the patient regarding options of uterine-sparing procedures must be undertaken. The presence of uterine or cervical pathology may also factor into consideration when discussing uterine preservation. If the patient is premenopausal, future fertility will need to be discussed. Should future pregnancies be desired, a hysteropexy may be discussed. There is evidence that hysterectomy performed for uterine prolapse carries a lower risk of apical recurrent prolapse [42]. Therefore, a detailed discussion regarding pros and cons of uterine preservation needs to be carried out with the patient.

Uterine Suspension

Preservation of the uterus via uterine suspension may be performed transvaginally and abdominally. The most common complications resulting from vaginal sacrospinous hysteropexy have been reported to be buttock pain and recurrent prolapse [43]. Most cases of buttock pain resolve, it resolved spontaneously. Some patients may require surgical intervention to release sutures related to pain. Complications are similar to that of vault suspension procedures, including risk of ureteral injury and nerve-related entrapment and pain. Women undergoing vaginal hysterectomy versus sacrospinous hysteropexy have been compared showing similar objective and subjective results for prolapse recurrence [44]. Few women did become pregnant with uterine preservation. Proponents for preservation of the uterus and cervix believe that it may have a role in libido and orgasm [45]. Some patients who underwent colposacropexy and hysterosacrocolpopexy found no difference in female sexual dysfunction [46]. Another study also did not reveal any difference in sexual function between patients who underwent transvaginal hysterectomy (TVH) versus SSLF [47].

Laparoscopic hysteropexy has been described and has shown feasibility for correcting uterine prolapse [48]. With any minimally invasive technique, there is a possibility of conversion to open surgery; however, this is rare. Robotic and laparoscopic hysteropexy carries the risks inherent to transabdominal surgery including risks of injury to bowels, bladder, ureter, and nearby blood vessels. As with other prolapse procedure, there is also risk of infection and recurrence of prolapse. In addition, dyspareunia and mesh-related complications are present.

Hysterectomy: Transvaginal and Transabdominal Complications

If patient is postmenopausal with a high grade apical prolapse, a hysterectomy may be performed prior to one of the above suspension procedures. Advocates for hysterectomy propose that there is a decrease in failure rate with removal of the uterus. There have not been any high quality randomized trials with or without hysterectomy versus in situ uterine prolapse repair and would likely be difficult to perform. Therefore, there are mostly retrospective or non-randomized studies evaluating the success of uterine prolapse and recurrence of vault or recurrent uterine prolapse. There is no standard guideline regarding uterine prolapse with treatment of hysterectomy or uterine preservation. Thus, a detailed discussion must be carried out with the patient.

Transvaginal Hysterectomy

In the short term, patients who underwent a vaginal hysterectomy for uterine prolapse versus an ASC with uterine preservation had improved postoperative pain, QOL, and better mobility at 6 weeks postoperatively [49]. A retrospective study of 66 women with stage 2–4 uterine descent was randomized to vaginal hysterectomy or sacrospinous hysteropexy [42]. The risk of recurrent prolapse stage 2 or more of the apical compartment at 1-year follow-up was 17 % in favor of the vaginal hysterectomy.

Complications related to TVH are similar to previously discussed transvaginal procedures. Intraoperative risks of TVH include injury to the bladder, bowels and rectum, ureters, and hemorrhage. TVH should be performed with a vault suspension procedure and the risks were described earlier in this chapter. Postoperative complications include dyspareunia, vaginal shortening, and complications related to previously described vault suspension procedures. Unrecognized injuries may lead to fistula formation.

Transabdominal Hysterectomy: Open, Laparoscopic

A hysterectomy may be performed with a concomitant vault suspension procedure. As the ureters are in close proximity to the cervix, uterine vessels, and infundibulo-pelvic-ligament, care must be taken to identify and preserve the ureters. Dissection between the cervix and the bladder poses a risk for cystotomy. Intraoperative injuries should be identified and repaired. Unrecognized injuries or ischemic injuries which present later in the postoperative period will give rise to vesicoureteral or vesicovaginal fistulas. Care must be taken to ensure adequate hemostasis, as a cuff hematoma may arise and infection may occur. A prospective cohort study in Finland investigated complications of hysterectomy for benign diseases and found that major complication rates were highest in laparoscopic hysterectomy (4.3 %), followed by abdominal hysterectomy (4.0 %), and vaginal hysterectomy (2.6 %), but logistic regression did not show major differences between approaches for any organ injury or major complication [50]. A wide range of complications were investigated. There was not a statistically significant difference in bladder, ureter, and bowel injuries between the three surgical approaches. Most were recognized and repaired intraoperatively. Pelvic infection was found to be higher in laparoscopic and vaginal hysterectomy than open abdominal hysterectomy by fivefold. Wound infection was higher in the open abdominal hysterectomy group by 1.6-fold.

Abdominal Sacral Colpopexy

A MEDLINE search by Beer et al. found that ASC and SSLF were the most commonly used vault procedures [51]. A review of the literature indicated that the ASC was associated with a lower rate of recurrent vault prolapse, less dyspareunia, longer operating time, longer recover period, and higher expense compared to vaginal sacrospinous colpopexy [52]. A recent Cochrane review evaluated the literature examining abdominal sacrohysteropexy for uterine preservation versus vaginal hysterectomy and repair. The trial with an 8-year follow-up revealed 87 % in the vaginal group versus 68 % in the abdominal group which reported that they had symptomatic prolapse improvement, providing some evidence that the hysterectomy group did better postoperatively. Unless there is a strong indication and desire to preserve the uterus, a hysterectomy may be performed concomitantly at the time of ASC.

Complications of Abdominal Sacral Colpopexy

In a Medline review of 1,571 procedures, common complications of ASC include bleeding (2 %), infections from cystitis (6 %), fever, secondary healing, dehiscence or abscess (6 %), and mesh-related problems. Organ perforation of the bladder, rectum, or intestines occurred in 1.6 % of cases. Urologic complications ranging from ureteral kinking, voiding disorders, urinary incontinence, and urgency were rare, occurring in only 1.9 % of cases. Mesh complications occurred in 2 % of cases. Total risk of reoperation for ileus, incisional hernia, or vesicovaginal fistula was at a rate of 2.9 %. One study reported graft erosion in 15 of its 273 patients [53].

A literature review of 2,178 patients who underwent ASC [54] revealed intraoperative complications, including hemorrhage in 4.4 %, cystotomy in 3.1 %, enterotomy in 1.6 %, and ureteral injury in 1.0 % of cases. Postoperative complications included UTIs in 10.9 %, wound infections in 4.6 %, ileus in 36 %, deep venous thrombosis or pulmonary embolus in 3.3 %, and small bowel obstruction requiring surgery in 1.1 % of cases. Some recommend reperitonalization of the mesh to prevent bowel obstruction. Mesh erosion was noted at 3.4 % of cases. Reoperation for prolapse and stress incontinence in series that reported these outcomes had rates of 4.4 % (range 0–18.2 %) and 4.9 % (range 1.2–30.9 %), respectively [54]. Potential complications include prolapse of other vaginal compartments, bleeding, sciatic nerve injury, and rectal laceration. Injuries to the presacral and perirectal vessels have been reported with life-threatening hemorrhage.

Paraiso et al. compared laparoscopic and open abdominal sacral colpopexies and there did not appear to be a significant difference in the encountered complications [40]. Noted complications included cystotomy or sutures noted within the bladder at the time of cystoscopy. Sutures which were detected at the time of surgery were removed and cystotomies were closed primarily. Intraoperative enterotomy was primarily closed. Postoperative enterotomy required washout and bowel diversion.

Risk of Mesh Erosion with Concomitant Hysterectomy

If a hysterectomy is performed at the time of ASC, a supracervical hysterectomy is recommended in order to avoid increased risk of mesh erosion through the vaginal apex. Patients who had a concomitant vaginal hysterectomy with ASC were found to have a mesh erosion rate of 23 % [55]. However, those who underwent supracervical hysterectomy were found to have the same expected rate of mesh erosion as that of patients who had undergone a prior hysterectomy.

With reports of higher rates of erosion at the vaginal cuff after concomitant hysterectomy, some recommend preservation of the cervical stump to prevent mesh erosion. However, a retrospective review comparing patients who underwent ASC and supracervical hysterectomy versus patients who had undergone prior hysterectomy, revealed that both were associated with a low incidence of mesh erosion ranging from 0.5 to 2.4 % at 7–8 months, which was not statistically significant [56]. Cundiff et al. [57] reported that risks factors contributing to mesh erosion into the vagina after abdominal sacral colpopexy include smoking (OR 5.2), use of gore-tex mesh (OR 4.2), and concurrent hysterectomy (OR 4.9).

Posterior Vaginal Repair Complications

Posterior vaginal wall prolapse repair, also called rectocele repair, is a common procedure performed concomitantly with other POP procedures. Rectocele repairs alone or combined with other compartmental procedures account for nearly 50 % of the surgical repairs for POP [1]. Surgical repair is indicated for symptomatic rectoceles with a less defined role of surgical repair for the management of asymptomatic rectoceles. It is known that the physical exam findings do not correlate with symptoms; therefore, careful questioning is important during patient evaluation. The symptoms associated with posterior vaginal wall prolapse can be categorized into three categories of bother involving vaginal prolapse, bowel issues, and sexual dysfunction. Patients' symptoms may include vaginal pressure, bulge, discomfort, and pulling. Defecatory dysfunction can range from constipation, incomplete emptying of rectum, manual splinting, and/or fecal incontinence. Sexual function may be compromised with lack of vaginal sensation or dyspareunia.

Posterior Vaginal Repair: Complications to the Transanal Approach

The goal of surgical repair is to restore the anatomical defect and to improve sexual, bowel, and prolapse symptoms while limiting the associated complications. Historically, posterior vaginal wall prolapse was repaired by the transanal approach, although this has largely been replaced by the transvaginal approach. Two randomized trials report that the transanal approach results in a higher recurrence rate of posterior prolapse compared to vaginal repair [58, 59]. Transanal repair is associated with significant complications of fecal incontinence with rates reported as high as 38 % [60] and the symptomatic outcome is better with the transvaginal approach. The transvaginal approach involves two main techniques, which are the midline fascial plication and the site-specific repair.

Intraoperative Complications

All transvaginal posterior approaches are associated with minimal operative complications such as bleeding requiring transfusion (2 %), infection (7 %), and isolated reports of rectovaginal fistula and rectal injury [61]. Identification of rectal injury by an intraoperative rectal exam is recommended by some pelvic surgeons. Narrowing of the vagina can occur with posterior repairs and should be prevented so that the introitus width should accommodate 2–3 fingerbreadths.

Postoperative complications resulting from posterior vaginal repair center on dyspareunia, recurrence, and defecatory dysfunction. A randomized trial compared anatomic success of the midline plication, site-specific, and porcine graft repairs at 1 year (86 %, 78 %, 54 %). They showed that the midline plication had the statically lowest recurrence rates [62]. There was no significant difference in complications or functional failures for each technique.

Dyspareunia

Dyspareunia rates were high at 36 % postoperatively, but this may be explained by the preoperative dyspareunia rate of 51 %, which was based on validated questionnaires. Although the dyspareunia rates were higher than other reports, the majority of patients reported they were better, and 93 % would choose the same treatment. De novo rates of dyspareunia range from 0 to 19 % [63, 64]. Dyspareunia rates in other studies have a wide range of 5–46 % depending on how they were reported [65, 66]. Dyspareunia is thought to be preventable and results from narrowing of the vagina by plication of the levator ani.

Recurrence

Recurrence rates are lower for the midline plication compared to the site-specific and porcine graft-augmented repair based on a randomized control trial. The midline plication technique has similar success compared to mesh-augmented repair based on two randomized trials [20, 67]. In studies where mesh-augmented repairs were performed for rectocele repair, there was a high rate of complications including dyspareunia and pain. Based on the evidence, the United States Food and Drug Administration (FDA) made the recommendation that vaginal mesh was not indicated in the posterior compartment, as there was no evidence for improved outcomes and because of the unique complications that are related to mesh [68]. Specific complications related to mesh are addressed later in the chapter.

Table 21.2 Midline fascial plication improvement of defecation

Midline fascial plication	Improvement of defecation
Singh et al. [64]	65 %
Milani et al. [63]	63 %
Maher et al. [65]	87 %
Paraiso et al. [62]	68 %
Abramov et al. [89]	66 %

Table 21.3 Site-specific repair and improvement of defecation

Site-specific repair	Improvement of defecation
Cundiff et al. [90]	63 %
Porter et al. [66]	44 %
Kenton et al. [91]	54 %
Glavind et al. [92]	85 %
Abramov et al. [89]	63 %

Defecatory Dysfunction

Defecatory dysfunction includes constipation, incomplete emptying, fecal and/or flatal incontinence, and the need to perform perineal or vaginal splinting. Most series support improvement of constipation, incomplete emptying, and the need to splint. Regardless of the surgical approach (midline fascial plication, site-specific, or mesh repair), the majority of studies report improvement in defecation (Tables 21.2 and 21.3). Fecal incontinence is not changed unless the anal sphincter is addressed.

Complications of Obliterative Procedures

Partial and complete colpocleisis are obliterative procedures that are minimally invasive and associated with low morbidity and low complication rate. This procedure addresses prolapse in all vaginal compartments, although avoids many of the complications with apical repair and has similar complications as anterior and posterior vaginal repair. Obliterative procedures are generally offered to elderly women that are no longer sexually active and do not wish to preserve coital function. Many elderly women are not sexually active, with a prevalence of 17 % within the age range of 75–85 years [69]. Some also propose this option for elderly patients who have comorbid conditions, who may not tolerate a more extensive procedure. As the population of the elderly is projected to grow, this procedure may be more utilized.

A complete colpocleisis is removal of the vaginal epithelium from the bladder neck to the vaginal cuff anteriorly and posteriorly. A partial or LeFort colpocleisis is similar except the vaginal epithelium on both sides is left intact to create bilateral tunnels that can drain vaginal secretions. These procedures can be performed with or without a concomitant hysterectomy. There are studies that suggest that a concomitant hysterectomy does not improve success and increases bleeding and operative time [70, 71].

The success rate for colpocleisis is 90 % or more in case series and prospective cohorts with overall low morbidity [72]. In a prospective cohort study at 1 year, 94 % of women reported that they were satisfied or very satisfied with the surgery. Although this is a minimally invasive surgery, there are associated complications. Body image may be compromised, with up to 13 % of patients having regret about loss of sexual function of the vagina [73]. Even amongst those who did express regret about the loss of sexual function, half of them still would have the procedure again [73].

Intraoperative Complications

Only about 5 % of cases involved major perioperative complications, such as blood transfusions as well as cardiac, cerebrovascular, thromboembolic, and pulmonary events [74]. The morality rate, 1 in 400, is acceptable, as many patients have preexisting comorbidities [74]. Just as in anterior and posterior vaginal compartment repairs, there are risks for bladder and bowel injuries with colpocleisis. Urinary or fecal fistulas secondary to colpocleisis are rare. Ureteric obstruction has also been reported [75].

Postoperative Complications

About 15 % of cases involve minor complications, such as fever, UTI, vaginal hematoma, and bleeding. UTI is the most common perioperative complication in one series [73]. Anatomical recurrence rates are low at 7 % with 94 % of women satisfied or very satisfied with their surgery at 1 year [73]. As with any vaginal surgery there are rare, but reported, complications that can occur and vary from bladder injury to rectal bleeding [70]. Bowel and bladder symptoms overall improve with colpocleisis, and development of de novo symptoms is uncommon [76]. Patients that have preoperative urinary retention achieve resolution in 90 % of cases [77]. Preoperative urge incontinence improves from 41 to 15 % postoperatively, and postoperative de novo SUI rates occur at approximately 15 % [73].

Colpocleisis is a reasonable alternative to elderly women with prolapse who either may have multiple comorbidities or do not wish to preserve coital function. The procedure is deemed safe and efficacious [78] and has high patient satisfaction with a minimal associated complication. A detailed discussion with the patient is imperative prior to surgery.

Mesh Kits on the Market: Mesh-Related Complications

Pelvic surgeons began implementing the use of mesh into the abdominal repair of POP surgery in the 1970s, as it had demonstrated good anatomic success for abdominal hernias since the 1950s. As this had successful outcomes for abdominal POP surgery, this was then adapted for surgery for SUI and transvaginal POP in the 1990s. Early on, mesh was fashioned for site-specific vaginal repairs. The FDA then approved mesh for the use of transvaginal SUI surgery in 1996 and for POP in 2002. Following that, there was an explosive growth of transvaginal mesh "kits" that were designed with the intention of providing the surgeon with a minimally invasive, safe, easily reproducible, and effective method to correct POP. Mesh kits received FDA approval through the 510(k) process, as mesh had demonstrated efficacy in the general surgery realm in abdominal hernia repairs. Therefore, companies were not required to perform clinical trials, as they had already undergone the FDA approval process.

The proliferation of mesh kits into the market was expansive, as more than a hundred mesh kits were introduced by various companies. Clinical studies that were performed on mesh kits were mostly retrospective with short follow-up. Over time, the Manufacturer and User Facility Device Manager (MAUDE) database demonstrated an increasing number of patients presenting with mesh-related complications. Though the mesh kits provide an "easy" way to perform the procedure, many providers were not prepared to treat the postoperative complications associated with blind trocar placement and mesh-associated issues with erosion and extrusion.

Mesh kits used for anterior, apical, and posterior repair have different routes of trocar passage and fixation points. Earlier generation anterior repair kits involved transobturator passage of mesh arms. These included the American Medical Systems (AMS) Perigee, Gynecare Prolift, and Bard Avaulta, to name a few. The posterior repair kits, including the AMS Apogee, Gynecare Prolift posterior, and Bard Avaulta utilized trocar passage through the ischiorectal fossa. The difference between the devices was the apical support fixation points. The AMS Apogee kit is anchored at the iliococcygeus muscle, the Prolift is anchored at the SSL, and the Bard Avaulta requires a separate vault procedure. The Elevate system is a trocar-less procedure that utilizes self-fixating tips. This was an attempt to lessen complication rates by using a trocar-less procedure. Further, the Prosima kit offered a sutureless placement of mesh with placement of a vaginal support device, much like that of a pessary which remained intact in the patient's vagina for a period of 3 weeks postoperatively. Despite the evolution of mesh kits, mesh complications have continued.

Due to the increase in reported complications encountered with mesh, the FDA updated their public health notifications (PHN) in July 2011. The FDA reported that surgical placement of mesh for POP may expose patients to greater risks than other surgical options, and that the greater risk did not show greater clinical benefit such as improved quality of life. Serious risks were not rare as previously reported. They recommend a proactive approach by patients in discussing the use of mesh with their surgeons. In addition, they are exploring regulatory solutions to evaluate the safety and efficacy in mesh use. Soon after the PHN was released, some kits including the Prolift and Avaulta were removed from the market. If performing a mesh-augmented repair, informed consent detailing the potential risks and outcomes needs to be discussed with the patient.

Exposure

Mesh exposure is one of the most common mesh complications. According to the MAUDE database, mesh exposure and erosion account for 35 % of the complications of vaginal mesh [79]. Smoking, total vaginal mesh, surgeon experience, young age, and sexual activity, parity, somatic inflammatory disease have been cited as risk factors for mesh exposure [81, 82].

Patients presenting complaints vary widely in this population. Patients may present with the complaint of vaginal bleeding, recurrent UTIs, vaginal pain, dyspareunia, and urinary symptoms. Sexual partners have also stated that they may feel a "scratching" sensation or pain described as "hispareunia." Early presentation may include vaginal induration or intraepithelial infiltration as the mesh is extruding out of the vaginal wall. This requires further evaluation with a vaginal examination and cystoscopy to ensure there is no urethral or bladder perforation. Various factors contribute to vaginal mesh exposure. Bleeding and separation of the suture line may cause vaginal mesh exposure. In addition, wound infection at the time of surgery or later may occur with resulting mesh exposure with chronic drainage. Placement of the mesh too superficially on the vaginal epithelium is another causative factor. A woman's vagina may become more atrophic with time, and the thinning, fragile vaginal epithelium may put the existing mesh at risk for exposure. Exposures have been reported as late as 10 years postoperatively.

Mesh exposure may be managed conservatively if asymptomatic with observation and estrogen cream. If the exposure is small, some physicians perform in-office excisions of the mesh. Often, these excisional attempts will fail, as more mesh will erode through the vaginal epithelium. Surgical excision in the operating room with multiple removal attempts may be required. Total mesh removal may be recommended in cases of multiple areas of exposure, pain, vaginal scarring, and stenosis. When the area of mesh is large and infiltrating a significant proportion of the vaginal wall, coverage of the vaginal wall with a rotational flap may be required.

Mesh Pain

Pain due to mesh is a complex disorder and dependent upon what type of procedure was performed. Due to the trocar devices designed to traverse the obturator foramen, muscles, tendons, and nerves may be injured during the passage. As a result, patients' presentation may be wide ranging varying from vaginal pain, dyspareunia, suprapubic pain, chronic pelvic or bladder pain, leg and groin pain, hip pain, and inability to walk. These symptoms may present immediately after surgery or may present as a delayed complication.

Evaluation of chronic mesh pain requires a detailed history and physical examination. History including the type of mesh and operative reports are necessary. It is helpful to query regarding pain complications by following the standard questions involving QRST: quality, radiation, site, and timing. In addition, localizing the pain and eliciting any aggravating or alleviating factors is imperative. For instance, when the patient is supine and still, is the pain present or aggravated? Is the pain aggravated with sitting or with movement? These are important questions to distinguish the etiology of the pain. A neurologic examination including motor and sensory responses is of utmost importance. This will help localize the nerve distribution of the pain and narrow the etiology of the pain. On physical examination, the examiner many times may feel the mesh as an indurated, cord-like structure. The mesh may also be exposed and palpation of this region may exacerbate the pain symptoms. Vaginal tissue quality, vaginal depth, and caliber are important to note. There are some patients where the pain has become centralized and does not follow any anatomic distribution of pain. Often times, these patients have failed pelvic floor physical therapy, vaginal injections, and are on narcotics.

Pain Due to Nerve Damage

Nerve damage can occur during mesh placement. This can occur when trocars are used for passage of the mesh. Injury may occur when trocars are used to traverse the obturator foramen or at the level of the SSL and iliococcygeus muscle. During transobturator trocar passage, there is risk of injury to the ilioinguinal nerve (L1), which provides sensation to the anterior labia majora and mons pubis. In addition, the anterior, lateral, and posterior femoral cutaneous nerves (L2–S3) are at risk of injury and provide sensation to the thigh and lateral perineum [83]. Around the SSL, the pudendal nerve, which passes posterior to the ischial spine, the sciatic nerve, or lumbosacral plexus may be injured. Presenting complaints may include buttock pain, posterior leg pain, or loss of sensory or motor function in those regions. Pudendal and sciatic nerve pain may also result from mesh placement into the ischiorectal fossa during posterior repair (Fig. 21.1).

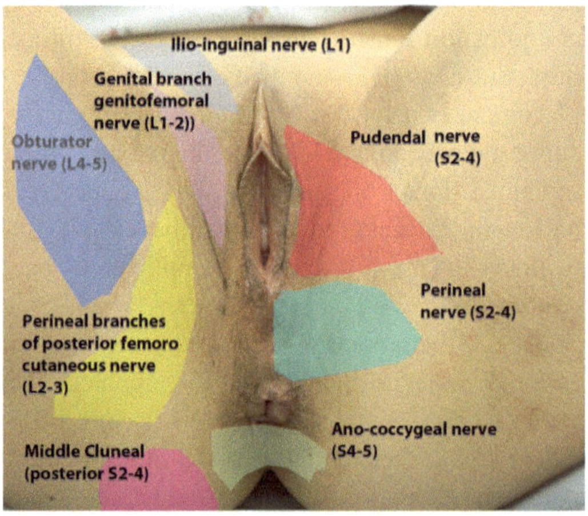

Fig. 21.1 Pudendal and sciatic nerve pain may result from mesh placement into the ischiorectal fossa during posterior repair

Pain Due to Bone

Patients may present with pain that is constant and/or exacerbated with palpation. Depending on mesh placement, bony structures at risk for injury include the inferior pubic ramus during transobturator trocar passage or sacral promontory due to ASC. The periosteum may be damaged, irritated, or infected during these procedures and may cause an inflammatory reaction and pain. As a result, osteitis or osteomyelitis may develop.

Pain Due to Muscle

Muscular pain due to mesh placement during prolapse surgery results from trocar passage or suspension sutures through muscular structures. Muscular pain can be direct due to restriction of movement by the mesh, fascial irritation, or secondary to the sensitized nociceptors of the vagina producing secondary activation giving rise to muscle spasm and pain. Muscles may be at risk for injury depending on the procedure performed. When performing anterior repairs involving transobturator passage, the hip adductors are at risk for injury. The fascia may also become inflamed contributing to pain symptoms. In addition, direct muscular penetration of the adductor longus, adductor brevis, adductor magnus, gracilis, and obturator externus, which all originate along the inferior pubic ramus and ischial rami, may produce pain. These muscles are involved in hip flexion, thigh adduction, and medial and lateral leg rotation. The pain may be exacerbated with movement of these muscles and alleviated with rest. The levator ani muscles may also be penetrated and may cause pelvic pain, dyspareunia, or pain with prolonged standing or activity [83]. During apical repairs, muscles that are at risk for injury depend upon the procedure performed. The piriformis muscle, which has its origin along the anterior sacrum, may be affected thereby inhibiting lateral thigh rotation. During vaginal vault suspension, the obturator internus, near the ischial spine, is at risk for injury. The obturator internus provides lateral thigh rotation during flexion. Mesh placement into the posterior compartment may injure the levator muscles, and pain may be exacerbated with sitting.

Pain Due to Viscera

Patients may experience diffuse pain within the abdominopelvic region. Important considerations include the presence of urinary or bowel issues, including hematuria, dysuria, obstruction, recurrent infections, constipation, and diarrhea. Mesh may be present in the bladder or urethra and cause symptoms of suprapubic pain, bladder spasms, dysuria, hematuria, OAB, and/or recurrent UTIs. During apical repairs, mesh may penetrate intra-abdominal and pelvic organs including the uterus, cervix, bladder, or bowel. Patients may present with complaints of vaginal/uterine bleeding and urinary or bowel obstruction. Posterior placement of mesh perforating the bowel may cause rectal pain, urgency, and possible bleeding and obstructive symptoms. We believe that the fundamental concept of treatment for mesh-related complications is mesh removal. The patient's presentation will guide the type of treatment and mesh removal.

Mesh Removal

Mesh Removal for Organ Erosion

For patients found to have penetration of mesh into the bladder, a transvesical or vaginal approach may be performed depending on the comfort level of the surgeon. The mesh must be removed from the hollow organ; otherwise, there will be future risks of stone formation and recurrent UTIs. Mesh perforation into the urethra will require additional coverage using a Martius flap to prevent future urethrovesical fistula formation. If suspicion for bowel or rectal perforation exists, patients should be evaluated by a gastroenterologist, and a colonoscopy should be performed. Mesh present in the rectum may be approached transvaginally depending on surgeon preference. An adequate amount of perirectal fascia is used for layered coverage, and an interpositional flap may be placed.

Mesh Removal for Pain

For armed polypropylene mesh placement causing vaginal pain, dyspareunia, or pain with ambulating requiring mesh excision, palpable, painful cords of contracted mesh can be removed to alleviate pain. For patients who have had mesh placed in a transobturator fashion who present with leg and groin pain, the mesh arms may be removed; however, there is no guarantee in pain relief. Mesh removal requires expertise, as it can be difficult to identify and completely remove mesh components.

Mesh Removal by Compartment

Mesh placed in a transobturator fashion may cause leg and groin pain. An attempt at removal may be performed, but as previously stated, may not be curative of pain. Generally, these arms are left in situ during mesh excision procedures unless causing intractable pain, as the risks may outweigh the benefits of removal.

Removal of mesh from ASC procedures of vaginal vault suspension requires expertise in pelvic anatomy. Indications for mesh removal for ASC procedures include vaginal bleeding, draining sinus tract, exposed mesh, and chronic abdominal pain. Mesh from the sacral promontory should be removed through a transabdominal approach. Many times the scarring that has resulted from the mesh placement may be enough to suspend the vault. However, if an additional vault procedure is needed at the time of mesh removal, a piece of autologous rectus fascia may be harvested to place from the vaginal apex to the sacral promontory. For vault suspension procedures, buttock and gluteal pain may be alleviated by releasing and removing the mesh from the point of attachment to the SSL or iliococcygeus fascia.

Placement of mesh for rectocele repairs involves either apical attachment or trocar placement through the ischiorectal fossa. Patients may complain of gluteal and buttock pain since this passage traverses the gluteal muscles and may be reproducible by palpation. The area of pain should be marked prior to the patient undergoing anesthesia to clearly define the region of pain. The levators are also at risk for injury during ischiorectal fossa trocar passage. Removal of posterior vaginal wall mesh is a delicate procedure that should avoid perforation into the rectum. If rectal perforation does occur, it may be repaired in two layers with overlying perirectal tissue. If there is not adequate perirectal fascia, an interpositional flap may be required to prevent formation of a rectovaginal fistula.

Mesh Contraction, Vaginal Stenosis, Mesh Folding

Vaginal pain and dyspareunia may be caused by several factors secondary to mesh. Mesh may contract up to 30 % based on ultrasound evidence and cause vaginal shrinkage, although there is divergent evidence for this issue [84, 85]. Vaginal mesh exposure may cause vaginal discomfort and/or pain, and may cause the sexual partner to feel discomfort, termed by some as "hispareunia." Folding is a complication by which the mesh is inserted flat but postoperatively becomes folded, creating areas of induration and "bumps" of irregularly elevated vaginal wall. A case series of women who underwent surgical intervention for symptomatic vaginal mesh contraction was evaluated where post-surgery a significant number of patients had improvement in vaginal pain and dyspareunia [86]. Their symptoms consisted of vaginal pain aggravated by movement, dyspareunia, and focal tenderness of the mesh. Many patients were also found to have mesh erosion, vaginal tightness, and vaginal shortening. Patients who suffer from vaginal stenosis and shrinkage may require a vaginoplasty to enlarge the vaginal caliber. Our preferred method is usage of a pudendal-based gluteal flap. We have found success in the gluteal flap to alleviate vaginal stenosis and dyspareunia associated with it.

Definition of Complications

The International Urogynecological Association (IUGA) and International Continence Society (ICS) jointly published a terminology and classification system for complications related to the insertion of mesh and grafts in pelvic floor surgery [87]. The classification is based on the category (C), time (T), and site (S). The CTS classification addresses all insertion and healing issues. The seven categories range from no epithelial separation but mesh prominence or contraction (category 1) to patient compromise including hematoma or systemic compromise (category 7). The categories are further classified by letter based on the presence of pain and/or infection. Time references the time when the complication was clinically diagnosed relative to the date of the procedure. The site defines the location of the mesh complication. The classification system was devised to more accurately report and standardize the reporting of mesh-related complications. However one study has shown the classification system to be highly complex, lacking clarity, and presenting poor inter-rater reliability [88].

Summary

A thorough conversation with the patient and physician should take place before embarking on POP surgery. Specifically, if mesh use is planned to augment a repair, the surgeon should provide full disclosure regarding the potential adverse effects related to mesh. Evaluation of a patient after a mesh complication requires a complete evaluation. Experienced, trained pelvic surgeons may be able to recognize and treat these conditions with fewer complications. With the patient's best outcome as the primary goal, all steps should be taken to prevent any complications.

References

1. Olsen AL, Smith VJ, Bergstrom JO, et al. Epidemiology of surgically managed pelvic organ prolapse and urinary incontinence. Obstet Gynecol. 1997;89:501.
2. Smith FJ, Holman CD, Moorin RE, et al. Lifetime risk of undergoing surgery for pelvic organ prolapse. Obstet Gynecol. 2010;116:1096.
3. Wu JM, Kawasaki A, Hundley AF, et al. Predicting the number of women who will undergo incontinence and prolapse surgery, 2010 to 2050. Am J Obstet Gynecol. 2011;205:230.e1.
4. Memon H, Handa VL. Pelvic floor disorders following vaginal or cesarean delivery. Curr Opin Obstet Gynecol. 2012;24:349.
5. Lavy Y, Sand PK, Kaniel CI, et al. Can pelvic floor injury secondary to delivery be prevented? Int Urogynecol J. 2012;23:165.
6. Kudish BI, Iglesia CB, Gutman RE, et al. Risk factors for prolapse development in white, black, and Hispanic women. Female Pelvic Med Reconstr Surg. 2011;17:80.
7. Swift SE. The distribution of pelvic organ support in a population of female subjects seen for routine gynecologic health care. Am J Obstet Gynecol. 2000; 183:277.
8. Gilmour DT, Dwyer PL, Carey MP. Lower urinary tract injury during gynecologic surgery and its detection by intraoperative cystoscopy. Obstet Gynecol. 1999;94:883.
9. Altman D, Vayrynen T, Engh ME, et al. Anterior colporrhaphy versus transvaginal mesh for pelvic-organ prolapse. N Engl J Med. 2013;364:1826.
10. Frankman EA, Wang L, Bunker CH, et al. Lower urinary tract injury in women in the United States, 1979–2006. Am J Obstet Gynecol. 2010;202:495.e1.
11. Harkki-Siren P, Sjoberg J, Tiitinen A. Urinary tract injuries after hysterectomy. Obstet Gynecol. 1998; 92:113.
12. Visco AG, Brubaker L, Nygaard I, et al. The role of preoperative urodynamic testing in stress-continent women undergoing sacrocolpopexy: the Colpopexy and Urinary Reduction Efforts (CARE) randomized surgical trial. Int Urogynecol J Pelvic Floor Dysfunct. 2008;19:607.
13. Wei J. A mid urethral sling prevents incontinence among women undergoing vaginal prolapse repair—the OPUS trial. Glasgow, Scotland: International Continence Society; 2011.
14. Ballert KN, Biggs GY, Isenalumhe Jr A, et al. Managing the urethra at transvaginal pelvic organ prolapse repair: a urodynamic approach. J Urol. 2009;181:679.
15. de Boer TA, Vierhout ME. Predictors for overactive bladder symptoms after pelvic organ prolapse surgery. Curr Opin Obstet Gynecol. 2011;23:366.
16. Diez-Itza I, Aizpitarte I, Becerro A, et al. Incidence of overactive bladder after vaginal hysterectomy and associated repairs for pelvic organ prolapse. Gynecol Obstet Invest. 2009;68:65.
17. Eilber KS, Kavaler E, Rodriguez LV, et al. Ten-year experience with transvaginal vesicovaginal fistula repair using tissue interposition. J Urol. 2003;169:1033.
18. Hendrix SL, Clark A, Nygaard I, et al. Pelvic organ prolapse in the Women's Health Initiative: gravity and gravidity. Am J Obstet Gynecol. 2002;186:1160.
19. Lentz G. Comprehensive gynecology. Philadelphia, PA: Elsevier; 2012. p. 462.
20. Sand PK, Koduri S, Lobel RW, et al. Prospective randomized trial of polyglactin 910 mesh to prevent recurrence of cystoceles and rectoceles. Am J Obstet Gynecol. 2001;184:1357.
21. Weber AM, Walters MD, Piedmonte MR, et al. Anterior colporrhaphy: a randomized trial of three

surgical techniques. Am J Obstet Gynecol. 2001; 185:1299.
22. Peterson TV, Karp DR, Aguilar VC, et al. Primary versus recurrent prolapse surgery: differences in outcomes. Int Urogynecol J. 2010;21:483.
23. Margulies RU, Rogers MA, Morgan DM. Outcomes of transvaginal uterosacral ligament suspension: systematic review and metaanalysis. Am J Obstet Gynecol. 2010;202:124.
24. Morgan DM, Larson K. Uterosacral and sacrospinous ligament suspension for restoration of apical vaginal support. Clin Obstet Gynecol. 2010;53:72.
25. Barber MD, Visco AG, Weidner AC, et al. Bilateral uterosacral ligament vaginal vault suspension with site-specific endopelvic fascia defect repair for treatment of pelvic organ prolapse. Am J Obstet Gynecol. 2000;183:1402.
26. Buller JL, Thompson JR, Cundiff GW, et al. Uterosacral ligament: description of anatomic relationships to optimize surgical safety. Obstet Gynecol. 2001;97:873.
27. Montoya TI, Luebbehusen HI, Schaffer JI, et al. Sensory neuropathy following suspension of the vaginal apex to the proximal uterosacral ligaments. Int Urogynecol J. 2012;23(12):1735–40.
28. Siddiqui NY, Mitchell TR, Bentley RC, et al. Neural entrapment during uterosacral ligament suspension: an anatomic study of female cadavers. Obstet Gynecol. 2010;116:708.
29. Karram M, Goldwasser S, Kleeman S, et al. High uterosacral vaginal vault suspension with fascial reconstruction for vaginal repair of enterocele and vaginal vault prolapse. Am J Obstet Gynecol. 2001; 185:1339.
30. Ridgeway B, Barber MD, Walters MD, et al. Small bowel obstruction after vaginal vault suspension: a series of three cases. Int Urogynecol J Pelvic Floor Dysfunct. 2007;18:1237.
31. Petri E, Ashok K. Sacrospinous vaginal fixation–current status. Acta Obstet Gynecol Scand. 2011;90:429.
32. Barksdale PA, Elkins TE, Sanders CK, et al. An anatomic approach to pelvic hemorrhage during sacrospinous ligament fixation of the vaginal vault. Obstet Gynecol. 1998;91:715.
33. Baumann M, Salvisberg C, Mueller M, et al. Sexual function after sacrospinous fixation for vaginal vault prolapse: bad or mad? Surg Endosc. 2009;23:1013.
34. Hefni MA, El-Toukhy TA. Long-term outcome of vaginal sacrospinous colpopexy for marked uterovaginal and vault prolapse. Eur J Obstet Gynecol Reprod Biol. 2006;127:257.
35. Aigmueller T, Riss P, Dungl A, et al. Long-term follow-up after vaginal sacrospinous fixation: patient satisfaction, anatomical results and quality of life. Int Urogynecol J Pelvic Floor Dysfunct. 2008;19:965.
36. Maher CF, Qatawneh AM, Dwyer PL, et al. Abdominal sacral colpopexy or vaginal sacrospinous colpopexy for vaginal vault prolapse: a prospective randomized study. Am J Obstet Gynecol. 2004; 190:20.
37. Morgan DM, Rogers MA, Huebner M, et al. Heterogeneity in anatomic outcome of sacrospinous ligament fixation for prolapse: a systematic review. Obstet Gynecol. 2007;109:1424.
38. Shull BL, Capen CV, Riggs MW, et al. Bilateral attachment of the vaginal cuff to iliococcygeus fascia: an effective method of cuff suspension. Am J Obstet Gynecol. 1993;168:1669.
39. Maher CF, Murray CJ, Carey MP, et al. Iliococcygeus or sacrospinous fixation for vaginal vault prolapse. Obstet Gynecol. 2001;98:40.
40. Paraiso MF, Walters MD, Rackley RR, et al. Laparoscopic and abdominal sacral colpopexies: a comparative cohort study. Am J Obstet Gynecol. 2005;192:1752.
41. Miranda CS, Carvajal AR. Complications of operative gynecological laparoscopy. JSLS. 2003;7:53.
42. Dietz V, van der Vaart CH, van der Graaf Y, et al. One-year follow-up after sacrospinous hysteropexy and vaginal hysterectomy for uterine descent: a randomized study. Int Urogynecol J. 2010;21:209.
43. Dietz V, de Jong J, Huisman M, et al. The effectiveness of the sacrospinous hysteropexy for the primary treatment of uterovaginal prolapse. Int Urogynecol J Pelvic Floor Dysfunct. 2007;18:1271.
44. Maher CF, Cary MP, Slack MC, et al. Uterine preservation or hysterectomy at sacrospinous colpopexy for uterovaginal prolapse? Int Urogynecol J Pelvic Floor Dysfunct. 2001;12:381.
45. Kilkku P, Gronroos M, Hirvonen T, et al. Supravaginal uterine amputation vs. hysterectomy. Effects on libido and orgasm. Acta Obstet Gynecol Scand. 1983;62:147.
46. Zucchi A, Costantini E, Mearini L, et al. Female sexual dysfunction in urogenital prolapse surgery: colposacropexy vs. hysterocolposacropexy. J Sex Med. 2008;5:139.
47. Jeng CJ, Yang YC, Tzeng CR, et al. Sexual functioning after vaginal hysterectomy or transvaginal sacrospinous uterine suspension for uterine prolapse: a comparison. J Reprod Med. 2005;50:669.
48. Price N, Slack A, Jackson SR. Laparoscopic hysteropexy: the initial results of a uterine suspension procedure for uterovaginal prolapse. BJOG. 2010;117:62.
49. Roovers JP, van der Vaart CH, van der Bom JG, et al. A randomised controlled trial comparing abdominal and vaginal prolapse surgery: effects on urogenital function. BJOG. 2004;111:50.
50. Brummer TH, Jalkanen J, Fraser J, et al. FINHYST, a prospective study of 5279 hysterectomies: complications and their risk factors. Hum Reprod. 2011;26:1741.
51. Beer M, Kuhn A. Surgical techniques for vault prolapse: a review of the literature. Eur J Obstet Gynecol Reprod Biol. 2005;119:144.
52. Maher CM, Feiner B, Baessler K, et al. Surgical management of pelvic organ prolapse in women: the updated summary version Cochrane review. Int Urogynecol J. 2011;22:1445.
53. Visco AG, Weidner AC, Barber MD, et al. Vaginal mesh erosion after abdominal sacral colpopexy. Am J Obstet Gynecol. 2001;184:297.

54. Nygaard IE, McCreery R, Brubaker L, et al. Abdominal sacrocolpopexy: a comprehensive review. Obstet Gynecol. 2004;104:805.
55. Tan-Kim J, Menefee SA, Luber KM, et al. Prevalence and risk factors for mesh erosion after laparoscopic-assisted sacrocolpopexy. Int Urogynecol J. 2011;22:205.
56. Ginath S, Garely AD, Condrea A, et al. Mesh erosion following abdominal sacral colpopexy in the absence and presence of the cervical stump. Int Urogynecol J. 2013;24(1):113–8.
57. Cundiff GW, Varner E, Visco AG, et al. Risk factors for mesh/suture erosion following sacral colpopexy. Am J Obstet Gynecol. 2008;199:688.e1.
58. Nieminen K, Hiltunen KM, Laitinen J, et al. Transanal or vaginal approach to rectocele repair: a prospective, randomized pilot study. Dis Colon Rectum. 2004;47:1636.
59. Kahn MA, Stanton SL, Kumar D. Posterior colporrhaphy is superior to the transanal repair for treatment of posterior vaginal wall prolapse. Neurourol Urodyn. 1999;18:70.
60. Arnold MW, Stewart WR, Aguilar PS. Rectocele repair. Four years' experience. Dis Colon Rectum. 1990;33:684.
61. Mathevet P, Valencia P, Cousin C, et al. Operative injuries during vaginal hysterectomy. Eur J Obstet Gynecol Reprod Biol. 2001;97:71.
62. Paraiso MF, Barber MD, Muir TW, et al. Rectocele repair: a randomized trial of three surgical techniques including graft augmentation. Am J Obstet Gynecol. 2006;195:1762.
63. Milani AL, Withagen MI, Schweitzer KJ, et al. Midline fascial plication under continuous digital transrectal control: which factors determine anatomic outcome? Int Urogynecol J. 2010;21:623.
64. Singh K, Cortes E, Reid WM. Evaluation of the fascial technique for surgical repair of isolated posterior vaginal wall prolapse. Obstet Gynecol. 2003;101:320.
65. Maher CF, Qatawneh AM, Baessler K, et al. Midline rectovaginal fascial plication for repair of rectocele and obstructed defecation. Obstet Gynecol. 2004;104:685.
66. Porter WE, Steele A, Walsh P, et al. The anatomic and functional outcomes of defect-specific rectocele repairs. Am J Obstet Gynecol. 1999;181:1353.
67. Carey M, Higgs P, Goh J, et al. Vaginal repair with mesh versus colporrhaphy for prolapse: a randomised controlled trial. BJOG. 2009;116:1380.
68. FDA. FDA safety communication: UPDATE on serious complications associated with transvaginal placement of surgical mesh for pelvic organ prolapse; 2011. http://www.fda.gov/medicaldevices/safety/alertsandnotices/ucm262435.htm
69. Lindau ST, Schumm LP, Laumann EO, et al. A study of sexuality and health among older adults in the United States. N Engl J Med. 2007;357:762.
70. Harmanli OH, Dandolu V, Chatwani AJ, et al. Total colpocleisis for severe pelvic organ prolapse. J Reprod Med. 2003;48:703.
71. Hoffman MS, Cardosi RJ, Lockhart J, et al. Vaginectomy with pelvic herniorrhaphy for prolapse. Am J Obstet Gynecol. 2003;189:364.
72. Abbasy S, Kenton K. Obliterative procedures for pelvic organ prolapse. Clin Obstet Gynecol. 2010;53:86.
73. Fitzgerald MP, Richter HE, Bradley CS, et al. Pelvic support, pelvic symptoms, and patient satisfaction after colpocleisis. Int Urogynecol J Pelvic Floor Dysfunct. 2008;19:1603.
74. FitzGerald MP, Richter HE, Siddique S, et al. Colpocleisis: a review. Int Urogynecol J Pelvic Floor Dysfunct. 2006;17:261.
75. von Pechmann WS, Mutone M, Fyffe J, et al. Total colpocleisis with high levator plication for the treatment of advanced pelvic organ prolapse. Am J Obstet Gynecol. 2003;189:121.
76. Gutman RE, Bradley CS, Ye W, et al. Effects of colpocleisis on bowel symptoms among women with severe pelvic organ prolapse. Int Urogynecol J. 2010;21:461.
77. Fitzgerald MP, Kulkarni N, Fenner D. Postoperative resolution of urinary retention in patients with advanced pelvic organ prolapse. Am J Obstet Gynecol. 2000;183:1361.
78. Koski ME, Chow D, Bedestani A, et al. Colpocleisis for advanced pelvic organ prolapse. Urology. 2012;80:542.
79. FDA. Surgical mesh for treatment of women with pelvic organ prolapse and stress urinary incontinence FDA executive summary; 2011. http://www.fda.gov/downloads/AdvisoryCommittees/CommitteesMeetingMaterials/MedicalDevices/MedicalDevicesAdvisoryCommittee/ObstetricsandGynecologyDevices/UCM270402.pdf
80. Elmer C, Falconer C, Hallin A, et al. Risk factors for mesh complications after trocar guided transvaginal mesh kit repair of anterior vaginal wall prolapse. Neurourol Urodyn. 2012;31(7):1165–9.
81. Withagen MI, Vierhout ME, Hendriks JC, et al. Risk factors for exposure, pain, and dyspareunia after tension-free vaginal mesh procedure. Obstet Gynecol. 2011;118:629.
82. Kaufman Y, Singh SS, Alturki H, et al. Age and sexual activity are risk factors for mesh exposure following transvaginal mesh repair. Int Urogynecol J. 2011; 22:307.
83. Rogo-Gupta L, Raz S. Complications of female incontinence and pelvic reconstructive surgery. New York: Humana Press; 2013. p. 87.
84. Dietz HP. Pelvic floor ultrasound: a review. Am J Obstet Gynecol. 2011;202:321.
85. Svabik K, Martan A, Masata J, et al. Ultrasound appearances after mesh implantation–evidence of mesh contraction or folding? Int Urogynecol J. 2011; 22:529.
86. Feiner B, Maher C. Vaginal mesh contraction: definition, clinical presentation, and management. Obstet Gynecol. 2010;115:325.
87. Haylen BT, Freeman RM, et al. An International Urogynecological Association (IUGA)/International Continence Society (ICS) joint terminology and classification of the complications related directly to the insertion of prostheses (meshes, implants, tapes) and grafts in female pelvic floor surgery. Neurourol Urodyn. 2011;30(1):2–12. doi: 10.1002/nau.21036.

88. Tunitsky E, Abbott S, Barber MD. Interrater reliability of the International Continence Society and International Urogynecological Association (ICS/IUGA) classification system for mesh-related complications. Am J Obstet Gynecol. 2012;206:442.e1.
89. Abramov Y, Gandhi S, Goldberg RP, et al. Site-specific rectocele repair compared with standard posterior colporrhaphy. Obstet Gynecol. 2005;105:314.
90. Cundiff GW, Weidner AC, Visco AG, et al. Am J Obstet Gynecol. 1998;179:1451.
91. Kenton K, Shott S, Brubaker L. Outcome after rectovaginal fascia reattachment for rectocele repair. Am J Obstet Gynecol. 1999;181:1360.
92. Glavind K, Madsen H. A prospective study of the discrete fascial defect rectocele repair. Acta Obstet Gynecol Scand. 2000;79:145.

22 Minimally Invasive Abdominal Surgery in the Management of Pelvic Dysfunction

Gamal M. Ghoniem and Jane Cho

Urinary incontinence continues to have a significant impact on the quality of life of women and is the chief complaint in more than 1.1 million office visits per year [1]. Pelvic dysfunction leading to incontinence occurs when there is a disruption in either the storage or voiding of urine and the etiology of incontinence can vary from overactive bladder, intrinsic sphincter deficiency, urethral hypermobility, and pelvic organ prolapse to vesical fistulas. The symptoms are often nonspecific and complete evaluation is necessary to completely characterize the incontinence.

Diagnostic Work-up

The standard evaluation of patients with incontinence includes a thorough and detailed history and can be done with the help of various validated questionnaires. Regardless of which questionnaire is utilized, it is important to characterize the incontinence by frequency of incontinence episodes, urgency, precipitating or exacerbating factors, severity, degree of bother, and, eventually, patient expectations of treatment [2]. Specific to pelvic organ prolapse, awareness of a bulge or discomfort should be assessed. Past medical and surgical history including gynecologic and obstetric history and medication list are also vital in the history of present illness. By defining these parameters, the etiology can be ascertained leading to proper treatment planning.

Physical examination includes a focused pelvic examination. Depending on the history of present illness, it may also include a stress test, where the bladder is filled with 250–300 ml of fluid prior to increase in abdominal pressures with either Valsalva or cough. While not pathognomonic for stress urinary incontinence (SUI), urethral hypermobility can also be assessed with a standard Q-tip test. Prolapse should be assessed with patient in both lithotomy and standing positions.

Most patients should undergo urinalysis with culture as well as uroflow and post-void residual measurement. Additional diagnostic studies include voiding diary, urodynamics (with or without fluoroscopy), cystoscopy, and radiographic imaging (especially in the setting of vesical fistula). While not standard, these tests can help elucidate the nature of incontinence when complex.

Indications

The main indication for the treatment of symptomatic incontinence is significant adverse effect on the quality of life of the patient (i.e., incontinence leading to social or hygiene issues).

G.M. Ghoniem, M.D., F.A.C.S. (✉) • J. Cho, M.D.
Department of Urology, University of California Irvine, 333 City Boulevard West, Suite 2100, Orange, CA 92868, USA
e-mail: gghoniem@uci.edu

G.H. Badlani (ed.), *Minimally Invasive Therapy for Urinary Incontinence and Pelvic Organ Prolapse*, Current Clinical Urology, DOI 10.1007/978-1-4939-0008-4_22,

Conservative therapies for incontinence depend on the etiology of the incontinence and may include physical therapy, and pessary use. Surgical intervention includes injection of bulking agents, fulguration of fistulas, neuromodulation, and various transvaginal procedures which are covered in other chapters.

While the first transvaginal procedure for SUI was described in 1913 [3], it was 35 years more until a transabdominal retropubic approach was described [4]. This procedure was later modified by Burch by placing sutures more laterally into Cooper's ligament [5] and was the gold standard transabdominal approach for the treatment of SUI. More recently, tension-free transvaginal slings (TVT) have become the gold standard secondary to their ease in placement as well as comparable results to colpopexy [6].

Abdominal sacrocolpopexy is often considered in the setting of isolated apical prolapse or enterocele. While open abdominal sacrocolpopexy is slowly going by the wayside to the laparoscopic and robotic approach [7], the principles have not changed.

Unlike SUI or pelvic organ prolapse, incontinence as a result of urinary fistula is often continuous and sudden in onset. In addition, the etiology is often iatrogenic and, as a result, often causes considerable distress. Therefore, surgery is often the primary treatment in these patients. Patient comorbidities, size, number, and location of fistula are important factors in the surgical approach. However, surgeon experience and preference often have the largest influence.

Advantages to an abdominal approach are:

- Familiarity of retropubic anatomy to most urologists.
- Excellent exposure.
- Reduction in dyspareunia risk.
- Opportunity to repair any coexisting abdominal disease through one incision.
- Increased efficiency in the setting of limited vaginal access.
- Less recurrence of prolapse.
- Maintenance of functional vaginal length in sexually active women.
- Avoidance of vaginal mesh complications and their medicolegal implications.

Disadvantages traditionally included a larger incision resulting in prolonged hospital stay, recovery, and increased pain. However, with the advent of minimal invasive technology, this disadvantage has been largely eliminated. There is also the added benefit of increased magnification. Disadvantages to laparoscopic approach include greater technical difficulty with a steeper learning curve and higher operating costs.

Laparoscopic Colposuspension

Laparoscopic colposuspension can be performed via an extraperitoneal or transperitoneal approach [8]. For all transabdominal procedures, patients perform bowel prep the day before surgery, and receive antibiotics 30 min prior to surgery. Five thousand units of subcutaneous heparin are also administered at the time of surgery. In transperitoneal approach patient is placed in low lithotomy position in slight Trendelenburg and the vagina and abdomen are prepped and draped in the usual sterile fashion. A 16 Fr Foley catheter is initially placed which decompresses the bladder and helps prevent trauma during initial port placement. The peritoneum is entered through a small infraumbilical incision using either the standard Veress needle or Hasson trocar. Once pneumoperitoneum is established up to 15 mmHg, a trocar is inserted infraumbilically. Two more working trocars are placed at the left lateral border of rectus muscle under direct vision. Care is taken to avoid any superficial inferior epigastric vessels by transilluminating the abdominal wall. The left-sided placement would allow the surgeons to not only operate with the laparoscopic instrument using their dominant hand but also be able to place the nondominant index finger in the vagina during the procedure, if necessary.

The space of Retzius is dissected by identifying the umbilical ligaments laterally and then incising the anterior parietal peritoneum over the bladder directly under the pubic symphysis. Once the pubic bone is identified, it can be followed into the space of Retzius. The bladder neck can be identified by the Foley balloon and the endopelvic fascia at the bladder neck and Cooper's ligament along the superior surface of the pelvic bone are then identified. With the surgeon's finger elevating the vagina toward the ligament, the endopelvic fascia is sutured to the ligament on both sides. This elevation of the bladder neck behind the pubic symphysis addresses the urethral hypermobility causing stress incontinence. However, it should be noted that the vaginal tissue should not be completely tacked up to the ligaments as this may result in overcorrection as well as kinking of the ureter. Instead, approximately 2 cm of space between the suture and Cooper's ligament is usually left. Once the fascia is sutured, intravenous indigo carmine is routinely given and cystoscopy is carried out to assure no bladder or urethral perforation as well as the patency of bilateral ureters.

Other complications that may occur include hemorrhage, bladder or urethral injury, and infection as in almost any other major surgical procedures. Specific to colposuspension, patients should be counseled on potential for postoperative voiding difficulty necessitating intermittent catheterization. Reported rates range from 3.5 % to as high as 32 %; however, most incidences were temporary and the risk for permanent urinary retention was estimated to be <5 % [9]. The presence of overactive bladder symptoms with stress incontinence (mixed with incontinence) preoperatively may resolve in most patients after suspension. Those with persistent overactivity may be treated with anticholinergic therapy, or even botulinum toxin therapy, neuromodulation, or augmentation cystoplasty. Another potential complication is the development or exacerbation of vaginal prolapse, especially apical and posterior. In one recent prospective study, 38 % of women who underwent colposuspension developed symptomatic prolapse by 7 years [10]. Regarding laparoscopic surgery, there have been some studies reporting higher incidences of complications with bladder injury being the most common with laparoscopic procedures. It should be noted, however, that the same study reported a decline in injury with experience [11].

Laparoscopic colposuspension procedures were first described in 1991 and since then multiple studies have been published comparing outcomes between open and laparoscopic colposuspension. These studies vary in follow-up data and methodology in assessing outcomes. One of the largest studies was a randomized trial carried out by Carey et al. [12]. They found no significant difference in urodynamic cure rate or patient satisfaction at 6 months, 24 months, and at a mean follow-up of 3.7 years. The COLPO trial found similar results with no difference in objective or subjective cure rates [13]. Of note, this trial found that while complication rates were low, more bladder and bowel injuries occurred in the laparoscopic arm and more wound infections occurred in the open approach [13].

Laparoscopic Sacrocolpopexy

Unlike colposuspension surgery, the principles of the abdominal sacrocolpopexy have not changed since its initial description. The laparoscopic approach is described as follows. Again, patients undergo a bowel prep and are administered intravenous antibiotics and subcutaneous heparin prior to the procedure. Patients are placed in low lithotomy and both the abdomen and vagina are prepped and draped in the usual sterile fashion. A 16 Fr Foley catheter is inserted to decompress the bladder. Pneumoperitoneum is achieved in the same manner described above with either the Veress needle or the Hasson trocar. Once 15 mmHg of pressure is achieved, the camera port is inserted infraumbilically. At this point, the port placement varies slightly depending on whether the procedure will proceed with pure laparoscopy or with robotic assistance. When utilizing the robot, either docking may occur between the patient's legs or side-docking to the left of the patient, allowing an assistant access to the vagina.

Once ports are placed in appropriate position, patient is placed in steep Trendelenburg, thereby keeping the small bowel out of the pelvis. The rectum is slightly retracted to the left, exposing the right paracolic gutter and sacral promontory. An incision is made in the posterior peritoneum over the sacral promontory, taking care to avoid any presacral and the middle sacral vein. Dissection is carried out until the anterior surface of the promontory is identified by the anterior longitudinal ligament. Attention is then turned to the vaginal cuff. An obturator (either a sponge stick or Deaver or anastomosis sizer) is placed in the vagina to identify the vaginal cuff. The peritoneum over the cuff is incised and carefully dissected off of the vaginal cuff. Care must be taken to avoid complete perforation resulting in loss of pneumoperitoneum.

A Y-shaped graft made of polypropylene macroporous monofilament must be utilized. The two short arms of the Y-shaped grafts are sutured to the exposed vaginal cuff using several permanent interrupted stitches, taking care to avoid the bladder. The long end of the graft is then secured to the promontory. Excessive tension must be avoided and any excess length is carefully trimmed. The peritoneum is then closed over the graft over the sacrum and vaginal cuff with running stitch.

Potential complications from this procedure include hemorrhage (especially secondary to sacral vessel injury), bladder or bowel injury, ureteral injury, mesh infection and vaginal erosion, and ileus, and rates vary from 6 to 16 % [14]. There has been a concern of mesh erosion especially in the setting of combined hysterectomy and abdominal sacrocolpopexy. However, this has not been reported in the laparoscopic approach.

Success rates for laparoscopic sacrocolpopexy are reported to be as high as 100 % in some series [15]. Very few studies compare laparoscopic sacrocolpopexy to the open abdominal approach but similar complication and success rates are reported [16]. There are multiple studies comparing transvaginal sacrospinous fixation with abdominal sacrocolpopexy with most reporting higher success rates with the abdominal approach [17]. In these studies, postoperative morbidity was higher in the transabdominal approach but one can argue that morbidity would decrease significantly given the minimally invasive nature of laparoscopy.

Laparoscopic Vesicovaginal Fistula Repair

The initial step in fistula repair is cystoscopy. During cystoscopy, bilateral ureteral orifices are identified and stented. If possible, the fistulous opening is identified and also stented in order to facilitate dissection later. A Foley catheter is placed and kept accessible. The patient is then placed in supine position. Pneumoperitoneum is established as previously described. Camera port placement is usually umbilical with one working port in each midclavicular line. An assistant port is often placed in the left lower abdomen for retraction as well as suction and irrigation. Once the bladder is dissected off of the anterior vaginal wall, the bladder is filled with fluid and the wall is incised in the midline up to the edge of the fistula. A sponge stick should be placed in the vagina, not only for assistance in traction but also to maintain pneumoperitoneum. The vaginal wall is further dissected and separated from the bladder approximately 2 cm beyond the fistula. The vaginal defect is closed in two layers using absorbable suture. At this time, if omentum can be mobilized, it is sutured over the vaginal repair. The bladder defect is then closed in multiple layers. The bladder is then refilled to confirm a watertight closure. A suprapubic catheter is placed extraperitoneally and an abdominal drain is also placed in the pelvis.

Potential complications from transabdominal and transvesical repair of vesicovaginal fistula include vascular injury and bowel perforation. Another complication unique to fistula repair is ureteral injury especially if the fistula is located in close proximity to the ureteral orifice. Therefore, initial cystoscopy with catheterization of bilateral ureteral orifices is essential. The most important complication of vesicovaginal fistula repair is recurrence of the fistula. However, it should be noted that regardless of approach, vesicovaginal fistula repair success rates are often reported to be greater than 90 % [18]. Radiation-induced fistula has the lowest reported success rates (only 67 %).

Laparoscopic repair was first described in 1994 [15] and robotic-assisted repair was described in 2005 [19]. To date, very little is published on the outcomes of these procedures with most being small case series. The largest series was by Sotelo et al. [20] who described 15 patients who underwent laparoscopic repair. In that particular study, one patient did develop recurrence.

Conclusion

Since its advent in 1901, laparoscopy has advanced in leaps and bounds and has become a viable option in the treatment of pelvic dysfunction. As increased concerns are raised over FDA warnings of vaginal mesh complications, there has been a rise in interest in alternative options such as transabdominal procedures. While transabdominal procedures have traditionally been attributed with increased patient pain and hospital stays, the application of laparoscopy has decreased these issues. The future role of laparoscopy and robotic-assisted laparoscopy in the treatment of pelvis dysfunction will continue to rise.

References

1. Litwin MS, Saigal CS, Yano EM, Avila C, Geschwind SA, Hanley JM, et al. Urologic diseases in America Project: analytical methods and principal findings. J Urol. 2005;173:933–7.
2. Langford CF, Elmissiry MM, Ghoniem GM. Do women have realistic expectations of treatment for stress urinary incontinence? Neurourol Urodyn. 2008; 27(6):480–4.
3. Kelly HA. Incontinence of urine in women. Urol Cutaneous Rev. 1913;17:291–3.
4. Marshall FV, Marchetti AA, Krantz KE. The correction of stress incontinence by simple vesicourethral suspension. Surg Gynecol Obstet. 1949;88:509–18.
5. Burch JC. Urethrovaginal fixation to Cooper's ligament for correction of stress incontinence, cystocele and prolapsed. Am J Obstet Gynecol. 1994;170: 1713–20.
6. Ward KL, Hilton P. UK and Ireland TVT trial group. A prospectus multicenter randomized trial of tension-free vaginal tape and colposuspension for primary urodynamic stress incontinence: two-year follow-up. Am J Obstet Gynecol. 2004;190(2):324–31.
7. Vancaillie TG, Schuessler W. Laparoscopic bladder neck suspension. J Laparoendosc Surg. 1991;1(3): 169–73.
8. McDougall EM. Laparoscopic management of female urinary incontinence. Urol Clin North Am. 2001; 28:145–9.
9. Chapple CR. Retropubic suspension surgery for incontinence in women. In: Wein AJ, Kavoussi LR, Novick AC, Partin AW, Peters CA, editors. Campbell-Walsh urology. 10th ed. Philadelphia: Saunders; 2012. p. 2047–68.
10. Auwad W, Bombieri L, Adekanmi O, Waterfield M, Freeman R. The development of pelvic organ prolapse after colposuspension: a prospective, long-term follow-up study on the prevalence and predisposing factors. Int Urogynecol J Pelvic Floor Dysfunct. 2006;17(4):389–94.
11. Paraiso MF, Falcone T, Walters MD. Laparoscopic surgery for genuine stress incontinence. Int Urogynecol J. 1999;10:237–47.
12. Carey M, Goh JT, Rosamilia A, Cornish A, Gordon I, Hawthorne G, et al. Laparoscopic versus open Burch colposuspension: a randomised controlled trial. BJOG. 2006;113(9):999–1006.
13. Kitchener HC, Dunn G, Lawton V, Reid F, Nelson L, Smith AR, COLPO Study Group. Laparoscopic versus open colposuspension—results of a prospective randomized controlled trial. BJOG. 2006;113(9): 1007–13.
14. Rassweiler J, Giovannalberto P, Gozen AS, Klein J, Teber D. Role of laparoscopy in reconstructive surgery. Curr Opin Urol. 2010;20:471–82.
15. Nezhat CH, Nezhat F, Nezhat C, Rottenberg D. Laparoscopic repair of a vesicovaginal fistula: a case report. Obstet Gynecol. 1994;83(5):899–901.
16. Paraiso MF, Walters MD, Rackley RR, Melek S, Hugney C. Laparoscopic and abdominal sacral colpopexies: a comparative cohort study. Am J Obstet Gynecol. 2005;192(5):1752–8.
17. Benson JT, Lucente V, McClellan E. Vaginal versus abdominal reconstructive surgery for the treatment of pelvic support defects: a prospective randomized study with long-term outcome evaluation. Am J Obstet Gynecol. 1996;175:1418–22.
18. Rovner ES. Urinary tract fistulae. In: Wein AJ, Kavoussi LR, Novick AC, Partin AW, Peters CA, editors. Campbell-Walsh urology. 10th ed. Philadelphia: Saunders; 2012. p. 2223–61.
19. Melamud O, Eichel L, Turbow B, Shanberg A. Laparoscopic vesicovaginal fistula repair with robotic reconstruction. Urology. 2005;65:163–5.
20. Sotelo R, Mariano MB, Garcia-Segui A, Dubois R, Spaliviero M, Keklikian W, et al. Laparoscopic repair of vesicovaginal fistula. J Urol. 2005;173(5):1615–8.

Index

G.H. Badlani (ed.), *Minimally Invasive Therapy for Urinary Incontinence and Pelvic Organ Prolapse*, Current Clinical Urology, DOI 10.1007/978-1-4939-0008-4,

MIX
Papier aus verantwortungsvollen Quellen
Paper from responsible sources
FSC® C105338

If you have any concerns about our products,
you can contact us on
ProductSafety@springernature.com

In case Publisher is established outside the EU,
the EU authorized representative is:
Springer Nature Customer Service Center GmbH
Europaplatz 3, 69115 Heidelberg, Germany

Printed by Libri Plureos GmbH
in Hamburg, Germany